*Compliance
in Health Care*

COMPLIANCE IN HEALTH CARE

Edited by R. Brian Haynes,
D. Wayne Taylor, and David L. Sackett

THE JOHNS HOPKINS UNIVERSITY PRESS
BALTIMORE AND LONDON

613
C 737

176624

Manufactured in the United States of America

The Johns Hopkins University Press, Baltimore, Maryland 21218
The Johns Hopkins Press Ltd., London

Library of Congress Catalog Number 78-20527
ISBN 0-8018-2162-2

Library of Congress Cataloging in Publication data will be found on the last printed page of this book.

To the Finchley Harriers,
Alvy Singer,
and Kilgore Trout

Contributors

Marshall H. Becker, Ph.D., M.P.H., Professor, Department of Health Behavior and Health Education, School of Public Health, The University of Michigan, Ann Arbor, Michigan

J. Allan Best, Ph.D., Associate Professor, Department of Health Studies, University of Waterloo, Waterloo, Ontario

Barry Blackwell, M.D., Professor and Chairman, Department of Psychiatry, School of Medicine, Wright State University, Dayton, Ohio

Maurice Bloch, M.A., Graduate Student, Department of Psychology, University of British Columbia, Vancouver, British Columbia

Howard D. Cappell, Ph.D., Associate Professor, Department of Psychology, Lecturer, Department of Pharmacology, University of Toronto, and Head of Psychology, Addiction Research Foundation, Toronto, Ontario

Robert H. Drachman, M.D., Associate Professor, Department of Pediatrics, School of Medicine, The Johns Hopkins University, Baltimore, Maryland

Jacqueline M. Dunbar, R.N., Ph.D., Assistant Professor, Department of Family Practice, College of Medicine, University of Iowa, Iowa City, Iowa

Alvan R. Feinstein, M.D., Professor of Medicine and Epidemiology, Yale University School of Medicine, New Haven, Connecticut, and Chief, Clinical Biostatistics and Cooperative Studies Program Support Center, Veterans Administration Hospital, West Haven, Connecticut

Edward S. Gibson, M.D., Director of Occupational and Environmental Health, Dominion Foundries and Steel Ltd., and Associate Member, Department of Clinical Epidemiology and Biostatistics, Faculty of Health Sciences, McMaster University, Hamilton, Ontario

Charles H. Goldsmith, Ph.D., Associate Professor, Department of Clinical Epidemiology and Biostatistics, Faculty of Health Sciences, McMaster University, Hamilton, Ontario

Leon Gordis, M.D., Dr. P.H., Professor and Chairman, Department of Epidemiology, School of Hygiene and Public Health, The Johns Hopkins University, Baltimore, Maryland

Lawrence W. Green, Dr. P.H., Professor and Head, Division of Health Education, Department of Health Services Administration, School of Hygiene and Public Health, The Johns Hopkins University, Baltimore, Maryland

Don P. Haefner, Ph.D., Professor, Department of Health Behavior and Health Education, School of Public Health, The University of Michigan, Ann Arbor, Michigan

R. Brian Haynes, M.D., Ph.D., Assistant Professor, Department of Clinical Epidemiology and Biostatistics and Department of Medicine, Faculty of Health Sciences, McMaster University, Hamilton, Ontario

Carol C. Hogue, R.N., Ph.D., Associate Professor, School of Nursing, Duke University, Durham, North Carolina

Mel F. Hovell, Ph.D., Research Associate, Laboratory for the Study of Behavioral Medicine, Stanford University School of Medicine, Palo Alto, California

Barbara S. Hulka, M.D., M.P.H., Professor, Department of Epidemiology, School of Public Health, The University of North Carolina, Chapel Hill, North Carolina

Albert R. Jonsen, Ph.D., Professor, Health Policy Program, School of Medicine, University of California, San Francisco, California

A. Benjamin Kelley, Senior Vice President, Insurance Institute for Highway Safety, Washington, D.C.

John P. Kirscht, Ph.D., Professor, Department of Health Behavior and Health Education, School of Public Health, The University of Michigan, Ann Arbor, Michigan

James M. McKenney, Pharm. D., Assistant Professor of Pharmacy and Director, Ambulatory Clinical Services, School of Pharmacy, Medical College of Virginia, Virginia Commonwealth University, Richmond, Virginia

Lois A. Maiman, Ph.D., Assistant Professor, Department of Social and Administrative Pharmacy, College of Pharmacy, University of Minnesota, Minneapolis, Minnesota

Gary D. Marshall, Ph.D., Research Associate, Laboratory for the Study of Behavioral Medicine, Stanford University School of Medicine, Palo Alto, California

Joan A. Marshman, Ph.D., Associate Professor, Faculty of Pharmacy, University of Toronto, and Head of Pharmaceutical Sciences, Addiction Research Foundation, Toronto, Ontario

David L. Sackett, M.D., M.Sc., Professor, Department of Clinical Epidemiology and Biostatistics and Department of Medicine, Health Sciences Centre, McMaster University, Hamilton, Ontario

Edward M. Sellers, M.D., Ph.D., Associate Professor, Department of Medicine and Division of Clinical Pharmacology, Faculty of Medicine, University of Toronto, and Director, Clinical Institute, Addiction Research Foundation, Toronto, Ontario

John C. Snow, B.A., Research Assistant, Department of Clinical Epidemiology and Biostatistics, Faculty of Health Sciences, McMaster University, Hamilton, Ontario

D. Wayne Taylor, M.A., Lecturer, Department of Clinical Epidemiology and Biostatistics, Faculty of Health Sciences, McMaster University, Hamilton, Ontario

Contents

Preface

This book is concerned with compliance, *the extent to which a person's behavior (in terms of taking medications, following diets, or executing life-style changes) coincides with medical or health advice.* It is the second book we have compiled on the subject and records the advances in the "state of the art" that have occurred in the three years since its predecessor (794) was published.

ORIGINS

D.L.S. became interested in compliance when it finally dawned on him that his hypertensive patients' unpredictable and often disappointing responses to therapy were the result of neither "resistant" disease nor inadequate drugs, but were due to low compliance. R.B.H. was a graduate student in D.L.S.'s department at the time and became involved in compliance work when it finally occurred to him that D.L.S. might be right. D.W.T., who was searching the horizon beyond experimental psychology, escaped from the lab in time to collaborate in the compliance research that ensued.

Our work in compliance began in earnest in 1972, when we initiated a search of the scientific literature to set the foundation for experimental studies of ways to improve compliance among ambulatory hypertensive patients. We were astonished at how little had been written on compliance and initiated our first generation of studies with a heady sense of exploring the unknown. However, when we started the *Compliance Newsletter* it quickly became apparent that scores of other researchers and concerned clinicians had gathered at the same frontier. We therefore scheduled a meeting for May 1974 (The McMaster Workshop/Symposium on Compliance with Therapeutic Regimens). We planned for 75 people but received applications, pleas, and threats from over 200, necessitating a rather delicate juggling act to balance professions, regional interests, and good will. The conference consisted of plenary sessions in which various students of the new field gave their versions of the compliance story, and workshops in which participants shared knowledge, protocols, and miseries. Upon urging from those assembled, the plenary sessions eventually became the first book (794).

Though we feel the initial book provided an accurate description of compliance knowledge at the time it was written, it quickly became dated by the rapid advance of intense compliance research. Sufficient progress had been made by 1977 to warrant another gathering of the students of compliance, and this time we planned for 200. We attempted to screen out the dabblers by requiring an abstract describing the past, present, or future compliance work of the applicant. Although the 240 abstracts we received produced a good match with the number of places planned, they were of much higher quality than we had anticipated, and we therefore quadrupled the number of evening sessions devoted to the presentation of original work. These, plus the morning plenary sessions and the afternoon workshops (the latter tailored to the interests of the participants) resulted in an exhausting but delightful and congenial affair. In addition, the rapid increase in compliance research (complete with its own heading in *Index Medicus*) made us realize that compliance has come of age as a subject of vigorous scientific scrutiny.

This book is mainly an outgrowth of the expert presentations in the plenary sessions of the most recent Workshop/Symposium. Only two chapters have survived the three years since the first book was published; both of them concern theoretical aspects of the influence of compliance on the design and interpretation of clinical trials (Chapters 19 and 20). The other chapters have been extensively revised or are entirely new. Among the new additions are three chapters on unhealthy lifestyles. Having barely started to come to grips with the difficult problems of medication compliance, one might well ask why we have dared to take on "bad habits." We, ourselves, certainly feel intimidated by the thought of trying to counter smoking, drinking, overeating, underexercise, and drug abuse; however, we previously underestimated the rate of progress in understanding medication compliance. We therefore felt it was appropriate to make amends now and get on with these other extraordinarily important problems.

We have many people to thank for help in preparing this book. We acknowledge with gratitude the excellent work of the contributors to the book and admire the forbearance with which they accepted our editorial whims. We feel very fortunate to have had the editorial assistance of John Snow, Jayanti Mukherjee, Joanne Carson, and Irene O'Byrne. Jane Wright merits special thanks for her painstaking preparation of many of the manuscripts and tables.

Hamilton, Canada   R.B.H.
                                                                        D.W.T.
                                                                        D.L.S.

*Compliance
in Health Care*

1

Introduction

R. Brian Haynes

Compliance has come of age as a topic of medical concern and scientific contemplation. When the predecessor of this book (794) was published we could claim with justification that we had captured most of the world's stock of written compliance knowledge in 245 scientific articles published before 1974. As shown in Figure 1.1, however, there has been an explosion of written reports since that time and their sheer volume has humbled our efforts to keep pace. Further testimony to the eminence achieved by the topic is seen in the following signposts (855): compliance has been entered on the map of the *Index Medicus* under the place names of "Patient Compliance" and "Patient Dropouts"; it has been added to the list of medical high crimes and misdemeanors by Ivan Illich (854); it now rates equal billing with renin at hypertension symposia; and it has replaced screening as a topic of interest to the gurus of medical economics (841).

With this conflagration of interest in compliance, how much is heat and how much is light? And which is which? It is to these questions that this book is addressed. In order to explore them we have challenged many of the world's most knowledgeable students of compliance with the task of describing the state of the art as they see it. Furthermore, we have asked them to couch their assessments in practical terms wherever possible so that practitioners can apply what is feasible and researchers can learn where and how to launch new investigations. We believe that the contributors to this book have fulfilled our requests well—but that is for the reader to judge.

The prime objectives of this introductory chapter are to define what compliance is (and what it is not), to provide a brief historical perspective (mostly for or in fun), to emphasize one or two recurring themes in the book, and to arm readers with tactics for matching their needs with the book's contents.

THE DEFINITION OF COMPLIANCE

Compliance in this book is defined simply as the extent to which a person's behavior (in terms of taking medications, following diets, or executing lifestyle

1

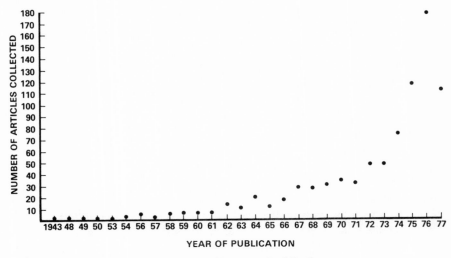

FIGURE 1.1. Compliance articles collected by year of publication.

changes) coincides with medical or health advice. The term *adherence* may be used interchangeably with *compliance*. The definition is intended to be non-judgmental; whereas in particular situations the therapist, patient, or circumstances may be appropriately blamed for noncompliance, the definition per se implies no fault. However, as was noted in the previous book (794), the term *compliance* is troublesome to many people because it conjures up images of patient or client sin and serfdom. Our attempts to defuse this concern (795) have been only partially successful; some still refuse to say the word and experience psychic pain when others do so. We accept their principles as laudable. Western society is rapidly redefining the relationship between health professionals and their clients and the connotation of compliance may seem to fly in the face of this evolution. Nonetheless, the term is now thoroughly rooted and we know of no acceptable alternative.* Moreover, the unhealthy connotations of the term keep ethical and social issues in compliance research and management up front where they belong, whereas a more neutral term might not. Thus, whether you believe the term is obnoxious or, as we do, merely utilitarian, we will use it with explanation but without apology.

COMPLIANCE AND ETHICS

The ethics of the investigation and manipulation of compliance are thoughtfully and thoroughly considered in Chapter 7 by Al Jonsen, a bioethicist. None-

---

*The coeditors' home base is an internationally renowned center for platelet research, and usurption of the term *adherence* is out of the question.

theless, the matter is of sufficient importance to warrant a brief exposition of our own views here. As stated by David Sackett in the first book on compliance:

> . . . the decision to apply strategies deliberately designed to change compliance behavior must meet at least three preconditions. First, the diagnosis must be correct; otherwise . . . the remainder of the exercise is futile. Second, the therapy must do more good than harm. Unless the clinical efficacy of the therapy has been clearly established, patients who undergo compliance modification will simply be exposed to increased treatment hazards, rather than treatment benefits. For the same reason, neither the illness nor the proposed therapy can be trivial. Finally, it must be established that the patient is an informed, willing partner in the execution of any maneuver designed to alter compliance behavior (795).

The individual in our society has a right to refuse to follow health advice in all but a few legally defined situations. However, we find that the people who actively refuse help with compliance are but a subset of all those who fail to comply. Thus, we see the study of compliance problems, aside from its phenomenological aspects, as a means to an end of assisting those who are seeking health and the benefits of modern medicine but who, for whatever reason, have difficulty sticking with the often inconvenient, stigmatizing, or expensive treatments currently in use. We now know that many of these people will volunteer for and respond to compliance-improving strategies, and we believe that we and other health professionals owe them the same efforts in this regard as we do for the other elements of diagnosis, therapy, and compassionate care.

COMPLIANCE SINCE EVE

The first recorded incident of human noncompliance in the Judeo-Christian tradition occurred in the Garden of Eden when Eve ate the fruit of the tree of knowledge. Although this action may have resulted from the alteration of her "health belief model" by a snake (and thus, in a sense, constitutes compliance with contrary advice), the snake appears in all of us occasionally and in some of us much of the time. In any event, Eve, not the snake, bears the blame, thus giving rise to the association of noncompliance with sin. A more charitable interpretation, in keeping with our definition of terms, is that noncompliance is simply one of the prices to be paid for free will and as such is an integral part of the human condition.

Among physicians, Hippocrates appears more astute than his modern counterparts in remarking (673, 725): "[The physician] should keep aware of the fact that patients often lie when they state that they have taken certain medicines." Unfortunately, he failed to relate how he discovered this axiom (see Chapter 3) or how he dealt with low compliance once detected.

Despite the admonition of Hippocrates, compliance appears to have received little systematic attention until its recent rediscovery by phthisiologists (137,

664, 665). (Those concerned with the ethics of compliance interventions will be reassured to learn that physicians did not take noncompliance very seriously until treatments of established efficacy were available.) The response in tubercular circles subsequently repeated itself in the mental health fraternity with the advent of the phenothiazines (223, 338, 394, 528). Unfortunately, however, there is little evidence of cross-fertilization between phthisiologists and psychiatrists, and much of the psychiatric effort went to rediscovery and reinvention rather than true advancement. It is also intriguing to note that both groups deal with disorders that pose a threat to the public. This may account for the draconian measure of incarceration (118, 255, 265, 387) and for the use of outpatient medication injections (255, 273), both of which have been introduced by these groups. It is hoped that the former strategy will be rendered obsolete by more readily accepted therapy and more appropriate compliance maneuvers. At the same time, adoption of the latter tactic in overcoming compliance problems in other illnesses would clearly benefit patients (692).

The last three decades have witnessed a proliferation of efficacious therapies for many infectious, endocrine, and hypertensive diseases; and compliance with short-term treatments is now easily assisted (see Chapter 8). On the other hand, the recognition of major compliance problems that accompany lengthy treatments such as those for hypertension has sensitized the health establishment to the subject. Thus, hypertension has served as a nidus for the crystallization of our understanding of compliance and its management, with the result that patients with a wide range of chronic illnesses may benefit.

Readers familiar with this book's predecessor (794) may be pleasantly surprised by the advance in knowledge that has occurred in the last three years. The determinants or causes of compliance are better defined (and even more plentiful) as reported in Chapters 4-6, and some highly practical maneuvers can now be employed by front line clinicians to combat low compliance with numerous regimens. Although some battles have been won, the compliance war is far from over. Some readers (especially those who seek easy, universal solutions to problems in understanding, measuring, and improving compliance) may be disappointed by what they find or do not find in these pages. Perhaps by the next edition . . .

But such a promise is premature because, having just achieved some success with compliance for long-term regimens, we have begun to fire the first rounds (or at least rattle sabers) in yet another war, this one against unhealthy lifestyles. Accordingly, we have added chapters on seat belt use and mass media (Chapter 12), cigarette smoking (Chapter 13) and alcoholism (Chapter 14). The toll from these "diseases of lifestyle" in Western society is awesome. However, a study of the contributions from Mr. Kelley and Drs. Best and Sellers and their coauthors reveals that we are far from achieving practical and effective strategies for changing these behaviors. Thus, these chapters demonstrate the limits as well as the progress made in managing these problems.

HOW THIS BOOK IS ORGANIZED

The authors of this book are seasoned compliance investigators with demonstrated expertise in understanding or managing one or more aspects of the compliance problem. Their specialized contributions are designed to cover all aspects of compliance without extensive overlap. Their contributions have been arranged to provide an orderly progression through what is currently known about compliance. The chapters fall into seven natural groupings.

I. The Magnitude and Measurement of Compliance

Chapter 2, on the magnitude of compliance problems, will be of interest to students of natural history and large aggregates. Its conclusions are distressing, and we long for the day that successful methods for maintaining and improving compliance become so common as to relegate these observations to the domain of history. Chapter 3, on measurement, is a must for anyone who wants to understand or modify compliance.

II. The Determinants of Compliance

The phenomenology of compliance is riddled with contradictions, and when we review our own prior perceptions of its determinants or those of newcomers to the field it is clear that compliance is one of the least understood yet most guessed-about topics in health care. Chapters 4 and 5 seek to clarify these murky waters, and Chapter 6 presents a debate that shows that even the experts cannot agree about some fundamental determinants of compliance behavior.

III. Strategies for Improving Compliance

This section begins with a discussion of the ethical issues in compliance intervention and research (Chapter 7) that should be read by all who contemplate the practical application of the information in this book. It is followed by an overview of controlled trials of compliance intervention (Chapter 8), which provides both an easy entry for the newcomer to the field and an updated review for the veteran. There follows a series of detailed discussions of individual modes of intervention. These emphasize practical suggestions both for implementing those strategies that work and for abandoning those that do not (Chapters 9-11).

IV. Altering Unhealthy Lifestyles

Chapter 12 through 14, on seat belt use, cigarette smoking, and alcohol abuse are included as an expanded foray into the perplexing problems posed by harmful lifestyles. They assess the state of the art and describe innovative treatment programs that have met with some success.

V. Compliance Providers and Places

Two groups of health professionals have taken the lead in exploring and dealing with compliance problems: nurses (Chapter 15) and pharmacists (Chapter 16). Although these chapters will be of particular interest to professional nurses and pharmacists, they should also be read by other professionals searching for ways to get on with the real work of monitoring and managing compliance problems.

These two chapters are followed by a thoughtful review (Chapter 17) of ways to organize providers and facilities to optimize compliance. The section concludes with a do-it-yourself primer (Chapter 18) for the clinician who wants to change compliance without necessarily mastering the theory and data presented in previous chapters.

VI. Research Applications and Future Research

This section is directed both to those involved in compliance research and to those whose research results are affected by variations in compliance. The final chapter provides a summary of research methods and pitfalls distilled from perhaps 200 man-years of compliance research experience, and should be helpful to those who seek to develop or validate new knowledge about compliance.

VII. Reference Materials

It is no longer possible to execute an exhaustive review of the scientific literature on compliance. Nonetheless, it has been possible to catalog most compliance articles published before our press time in 1978. The bibliography has two special features that extend its usefulness beyond the date of publication. First, the methodological merit of each investigation has been assessed and is summarized below each citation as a series of scores. These entries will assist the design of future investigations of the same topics. Second, the findings of each article have been entered in a series of tables at the end of the bibliography. The latter feature will be useful in determining where to start in learning about specific compliance issues, ranging from the influence of the patient's personality on compliance (Table 8) to the chemical reagents required to measure thiazide diuretics in urine (Table 11). These tables will also speed the updating of an area previously mastered. The bibliography thus permits the user to be both selective and efficient in further reading (more guides to the use of the reference materials appear in the introduction to Appendix I).

HOW TO USE THIS BOOK

We suspect that few people will read this book from cover to cover. It is a reference, not a novel. The preceding outline, the table of contents, and the index should guide readers in tailoring the use of the book to their own interests. Nonetheless, we do have a suggestion for those practitioners who find themselves reading the book more from duty than desire. The quick tour through the practical aspects of compliance measurement and management begins in whatever chapter in Part V (Compliance Providers and Places) best coincides with the reader's setting and ends in Chapter 3 on measurement and 7 on ethics.

I
THE MAGNITUDE
AND MEASUREMENT
OF COMPLIANCE

2

The Magnitude
of Compliance
and Noncompliance

David L. Sackett and John C. Snow

INTRODUCTION

The gap between the regimen recommended by the clinician and that adhered to by the patient is distressingly wide. It is one of the paradoxes of compliance that the former partner in this relationship is frequently the last to know. True, clinicians often believe that individuals under their care are noncompliant, but, as is shown in Chapter 3, they substantially overestimate the compliance of their own patients (though not necessarily that of other therapists' patients), and they have been shown to be unreliable predictors of whether their patients will comply.

For many students of compliance, an initial awareness of the extent of noncompliance came in the form of awe-struck disbelief at reading the work of pioneers such as Bergman and Werner (42) in North America and Porter (405) in Great Britain. As more reports have appeared it has become apparent that noncompliance is a protean feature of all regimens that involve self-administration. This chapter will document what is known of the magnitude of noncompliance by cataloging and summarizing representative studies from a variety of clinical situations and settings.

THE PRESENT STATE OF KNOWLEDGE

Methods of Assessing the Evidence

The strategies and tactics of our selection and methodologic assessment of the compliance literature are described in detail in Appendix I. For the purpose of this chapter, it is sufficient for the reader to know that each of the 537 original studies uncovered in our search has been assessed and scored with respect to the rigor with which it recognized and dealt with six methodologic issues of central importance to the investigation of compliance: study design, sample selection and specification, description of the illness, description of the therapeutic regimen, completeness of the definition of compliance, and the adequacy of the measurement of compliance.

Since the central focus of this chapter is the magnitude of the problem, it might seem that those methodologic criteria of greatest importance would be the definition and measurement of compliance. However, no measurement, regardless of its sophistication, can produce useful or universal results when it is applied to a thoughtlessly gathered sample of patients. To illustrate the importance of this point, consider the effect that the duration of therapy has upon the level of compliance with that therapy. If challenged to design an investigation to study this problem, most readers would select all the members of a group of patients who were just beginning a therapeutic regimen and would measure their compliance at appropriate intervals thereafter. Indeed, most of the studies reporting marked deterioration in compliance as the duration of therapy continues (42, 95, 192, 246, 265, 345) incorporated such a sampling strategy. However, it is often difficult and costly to track down all members of such an *inception cohort* (1408). Many investigators have therefore opted for the much easier strategy of taking all patients currently attending an appropriate clinic, measuring their compliance, and relating this measurement to the time elapsed since their therapy was started. The appropriateness of this second strategy can be assessed by considering whether its execution would result in the exclusion of the following members of the inception cohort: the patient who dislikes the regimen, stops, it, and seeks care elsewhere; the patient who dislikes the regimen, admits noncompliance, and is switched to an alternative regimen; the patient who dislikes the regimen, stops complying, raises hell, disrupts the clinic, and is told to seek care elsewhere; the patient who dislikes the regimen, stops complying, and succumbs to the illness. Clearly, the cross-sectional survey of such a clinic would miss these compliance failures and produce a spuriously high estimate of compliance that obscured the effect of time. That this attention to sampling is not merely of theoretical concern is confirmed by the finding that most of the reports that concluded that the duration of therapy has no important effect upon compliance (40, 127, 137, 405, 441) were performed upon cross sections of groups of patients who happened to be attending a given health facility at the time of the investigation.

For this reason, in preparing this chapter, the compliance articles were first screened for their attention to the selection and specification of the sample of patients studied. This screening process, which rejected articles with sample scores of 0, 1, or 2* (convenience samples—see Appendix I), reduced the refer-

---

*Readers of our earlier book (794) may note that we have raised the requirement for inclusion in this chapter.

TABLE 2.1. A guide to studies of the magnitude of compliance

Intent of recommendation	Type of Recommendation				
		Medications			
	Appointment-keeping	Short-term	Long-term	Diets	Others
Prevention	Table 2.2	2.4	2.6		2.9
Management or cure	2.3	2.5	2.7	2.8	

ence pool from 537 reports to fewer than 40. These were then grouped into clinically meaningful categories (Table 2.1) and reviewed for other methodologic standards and for their conclusions.

Despite this screening process, the reliability of the compliance rates provided here is frequently uncertain, and the reader is advised to bear the following restrictions in mind when interpreting them.

1. Strict limitation of this review to studies of inception cohorts would narrow its scope to a handful of randomized pharmacologic trials, the samples in which are frequently unattractive for other reasons (indeed, they are sometimes generated by tactics that weed out noncompliers before the trial begins). Thus, many of the compliance rates reported here are based on studies of "survivors" and may, as a result, overestimate the magnitude of compliance.

2. Bad news sells newspapers, and perhaps scientific journals as well. Reassuring or otherwise "bland" compliance rates may therefore be less likely to be submitted, and accepted, for publication. To the extent that they are affected by this factor, published rates will underestimate the magnitude of compliance.

3. Those who create the scientific literature base their reports, for the most part, on highly unusual groups of patients. The subjects of these reports are frequently referred to, sometimes attracted by, and usually tolerant of centers of clinical care with strong academic and research orientations. In generating large numbers of nonrepresentative patients with unusual disorders (an absolute prerequisite for the advancement of certain areas of knowledge), it is possible that these patients are also nonrepresentative of usual compliance patterns. Add to this the fact that the clinicians-in-training who care for these patients exhibit a high turnover (a factor which, as revealed in Chapter 4, is associated with decreased compliance), and the need for caution in interpreting these compliance rates is reinforced.

4. Finally, the reports summarized here have employed many definitions of, and measurements for, compliance. As shown in Chapter 3, it is difficult to be confident of conclusions drawn from studies using different definitions of compliance and measurement techniques of varying accuracy.

Having thus armed the reader with cautions and disclaimers sufficient to temper the interpretation of individual findings (but we hope not so many as to render the interpretation paretic or nihilistic), we are ready to proceed.

Results of the Assessment

Tables 2.2-2.9 provide an annotated listing of compliance rates in a number of situations and settings. A standard format has been followed for each entry in these tables, beginning with the reference number for the study and followed by a brief description of the regimen, the sample, the measure and definition of compliance that were applied, and, finally, the degree of compliance observed. Wherever appropriate, the methodologic scores for individual study components are included at the beginning of each entry.

Compliance with Scheduled Appointments.

Tables 2.2 and 2.3 describe the levels of compliance with appointment-keeping that have been observed in several different clinical settings. A review of these tables suggests that when appointments are initiated by health professsionals (Table 2.2 and the upper portion of Table 2.3) compliance with appointments is only about 50%; the exceptions occur when children are involved. On the other hand, when the appointment is initiated by the patient (as in the last two entries in Table 2.3), compliance rises to roughly 75%. This same trend was noted in our earlier review and suggests that readers who wish to compare these published results with those observed in their own settings would do well to distinguish between appointments initiated by patients and those initiated by their clinicians.

Compliance with Medications Prescribed for Short Periods of Time.

A scrutiny of the citations listed in Tables 2.4 and 2.5 suggests a repetition of the pattern found in Tables 2.2 and 2.3, but the number of entries is small. Raising the methodologic requirements for inclusion in these tables led to the rejection of several articles concerning short-term oral penicillin which revealed rapid declines in compliance even over the first ten days of therapy (32, 42).

Compliance with Medications Prescribed over Long Periods of Time.

Despite moderate variation (Tables 2.6 and 2.7), rates of compliance with different long-term medication regimens for different illnesses in different settings tend to converge to approximately 50%. Exceptions appear in the form of higher rates when based upon either the reports of clinicians or self-reporting by patients; the shortcomings of these alternative approaches to measuring compliance must be borne in mind, and they are fully discussed in Chapter 3.

An interesting issue arises here in considering "average" rates. Though the average compliance rates in long-term medication studies appear to be fairly

TABLE 2.2. Appointment-keeping for prevention

Citation	Regimen	Sample	Measure	Definition	Compliance
36	(2) Keeping an appointment for a Tay-Sachs screening test	(3+1) 30,000 individuals 16-45 years old (USA)	(3) Interview	(2) Showing up	10%
259	(2) Keeping an appointment for a Pap smear	(2+1) 23,000 welfare recipients (USA)	(3) Record review	(1) Showing up	52%
167	(1) Keeping an appointment for breast cancer screening	(2+1) (a) 4,972 women from a medical group practice and (b) 2,853 women from hospital clinics	(2) Record review	(1) Showing up	(a) 65% (b) 44%
221	(1) Keeping an appointment following hearing and vision screening	(2+1) 6,731 school children in 128 schools (USA)	(1+1) Record review	(1) Showing up	Hearing clinic: 32% Eye clinic: 39%
173	(0) Keeping an appointment following discovery of hypertension	(2+1) 291 patients seen in an emergency room (USA)	(2) Record review	(1) Showing up	58%
87	(1) Keeping an appointment following hypertension screening	(2+1) 533 individuals in a door to door survey (USA)	(2) Record review	(1) Showing up	65%
520	(0) Keeping an appointment following hypertension screening	(3) 6,012 individuals screened for hypertension (USA)	(1+1) Telephone interview	(2) Keeping a follow-up appointment	51%
374	(2) Keeping an annual follow-up appointment	(2+1) 300 patients with inactive tuberculosis (Canada)	(2+1) Record review	(2) Showing up for each of 3 annual exams	Indians: 16% Non-Indians: 44%

TABLE 2.3. Appointment-keeping for management or cure

Citation	Regimen	Sample	Measure	Definition	Compliance
180	(0) Keeping an appointment for recommended care	(3+1) 241 families of 4th grade school children (USA)	(2) Interview	(1) Kept appointments for care	79%
472	(0) Keeping an appointment for dental care	(1+1) 2,662 preschool children (USA)	(1) Interview	(0) Planned to use dental services	84%
446	(2) Keeping an appointment for dental care	(2+1) 108 children (Denmark)	(3) Direct observation	(2) Showing up and accepting care	60%
152	(1) Keeping appointments at a child guidance clinic	(3+1) 253 children (USA)	(3) Questionnaire	(2) Showing up and accepting care	55%
241	(1) Keeping appointments in a psychiatric clinic	(2+1) 91 adolescents (USA)	(2) Record review	(2) Showing up	60%
260	(1) Keeping appointments in a prepaid group practice	(3+1) 10,466 patients in the practice	(2) Record review	(2) Showing up	77%
443	(2) Keeping appointments for treatment of peptic ulcer	(3) 160 patients in an out-patient clinic	(2) Record review	(1) Showing up	71%

TABLE 2.4. Short-term medication for prevention

Citation	Regimen	Sample	Measure	Definition	Compliance
76	(0+1) Receiving recommended immunizations	(3) Children in 784 welfare families (USA)	(1) Record review	(2) Received all recomcomended immuziations	60%
247	(3+1) Receiving recommended immunizations	(3+1) 66 children born in a given county (USA)	(3) Interview plus record review	(2) Received all recommended immunizations	64%

TABLE 2.5. Short-term medications for treatment or cure

Citation	Regimen	Sample	Measure	Definition	Compliance
371	(1) Several regimens prescribed at discharge from hospital	(3+1) 96 patients recently discharged from hospital (USA)	(2+1) Pill counts	(1) Taking > 90% of prescribed medications	77%
138	(1) Various medications	(3+1) 82 patients recently discharged from hospital (USA)	(1) Interview	(1) Taking medication as as prescribed	78%

TABLE 2.6. Long-term medications for prevention

Citation	Regimen	Sample	Measure	Definition	Compliance
200	(1) Penicillin prophylaxis for rheumatic fever	(3) 103 children on long-term prophylaxis (USA)	(4) Urine assay	(2) Medication present in urine	33%
230	(1) Antihypertensive drugs	(2+1) 2,322 men surveyed for hypertension (Sweden)	(2) Record review	(2) Remaining in care and on therapy	1 year: 94% 2 years: 65% 3 years: 34%
301	(0) Antihypertensive drugs	(2+1) 185 patients surveyed for hypertension (USA)	(1) Questionnaire	(1) Remaining in care and on therapy	69%
449 and 228	(1+1) Antihypertensive drugs	(2+1) 230 hypertensive steel-workers (Canada)	(2+1) Pill count	(2) Taking > 80% of medication	6 months: 53% 12 months: 53%

TABLE 2.7. Long-term medications for treatment or cure

Citation	Regimen	Sample	Measure	Definition	Compliance
455	(0+1) Various medications	(2+1) 178 elderly ambulatory patients (USA)	(1) Interview	(1) Taking medications correctly	41%
256 and 258	(1+1) Various medications	(3+1) 357 patients with diabetes or congestive heart failure (USA)	(1) Interview	(2) Taking medications correctly	42%
236	(1) Various medications	(3+1) 217 patients in homes for the aged (Finland)	(1) Interview	(2) Taking medications correctly	69%
6	(1) Antituberculous chemotherapy	(3+1) 1,000 tuberculous patients (Canada)	(3+2) Interview and urine testing	(1) Taking drugs throughout follow-up	55%
141	(1) Antituberculous chemotherapy	(3+1) 1,828 tuberculous patients (Canada)	(3) Record review	(2) Continuing in therapy	63%
240	(0) Chemotherapy for leprosy	(3+1) 8,655 patients with leprosy (Tanzania)	(2) Record review	(2) Continuing in therapy	68%
315	(2+1) Tranquillizers in a randomized trial	(3) 254 neurotic out-patients (USA)	(2+1) Pill counts	(2) Pill counts within 25% of prescribed amount	54%
246	(1) Tranquillizers	(3+1) 374 schizophrenic outpatients (USA)	(1) Interview	(1) Taking medications correctly	42%

similar in different clinical settings, it is important to take into consideration the distribution of individual patient's compliance rates as well. Few studies have provided this information. Fortunately, Gordis et al. (200) provided valuable data from which a frequency distribution of compliance rates can be constructed for children on long-term oral penicillin prophylaxis for rheumatic fever. As discussed in Chapter 19, this compliance distribution is roughly U-shaped, with one-third of the patients taking virtually no medications, one-third almost all, and the rest scattered in between. A similar pattern has been found by our group among steelworkers on antihypertensive drugs (228, 449). If these distributions typify the compliance habits of other patient populations, the practical implications will be much different than would be the case if a statistically "normal" (or bell-shaped) distribution of rates applied, as discussed in Chapter 21. Is this U-shaped distribution the general pattern for compliance with medications? Do the individual determinants of compliance act through this range? We will not know until we look; so far, almost no one has.

Compliance with Diets and with Other Regimens.

The entries in Tables 2.8 and 2.9 are clearly morsels, not a feast; the tactics of our survey of the compliance literature favored medications at the expense of other therapeutic recommendations. Furthermore, although compliance with dietary recommendations (Table 2.8) is a key issue in preventive cardiology, studies that will produce dietary compliance rates applicable to the general public are only now getting underway. A second striking feature of compliance with diets is the sharply different estimates of dietary adherence achieved when "hard" measures of compliance (133) rather than the assessments of the clinical staff (58) are used.

Table 2.9 summarizes a handful of the very small number of methodologically sound studies of compliance with other preventive health regimens; antismoking regimens are described in detail in Chapter 13 and those for alcohol in Chapter 14. Low compliance with these "lifestyle" regimens constitutes a major impediment to their impact, and the paucity of careful studies in this field is profound.

To the extent that there is consistency in the compliance rates reviewed here, they can be summarized in three sentences. First, patients will keep approximately 75% of the appointments that they make, but only about 50% of those made for them. Second, compliance with short-term regimens declines rapidly. Finally, about one-half of patients on long-term regimens are compliant. This stark summary emphasizes the serious nature of the problem of compliance, and in its brevity also serves to underscore our continuing ignorance about the problem.

TABLE 2.8. Diets

Citation	Regimen	Sample	Measure	Definition	Compliance
182	(1) Weight reduction diets	(2+1) Members of 21 chapters of TOPS (USA)	(4) Body weights	(2) Weight loss of (a) ⩾ 20 lbs. or (b) ⩾ 40 lbs.	a: 29% b: 8%
133	(1) Special hemodialysis diet	(3+1) 136 patients with chronic renal failure (Israel)	(4+2) Interview plus measures of weight and blood chemistries	(2) Weight gain < 1 Kg and K+ < 6 mEq and BUN < 70 mg% predialysis	28%
58	(1) Special hemodialysis diet	(3+1) 661 patients with chronic renal failure (USA)	(1) Staff assessments	(2) Staff rating of excellent or adequate adherence	70%

TABLE 2.9. Other Preventive Regimens

Citation	Regimen	Sample	Measure	Definition	Compliance
431	(2) Seat belt use	(2+1) 162,835 drivers in several locations (USA)	(4) Direct observations	(2) Driver wearing seat belt	15% overall (5% in winter)
433	(1) Seat belt use	(2+1) 13,593 drivers in several locations (USA)	(3+1) Direct observations	(2) Driver wearing seat belt	23%–59%
487	(1) Wearing safety gloves	(3) 115 sugar cane cutters (Puerto Rico)	(2+1) Interview	(2) Acceptance of gloves	50%
267	(2) Cessation of smoking*	(2+1) 58 heavy cigarette smokers (Sweden)	(3+1) Carboxyhemoglobin measurement	(2) COHb <1% at 8 months	29%
346	(0) Appropriate use of safety containers for medications	(3) 636 patients with several regimens	(1) Interviews	(1) Using safety dispenser properly	78%

*The success of antismoking programs is discussed in detail in Chapter 13.

PRIORITIES FOR FUTURE RESEARCH

Four specific suggestions flow naturally from this review of the magnitude of compliance and warrant special mention here.

1. The Need for Studies of Inception Cohorts

Much work, by many investigators, has been seriously compromised through the failure to follow all patients who were started on a given therapeutic regimen. It is only through accounting for every patient who was present at the inception of therapy that the determination of group compliance at a later point in time is meaningful. The systematic loss to analysis of the least compliant patients (those who drop out entirely or rarely keep appointments) invalidates the conclusions of a large number of compliance investigations, and this failure cannot be overcome by statistical or pharmacologic maneuvers.

The issue here is not sophistication in sampling, but completeness. Nor does it restrict research workers to sitting on their haunches waiting for freshly diagnosed and newly treated patients to ripen for years before determining the long-term compliance rate. If a complete listing is available of all patients in a given facility who were placed on treatment at a fixed earlier point in time, the patients can be located and studied without delay. Indeed, the key issue in such an investigation concerns those among the inception cohort who either no longer come to the original facility or no longer attend any treatment facility at all, for their evaluation will produce crucial data.

2. The Need for Reporting Complete Compliance Distributions

As our understanding of compliance increases, simple measures such as the mean number of pills consumed or the percentage of patients who complied with all recommendations no longer provide sufficient information. Since some determinants may have important effects upon compliance only when it is relatively high, and others only when it is relatively low, compliance reports should include tables and graphs showing the distribution of compliance across all patients. The publication of these compliance distributions will permit comparisons between centers and regimens, yet still leave their authors free to use summary measures for other analyses of more direct pertinence to their experiments.

It must be recognized that some journals, through the pressures of tradition or space, will refuse to add further data on compliance distributions to published articles; when this occurs, use should be made of documentation* which, when

---

*One such service is The National Auxiliary Publications Service, c/o Microfiche Publications, 305 E. 46th St., New York, N.Y. 10017.

referred to by footnote in the published article, can supply other interested investigators with copies of any material submitted to them by the authors.

3. The Need for Coupling Compliance to the Achievement of Treatment Goals

Reports should recognize that the degree of compliance required for the achievement of the desired treatment goal probably varies from one regimen to another. For example, Leon Gordis points out in Chapter 3 that children taking as little as 30% of their prescribed prophylactic penicillin enjoy substantial protection from recurrences of rheumatic fever. On the other hand, we have found that hypertensives must take at least 80% of their medications before they will exhibit systematic blood pressure responses to therapy. What is the case for other regimens prescribed for other illnesses?

When reporting a compliance investigation to an applied audience, the relationship between compliance levels and the achievement of the treatment goal should be described. This can take the form of a two-way plot, and the treatment goal can perhaps best be expressed as a proportion of target outcomes achieved (e.g., percentage of sputa that no longer contain tubercle bacilli or percentage of patients who achieve goal blood pressures).

4. The Need for a Precise Description of the Study Design

Finally, publications of compliance research should describe in detail those strategies used in generating the study sample and should define precisely the illnesses and therapeutic regimens under investigation, as well as the definitions and measurements used in determining compliance and noncompliance. These descriptions should be presented with a degree of clarity that would permit a second research group to replicate the investigation with precision. Indeed, such precise replications, by other investigators in other settings, are crucial to the development of new knowledge concerning compliance with therapeutic regimens.

3

Conceptual
and Methodologic
Problems in Measuring
Patient Compliance

Leon Gordis

INTRODUCTION

It is perhaps a truism in medical or biological research that the quality of the research and the validity of the inferences that can be derived from it can be no better than the research design and measurement methods employed. This is particularly relevant to investigations of patient compliance in which global inferences are often made that are disproportionate to the quality of the research methods employed and yet are often used as the basis for programmatic intervention. It is therefore highly appropriate that a major focus of any discussion of compliance be on the methodologic aspects of measuring compliance and on the conceptual issues involved in the classification of patients' compliance behavior.

It is not the purpose of this chapter to review the details of specific techniques of measuring compliance, but rather to raise some key concerns about the reporting and interpretation of results derived from such techniques. Those readers who are interested in the practical application of existing techniques in busy clinical settings are also referred to Chapter 18 and to Table 2 in the annotated bibliography (Appendix I of this book), that categorizes citations according to objective methods of measuring compliance.

REASONS FOR MEASURING COMPLIANCE

Why measure compliance in the first place? There are a number of reasons for embarking on such a project. Basically, compliance is measured for either research or clinical purposes. In research studies, the focus may be on the extent

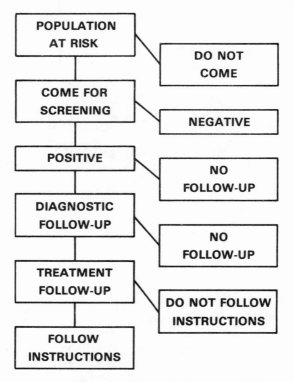

FIGURE 3.1.   Flow chart illustrating problem of defining noncompliance in a screening
              program.

of noncompliance, the effect of noncompliance on outcome, and/or the dynamics of noncompliance. In a clinical setting, there is interest in monitoring compliance as well as intervention, which may entail the substitution of an alternate medical regimen or some form of behavior modification to induce better compliance. However, regardless of whether the purpose is clinical care or research, a valid method of measuring compliance is essential.

PROBLEMS IN DEFINING NONCOMPLIANCE

Types of Noncompliance

Noncompliance may be manifested in a number of forms such as delay in seeking care, nonparticipation in health programs, breaking of appointments, or failure to follow physicians' instructions. This chapter will focus on the last form of noncompliance and specifically on the use of medications. Before addressing this subject, however, it is important to note that in many areas not discussed in this chapter the problem of defining noncompliance may be extremely difficult. Consider, for example, the question of noncompliance in a screening program (Figure 3.1) where there is at risk a population of which some members come for screening and some do not. Some of those who come have positive test results and some negative; some of the positives come for definitive diagnostic evaluation and others do not; some of those positively diagnosed come for treatment and others do not and of those who come, some follow therapeutic and/or preventive instructions and others do not. What numerators and denominators should be employed for calculating rates of noncompliance in this population? Specifically, what is meant by noncompliance? Are we talking about "no shows" in general, or are we talking only about the last group of people who do not follow physicians' recommendations? Each time a study of noncompliance with screening programs is carried out, the definition employed for noncompliance in that study must be explicit. Indeed, this same requirement holds for studies of any form of noncompliance in any setting.

NONCOMPLIANCE OR MEDICATION ERRORS

It is important to distinguish between noncompliance and medication errors. In the case of medication errors, the patient's intent is to comply but the complexity of the regimen, the patient's intellectual limitations, or other circumstances may have confused him so that he does not or cannot follow the instructions. On the other hand, noncompliance implies an intent not to follow instructions and therefore the dynamics involved and the intervention approaches that might be effective in each circumstance may be quite different. Long ago, Samuel Butler commented: "He that complies against his will, is of his own opinion still." Perhaps the patient's opinion may not be too important as long as he follows instructions. On the other hand, an important and practical question is whether noncompliant patients can be converted to across-the-board compliers in the clinical setting so that noncompliance will no longer be a repeated problem each and every time a new medication is prescribed. In other words, can patients be characterized accurately as noncompliers, and if they comply in one instance, should they then be characterized as compliers and can it be assumed they will comply in other settings as well? This is an important issue from the practical standpoint and one that requires appropriate methods of measurement.

METHODS FOR MEASURING COMPLIANCE

Let us now turn to some of the specific methods available for measuring compliance and in particular those for measuring compliance with medications.

TABLE 3.1. Ways of measuring medication compliance

A. *Direct*
  1. Blood levels
  2. Urinary excretion of
    a. medication
    b. metabolite
    c. marker (tracer)

B. *Indirect*
  1. Therapeutic or preventive outcome
  2. "Impression" of physician (predictability)
  3. Patient interview
  4. Filling of prescription
  5. Pill count

The latter is perhaps the area which has been studied most thoroughly and is most amenable to careful quantification. As seen in Table 3.1, it may be assessed both directly and indirectly.

Direct Methods

For accuracy, direct ways of measuring patient compliance are essential, but the available methods (see Table 11 in Appendix I) are not without difficulties. The problems are twofold: first, there are the technical aspects of the test itself, including its sensitivity and specificity as a method of detection; second, there are the conceptual questions of how to define or classify a patient as a complier or a noncomplier.

Detection Methods.

Figure 3.2 shows a method for detecting penicillin in the urine of patients on oral prophylaxis against rheumatic fever (862). A filter paper strip is dipped into the urine of the patient who is supposed to be taking penicillin and the end of the paper strip is cut off and applied to an agar plate streaked with *Sarcina lutea*, an organism highly sensitive to penicillin. When penicillin is present in the urine it diffuses out into the surrounding medium and inhibits the growth of the organism. In carrying out such a test, it is important that one know the absorption and excretion pattern of the agent. For example, when children were administered oral penicillin in a monitored hospital setting, almost 100% of the patients had positive urine tests for about four to five hours following ingestion of the penicillin. It is therefore critical that if a urinary test for penicillin compliance is to be used in nonhospital populations, it be carried out during the period when penicillin could be detected in the urine. A test carried out beyond this period would produce negative results even for true compliers.

Often it is not possible to detect either the medication or any by-product of the medication directly, and it may be necessary to add a detectable label to the

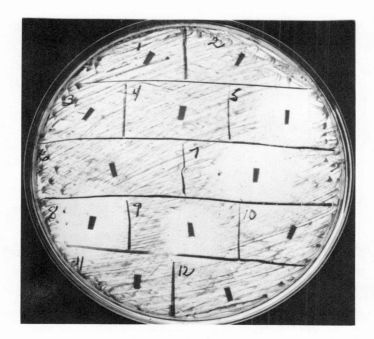

FIGURE 3.2. Assessment of the presence of penicillin in urine through *Sarcina lutea* inhibition.*

*Penicillin is present in urine in filter strips in cells 5, 7, 8, and 9, as is evidenced by zones of inhibited growth of *Sarcina lutea* surrounding these strips.

medication. Several years ago, Porter listed the requirements for an effective label for testing patient compliance (Table 3.2), and these remain an excellent guide today.

An important issue in measuring patient compliance is that of *pharmacokinetic variations*—differences among individuals in absorption, distribution, metabolism, and excretion of drugs. Two basic classes of factors enter into these differences: one is the bioavailability of a drug and the other is genetic differences among individuals in how they metabolize and excrete a drug. *Bioavailability* is defined as the amount of drug absorbed from a certain formulation

TABLE 3.2. Requirements for a urine marker to assess patient compliance in taking medication

A. Nontoxic; pharmacologically and chemically inert
B. Unaffected by physical and chemical properties of urine (pH, temperature, etc.)
C. Quickly and freely excreted; noncumulative
D. Simple, sensitive, and specific detection methods available
E. Patient unaware of the marker

SOURCE: Adapted from Porter 1969 (405).

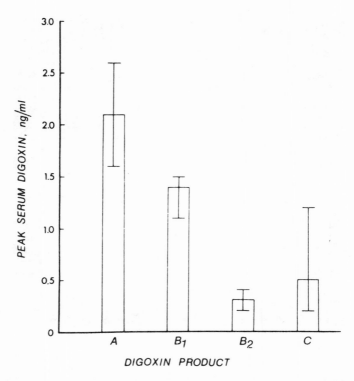

FIGURE 3.3.   Mean peak serum digoxin concentrations attained after oral administration
of 0.5 mg of each of four digoxin products to four subjects. The crossbars
represent the range of observations in the four volunteers.

SOURCE: Lindenbaum et al. 1971 (860).

of the drug relative to the amount of drug absorbed from a standard reference
formulation (858). The form in which the drug is administered—whether the
drug is in capsule or tablet form—will have a major effect on its absorption. The
rate of release of a drug upon oral administration will vary, with slowest rates
for coated tablets and most rapid rates for aqueous solutions and syrups. Furthermore, different formulations of the same drug have been shown to differ in
their bioavailability. For example, Lindenbaum et al. (860) showed marked
variations in the biologic availability of digoxin from four preparations (Figures
3.3 and 3.4). All these characteristics of the agent must therefore be taken into
consideration when assessing patient compliance, for when groups of patients
differ in the proportion who have positive tests, it is not always clear whether
variations in compliance or variations in the bioavailability of the drugs prescribed and taken are being identified.

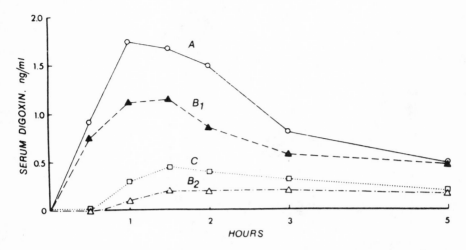

FIGURE 3.4.   Mean serum digoxin levels over a five-hour period after oral administration
of four digoxin products to four volunteers. Each line represents the mean of
four curves.

SOURCE: Lindenbaum et al. 1971 (860).

A second aspect of the pharmacokinetic variation associated with a given drug
is biologic variation in how an agent is handled among different individuals given
the same dose of a drug. For example, Brodie and co-workers (857) reported
significant interindividual variations in how biscoumacetate was metabolized by
eight normal subjects after a single intravenous dose of 20 mg/kg (Figure 3.5).
Of particular interest is the fact that genetic determinants are extremely important in the rate of metabolism of drugs. For example, Vessell (863) compared
the decline of antipyrine in three sets of identical and three sets of fraternal
twins (Figure 3.6). It will be observed that the curves for the identical twins over
time are quite close, but there is a significant divergence in the rates of metabolism of the drug among the sets of fraternal twins.

Another interesting consideration in compliance testing has to do with
whether the drug tested is being given over a short term or administered repeatedly over a long period. Repeated administration of certain drugs enhances their
metabolism by inducing hepatic microsomal enzyme systems. Consequently,
chronic administration could substantially decrease the blood level of these
drugs. On the other hand, some drugs such as dilantin produce metabolites
that inhibit biotransformation of the parent drug, thereby tending to increase
blood levels of the parent compound during its chronic administration.

It is thus clear that any study of compliance must take into account a number
of characteristics related to pharmacokinetic variation among patients and

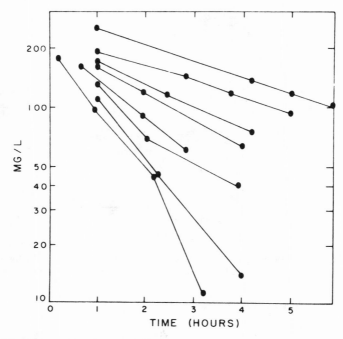

FIGURE 3.5.   Decay of ethyl biscoumacetate in the plasma of eight normal volunteers after a single intravenous dose of 20 mg/kg.

SOURCE: Brodie et al. 1952 (857).

other variables related to the drug preparation itself. Failure to consider these factors could lead to serious errors in inference regarding compliance levels of different groups of patients.

Indirect Measures of Compliance

Outcome as an Indirect Measure.

A frequently used indirect measure of compliance is the outcome of the treatment or preventive regimen. At first glance, outcome would appear to be a reasonable measure of compliance if we have sufficient faith that the recommended regimen, when adhered to, is truly effective. Several reports do indeed document a relationship between noncompliance and a lack of preventive or therapeutic effectiveness. For example, in rheumatic fever patients on oral penicillin prophylaxis, antistreptolysin O titers were determined at two-month intervals and correlated with levels of compliance (Figure 3.7). Although the groups were small, the data suggest that patients complying less than one-third of the time

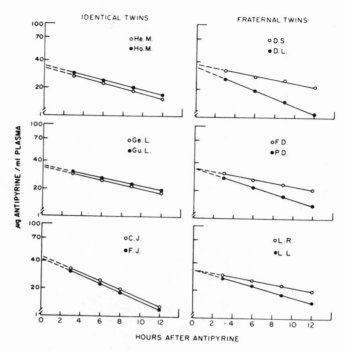

FIGURE 3.6. Decline of antipyrine in the plasma of three sets of identical twins (left) and of three sets of fraternal twins (right) after a single oral dose of 18 mg/kg.

SOURCE: Vessell 1974 (863).

had a higher risk of streptococcal infection than the remaining patients (861). Further evidence relating noncompliance to suboptimal outcome has been reported in patients with epilepsy who were not responding to diphenylhydantoin. Kutt and co-workers found that, in twelve of sixteen such patients, noncompliance was a significant problem; when the medication was administered to them under rigidly monitored hospital conditions, adequate blood levels of the drug were achieved and a good therapeutic response resulted (297).

There are, however, a number of conceptual problems in using outcome as a measure of compliance. The use of outcome for this purpose is predicated on a simple model in which the effect of good medical care in improving the patient's outcome is mediated through compliance (Figure 3.8a). However, some components of effective medical care are not necessarily mediated through compliance. For example, a patient on antihypertensive medication may also receive reassurance by his physician, with consequent reduction of stress that in itself may have a beneficial effect. Thus, the outcome in such a patient may

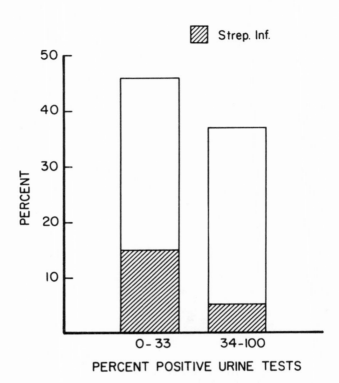

FIGURE 3.7. Comparison of the number and proportion of patients experiencing streptococcal infections while on penicillin prophylaxis, by a level of compliance.

SOURCE: Markowitz 1970 (861).

be the product of medical care factors mediated by compliance, combined
with medical care factors that do not require any such mediation (Figure 3.8b).
Another problem is that a patient may be on multiple medications and compliance with the medication being studied may differ from compliance with other
medications that, though not being investigated, are effective. If the patient
were a poor complier for the specific medication being studied yet a good complier for the other medications not being studied, a good outcome could result
in the face of poor compliance.

Yet another problem in using outcome measures as indexes of compliance is
that outcome is frequently affected by many external factors in addition to the
medical care provided (Figure 3.8c). Socioeconomic and cultural factors and
occupational exposures are but a few of these. Thus, the relationship of compliance to outcome becomes increasingly complicated. Indeed, these external
factors may modify not only the outcome but also compliance itself. The result

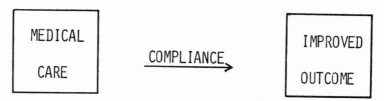

FIGURE 3.8a. Ideal model in which improved patient outcome is solely mediated by compliance with prescribed therapy.

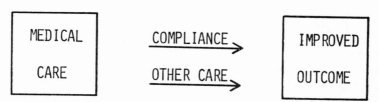

FIGURE 3.8b. Model in which improved patient outcome depends on both compliance with therapy and other medical care factors.

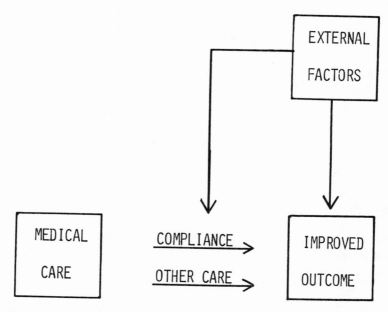

FIGURE 3.8c. Model in which improved patient outcome is also directly affected by external factors.

TABLE 3.3. Compliance with thiazide prescriptions and blood pressure control
during 207 clinic visits

| | | Urine thiazide test | | | |
| | | Positive | | Negative | |
		No.†	%	No.†	%
Blood pressure	Controlled‡	59	44	12	16
	Not controlled	75	56	61	84
	Total	134	100	73	100

SOURCE: Lowenthal et al. 1976 (319).
†Numbers refer to individual visits.
‡Controlled = < 145/95 at that visit; $P < 0.001$.

is a complex set of interactions in which compliance is only one of many factors relating to improved health. Viewed within this framework, differences in outcome are, in general, of limited value as measures of patient compliance.

Finally, even if there is a direct relationship between compliance and outcome, the nature of this relationship must be clarified. Although the compliance-outcome relationship may be comparable conceptually to a dose-response relationship, the configuration of the curves describing these relationships may differ. Is the compliance-outcome curve linear or exponential? Is it the same in different diseases and for different therapeutic or preventive agents? The compliance-outcome relationship is highly dependent upon the dose prescribed. For example, the effect of noncompliance will depend on how closely the prescribed dosage approximates the minimum dosage required for optimal therapeutic effect and on the margin of safety between the minimum effective dosage and that which produces toxicity. If, for example, the prescribed dosage substantially exceeds the minimum effective dosage, low compliance may not reduce the effectiveness of therapy at all; indeed, it may even serve to protect patients from toxicity due to overdosage.

An example of the problems inherent in this approach is seen in a study of compliance for antihypertensive medication (319). The results are shown in Table 3.3. Two groups of patients, those whose blood pressure was controlled and those whose blood pressure was not controlled, are compared using the results of a test for the presence of thiazide in the urine. As the data show, the relationship between positive versus negative thiazide tests and whether or not the blood pressure was controlled is statistically significant. However, the relationship is a limited one, for 56% of those with positive thiazide tests were not controlled, whereas 16% of those with negative tests were controlled. Viewed differently, the sensitivity is low—44%, whereas the specificity is fairly high—84%. Thus, in this instance, as in many others, depending on the purpose for which compliance testing is being carried out, outcome as defined by control of hypertension may not be an adequate reflection of actual compliance for thiazides.

Additional data are therefore needed to determine which relationship holds

TABLE 3.4. Comparison of compliance in children on penicillin prophylaxis by interview and by pill count

	By interview (N=113)	By pill count (N=109)
Good	73%	55%
Questionable	19%	35%
Poor	8%	10%
	100%	100%

SOURCE: Adapted from Feinstein et al. 1959 (160).

between compliance and outcome and whether the same relationship applies to different diseases and to different medications or regimens. Although outcome is a poor measure of the rate of compliance it does have one important use in nonresearch clinical settings: if it is impractical to assess the compliance of all patients by a means better than outcome, yet possible to measure compliance for some, the compliance assessments can be directed most efficiently and appropriately towards those who fail to reach the therapeutic goal. The implementation of this tactic is described further by Dave Sackett in Chapter 18.

The Interview as an Indirect Measure of Compliance.

In view of the difficulties involved in obtaining blood or urine specimens, particularly at unannounced but regular intervals, it is tempting to substitute an indirect but more practical measure of compliance such as asking the patient himself whether he has complied. Surprisingly, although Hippocrates observed that "[the physician] should keep aware of the fact that patients often lie when they state that they have taken certain medicines," it is only recently that the patient's reliability in reporting his own compliance has been scientifically investigated.

How valid are interview data as a measure of compliance? Data are available comparing interview responses with pill counts and with urine tests. Feinstein and his co-workers (160) compared compliance in children on penicillin prophylaxis by interview and pill count, as shown in Table 3.4. Although there was good agreement between the two methods among those classified as poor compliers, there was a considerable discrepancy among those classified as good compliers.

In another study, Park and Lipman (392) compared compliance estimates by interview and pill count in psychiatric outpatients on imipramine therapy (Table 3.5). By patient interview, 100 patients would be considered compliers, but by pill count only 57 were so classified. Conversely, of 14 patients who were noncompliers by pill count, only 7 of these admitted noncompliance at interview. Looking at the data in a different way, interview and pill count methods agree in only 68 of 117 patients.

TABLE 3.5. Comparison of compliance estimates by interview and pill count in psychiatric outpatients on imipramine therapy

		By patient interview			
		Compliers	Intermediates	Noncompliers	Total
By pill count	Compliers	55	2	0	57
	Intermediates	39	6	1	46
	Noncompliers	6	1	7	14
	Total	100	9	8	117

SOURCE: Adapted from Park and Lipman 1964 (392).

Rickels and Briscoe (426) compared 675 pill count and verbal reports in a group of neurotic outpatients. As before, verbal reports indicated generally less deviation from the prescribed dosage than did pill counts. However, the discrepancy between patients' reports and pill counts was greatest when deviation from prescribed dosage was small, and the discrepancy was relatively small when the deviation was large.

In a study of an outpatient pediatric clinic, Francis and co-workers (174) assessed compliance—in this case the degree to which mothers follow through on physicians' advice—primarily on the basis of responses to interviews. In addition, they were able to carry out pill counts among 129 of the 330 patients who had prescriptions for oral medication. Although the interpretation of these data is limited by this selection factor, in only 11 instances was there a discrepancy between interview assessment of noncompliance and pill count; in each case, the pill count suggested noncompliance when the interview responses had implied compliance.

Gordis et al. compared interview data with urine tests in children with rheumatic fever on oral prophylaxis (199). Figure 3.9a compares compliance estimates based on mothers' responses with estimates based on urine tests obtained at the time of clinic visits, and Figure 3.9b compares urine tests with the responses of children themselves. In both cases compliance was overstated and noncompliance understated by the respondents.

The inaccuracy of interview data in measuring patient compliance is also documented in the work of Sheiner and his co-workers, who found that the average outpatient took only 72% of the number of digitalis tablets which he claimed to have taken (578). Futhermore, Chaves reported that urine tests were negative in 27% of the patients who stated that they took their PAS (541). Finally, in a study by Preston and Miller (410), ambulatory tuberculosis patients were investigated to compare compliance based on their own statements with that shown through urine tests (Table 3.6). Twenty-four of 25 patients claimed to have taken their medication, when only 18 had done so according to urine tests.

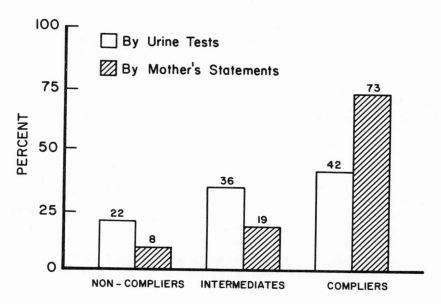

FIGURE 3.9a. Clinic compliance based on mother's statement compared with urine tests. (N=45)

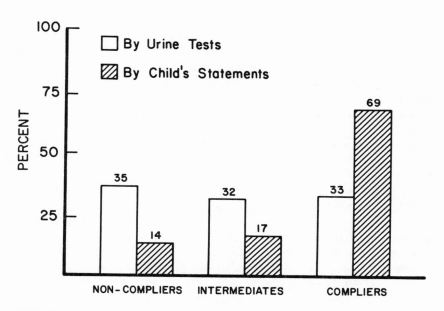

FIGURE 3.9b. Clinic compliance based on child's statement compared with urine test. (N=103)

TABLE 3.6. Compliance in ambulatory tuberculosis patients

| | Compliance | |
	No. †	%
By own statement	24	96
By physician assessment	20	80
By urine test	18	72

SOURCE: Preston and Miller 1964 (410).
†N=25.

In all these studies, there is little or no evidence to suggest that complying patients misrepresent themselves as noncompliers, nor is there evidence that those who profess noncompliance at interview are lying. Thus, although there are serious questions regarding the validity of interview responses, if the only objective of the interview is to identify noncompliers, many can be identified by this indirect measure. The degree to which this kind of information will be adequate depends upon the consequences to those noncompliers who are missed at interview because they profess to be compliant. Another important consideration, elaborated upon in Chapter 18, is that patients who admit to their noncompliance on questioning may respond better to efforts at improving compliance than will noncompliers who claim to be compliant.

The Pill Count as an Indirect Measure of Compliance.

The pill count or, more accurately, the comparison between the amount of medication remaining in the patient's bottle and the amount that should have remained (the latter calculated from the prescription and the length of time for which the medication had been prescribed) has frequently been used as a method of assessing compliance. Several studies have investigated the validity of this indirect measure.

Roth and his co-workers reported a two-year follow-up study of 105 patients with peptic ulcers (442). In order to study compliance with taking liquid antacids, sodium bromide was added to the antacid as a tracer. Of the 105 patients, 10 consistently returned more empty bottles than was justified on the basis of the bromide level in their blood. For these patients, the bottle counts were considered completely misleading by the investigators. Among the remaining patients, these investigators concluded that the bottle count was generally adequate, although it tended to overestimate compliance.

Bergman and Werner presented distribution data on both urine tests and pill counts in their study of children on ten-day penicillin therapy for streptococcal pharyngitis (42). The data, combined in Table 3.7, are marginal and therefore do not permit the identification of specific individuals in terms of both tests. By the ninth day, on the basis of urine tests, only 8% of the population was taking

TABLE 3.7. Comparison of compliance by urine test and pill count in children prescribed ten days of penicillin

On day	Percent complying by	
	Urine test	Pill count
3	46	44
6	31	29
9	8	18

SOURCE: Adapted from Bergman and Werner 1963 (42).

penicillin whereas on the basis of pill count 18% would have been considered compliant at that time.

Comparative data on the validity of pill counts therefore suggest serious problems of overestimation in using pill counts as indirect measures of compliance. Such problems would be even greater when the medication prescribed might be used by other members of the family as well as by the patient. For example, penicillin might be used by other family members for minor infections and antacids for a host of gastrointestinal complaints, whereas other agents, such as digitalis, would be less likely to present this problem. Thus, the limited data presently available suggest that the validity of pill counts as an indirect measure of compliance is open to serious question.

Physician Assessments of Compliance.

Another indirect measure of patient compliance is the physician's estimate. How valid is such a measure? How good is the physician at assessing compliance in his patients, identifying the noncompliers, and predicting noncompliant behavior?

Caron and Roth studied the ability of physicians to identify the noncompliant patient (90). Twenty-seven ward residents were asked to assess patient compliance with antacid regimens. The study showed that these physicians could not estimate their patients' drug intake any better than they might have by chance. The actual median patient compliance was 46% and the median physician error 32%. Twenty-two of the 27 physicians overestimated patient compliance. Even when their assessment was limited to patients about whom they felt fairly confident, the physicians were unsuccessful in identifying noncompliant patients. A similar study by Mushlin and Appel (370) investigated the ability of interns and residents at Baltimore City Hospitals to predict patient compliance in returning for follow-up appointments and in taking their dosage of digitalis and diuretics regularly. Table 3.8 shows some of Mushlin's data on the ability of residents to predict patient return. Although the physicians were correct in 145 of 187 patients, it is perhaps most signficant that the resident's predictions were accurate for only 14 of the 40 patients who failed to return for

TABLE 3.8. Predictions by medical residents of patient return for follow-up visit

| | | Returned | | Total |
		No	Yes	
Predicted return	No	14	16	30
	Yes	26	131	157
	Total	40	147	187

SOURCE: Mushlin and Appel 1977 (370).

their follow-up appointment. Furthermore, the data from this study indicate an even poorer ability to predict compliance with medications.

These data indicated that the physician's estimate of patient compliance is of very limited value, both in research studies of compliance and in practical applications in the day-to-day delivery of health services.

CLASSIFICATION OF COMPLIERS AND NONCOMPLIERS

It is clear from the foregoing that current methods of measuring compliance leave much to be desired. Nevertheless, the direct methods often permit an approximation of compliance. Given an adequate detection test, how should a patient be classified as complier or noncomplier? This question raises several fundamental conceptual issues relating to compliance research, and some of them have not been adequately examined at the present time. A number of factors may influence compliance testing, and if the results of the tests are to be used for labeling patients as compliers or noncompliers, these variables must be taken into consideration.

Although compliance can be studied as a continuous variable without characterizing individual patients as compliers or noncompliers, in most practical settings and for most research studies, classification of individual patients as compliers or noncompliers is essential. One approach to classifying a patient is to carry out a series of tests and calculate the percentage of tests which are positive. The population may then be dichotomized into compliers and noncompliers. Ideally this could be done on the basis of a biologic rationale such as the level of compliance required to achieve a therapeutic response, but often the necessary data for such a classification are not available. In lieu of this information, the dichotomization may be done on a statistical basis, for example, by using the median level of compliance in a group of patients as a cutoff between compliers and noncompliers. A more common method is to select an arbitrary level so that a certain percentage of positive tests is defined as evidence of adequate compliance.

There is, however, a very important problem in nonbiological approaches to defining compliance and noncompliance. Let us consider, for example, what is

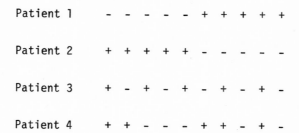

FIGURE 3.10. Hypothetical results of sequential tests in four "50% compliers."

meant by 50% compliance. It is important to realize that there are many varia-tions within this characterization of 50% compliance. Figure 3.10 shows possible sequences of 10 urine tests for a certain medication in four patients. Note the tremendous variation in test patterns among these four patients, although each is a 50% complier. In the first patient, the first five tests were negative and the next five were positive, suggesting that some environmental influence was brought to bear on the patient and modified his behavior. In the second patient, the first five tests were positive and the next five were negative suggesting that some factor converted him to noncompliance. In the third patient, positive and negative tests alternated throughout the period of the study, and in the fourth, there was what might be a random distribution of positive and negative tests.

The biological effects of these forms of noncompliance may be quite differ-ent. For example, if the drug is an antibiotic used for rheumatic fever prophy-laxis, the third patient might be protected even though he took his medication on alternate days. However, the first and second patients have long periods of negative tests during which they probably would not be protected. Thus, in each of these patients, all of whom are 50% compliers, the impact of noncompliance might be quite different. Is it reasonable, therefore, to group all these patients together as 50% compliers? Conceptually it may be neither legitimate nor useful—not only from the standpoint of the health hazard posed by noncompli-ance but also because the dynamics that may be operating to make them 50% compliers may not be the same. Since the behavior pattern in each case seems to be quite different, one might presume that the dynamics producing each behavior pattern might also vary considerably from one patient to another.

PREDICTING COMPLIANCE

Conducting long-term compliance studies using direct measures can be ex-tremely difficult administratively and logistically, and it often requires eliciting repeated or continuous patient cooperation. It would be desirable, therefore, to

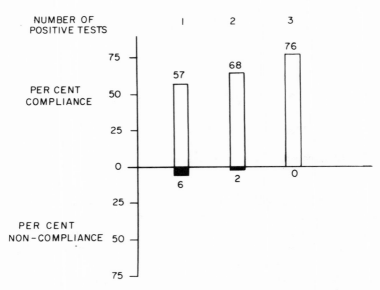

FIGURE 3.11. Probability of compliance and noncompliance after all positive initial urine
        test sequence.

NOTE: Compliance: ⩾ 75% of tests positive
        Noncompliance: ⩽ 25% of tests positive
        (Intermediates [26% - 74% of tests positive] are not shown.)

characterize a patient's compliance level over a long period of time using only a
short sequence of urine or blood tests. Moreover, if this were possible, it would
provide the basis for predicting the future course of a patient's compliance
behavior on the basis of a short-term study; obviously, this would have major
practical implications in the clinical setting. This possibility has been examined
in a study of children on oral penicillin prophylaxis. An initial sequence of
three weekly urine tests was found to be related to the overall level of compliance over a five-month period. As seen in Figure 3.11, this initial sequence of
one, two, or three positive urine tests was highly predictive of compliance,
and an initial sequence of negative tests was highly predictive of noncompliance
(Figure 3.12). These data suggest that by characterizing patients on the basis of
a short sequence of urine or blood tests, and perhaps by repeating this process
periodically, it may be possible to minimize the difficulty inherent in measuring
compliance directly.

PHYSICIANS' COMPLIANCE

Although in this book attention is focused on the question of patient noncompliance, it is appropriate to keep in mind that the doctor-patient interaction

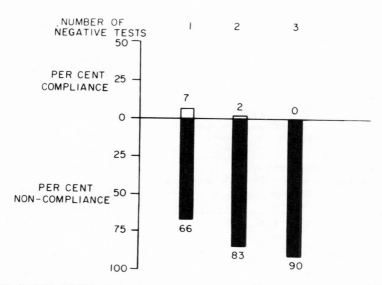

FIGURE 3.12. Probability of compliance and noncompliance after all negative urine test sequence.

NOTE: Compliance: ≥ 75% of tests positive
       Noncompliance: ≤ 25% of tests positive
       (Intermediates [26% - 74% of tests positive] are not shown.)

that determines the relative success of therapy in terms of outcome depends as much on the physician's compliance as on that of the patient. The physician must first of all know what is considered appropriate and proper care and, second, he must comply with current expert opinion and provide such care. Therefore, an important area for investigation in coming years will be that of *physician* compliance or noncompliance with accepted recommendations and the reasons for his noncompliance.

Some time ago we studied physicians' management of acute sore throats on the basis of their responses to mail questionnaires (859). As seen in Table 3.9, 91 pediatricians and 199 general physicians were surveyed. A marked difference in response rates was noted, with 79% of the pediatricians and only 36% of

TABLE 3.9. Response rates for pediatricians and general physicians

	Pediatricians	*General Physicians*
Number surveyed	91	199
Adult practice only		25
Eligible for study	91	174
Inadequate or no response	19	111
Responses analyzed	72	63
Response rate	79%	36%

SOURCE: Gordis et al. 1976 (859).

TABLE 3.10. Physicians' approaches to diagnosis and treatment of children
          with sore throats

Approaches	Pediatricians (N=72)	General physicians (N=63)
Below generally accepted standards	21%	76%
1. Treat all (no cultures)		17
2. Treat on clinical grounds (no cultures)	9	22
3. Culture, treat with full course on clinical grounds regardless of culture results	6	9
Acceptable treatment	79%	24%
4. Treat only after culture results	7	1
5. Culture, treat on clinical grounds, discontinue if culture is negative	25	4
6. Other, including 4 or 5	25	10

SOURCE: Gordis et al. 1976 (859).

the general physicians responding. As seen in Table 3.10, there was a marked
difference between pediatricians and general physicians in the appropriateness
of their approach to diagnosis. Seventy-six percent of the general physicians
did not use cultures in diagnosing sore throats in children or, when they took
cultures, did not use the results in their decisions regarding treatment. This
compares with only 21% of the pediatricians. When the specific therapy employed was examined (Table 3.11), there were significant differences between
pediatricians and general physicians in the percentage who used appropriate antibiotics, employed an adequate dosage, and prescribed the medication for an

TABLE 3.11. Antibiotic treatments for streptococcal pharyngitis

Treatment	Pediatricians (N=72)		General physicians (N=63)		P
Antibiotic					
Penicillin	56 ⎤		35 ⎤		
Erythromycin	1 ⎬	97%	⎬	67%	< .001
Penicillin and erythromycin	13 ⎦		7 ⎦		
Other agents	2		21		
Dosage					
Adequate	64	89%	40	65%	< .01
Inadequate	8		23		
Duration					
< 10 days	4		13		
10 days	66	92%	30	48%	< .001†
No response	2		20		
Overall assessment (antibiotic + dosage + duration)					
Adequate	63	88%	26	41%	< .001
Inadequate	9		37		

SOURCE: Gordis et al. 1976 (859).
†Excluding "No response," P< .02.

adequate duration. A composite rating based on these three characteristics showed that 88% of the pediatricians reported using what is currently considered appropriate therapy compared to only 41% of the general physicians. This preliminary study indicates the need for examining a variety of factors in the failure of physicians to comply with generally accepted diagnostic and treatment recommendations. Investigations in this area are a logical and important extension of present-day compliance research.

CONCLUSIONS

There are critical challenges in research related to compliance measurement. These require the input of clinical pharmacologists, biostatisticians, clinicians, and others, all working together. In general, there has thus far been too little interest in methodology and perhaps too much emphasis on premature applications such as intervention in the absence of a sufficient foundation of knowledge. In addition, on the practical side, dip sticks and other simple detection tests should be developed for many drugs commonly prescribed in private practice so that compliance research and monitoring can be encouraged and facilitated in the private practice setting. Finally, if the full benefits of compliance research are to be reflected in improved patient health, compliance research should be directed at the issue of noncompliant health providers as well as noncompliant patients.

II
THE DETERMINANTS
OF COMPLIANCE

4

Determinants of Compliance: The Disease and the Mechanics of Treatment

R. Brian Haynes

INTRODUCTION AND METHODS

This chapter is the first in a series of three which delve into the nature of patient noncompliance with therapeutic and prophylactic regimens. It will focus on compliance from the point of view of the therapist concentrating upon the disease as he diagnoses and perceives it, the setting in which the therapist provides care, and the regimen that he prescribes. Although this is a useful perspective, it ignores the most important participant in the process, the patient. The next chapter in the series deals with the patient and his interaction with the therapist. Finally, the last chapter in the set considers the Health Belief Model, which provides a multidimensional description of the problem. The main purpose of these chapters is to expose the problem rather than solve it. Such exposure will certainly suggest solutions, but it is the later sections of the book that bear the main responsibility for the implementation and evaluation of these potential solutions.

Before accepting an author's claim that a particular factor is correlated with compliance, the arbitrary but useful standard of statistical significance has been imposed. For a fictitious example, an investigator who reported that coughing was correlated with compliance would have had to demonstrate that coughers were statistically significantly ($P < .05$) more compliant than noncoughers, or that compliers coughed significantly more frequently than noncompliers. The author need not have performed the statistical test himself, provided that he presented sufficient information for the test to be made.

This chapter is based on a review of relevant articles in the annotated bibliography (Appendix I, Tables 2-4).

Findings that failed to meet the standard of statistical significance were categorized as showing *no correlation* with compliance if there were at least 50 subjects in each of the groups being compared. Studies were excluded entirely from the analysis if the sample size was smaller than this. Readers interested in the justification and implications of these criteria are invited to read the extract below. Those not so inclined are urged to skip to the next section.

Three important problems must be recognized in applying these statistical criteria. First, most investigators executing descriptive studies examined several factors at once but presented their analysis for each factor in isolation. Thus, a failure to control for the influence of confounding factors could result in a false conclusion. Second, by the very nature of "statistical significance," the likelihood that findings will be judged "significant" by a series of mutually independent tests is strongly influenced by the number of significance tests performed (quite apart from any real differences in the data). Thus, if ten factors are studied and ten comparisons are performed, the probability that one of these comparisons will yield a "statistically significant" result *by chance alone* is not 0.05, but 0.40. Although there are several statistical tools for carrying out such multiple comparisons appropriately, few authors know of them or apply them, and no attempt has been made here to do it for them. The third problem, perhaps less serious than the former two, is the risk of failure to detect a true difference in the data. In statistical terms, this is called a *type 2* or β error and is determined by the magnitude of the difference observed between groups, the amount of "noise" in the system, and sample size. In assessing the material reviewed here, this third problem was handled as follows: all no correlation findings were analysed except those derived from samples with less than 50 subjects per comparison group. This number is based on the criterion that a study should include sufficient numbers to detect, with 80% assurance $(1 - \beta = .80)$, an absolute difference of 25% in compliance associated with presence of the factor in question. Returning to the previous example, if coughing were associated with 25% greater compliance, studies with 50 coughers and 50 noncoughers could detect this clinically important difference on 80% of occasions. These guidelines are generous for a 25% difference in compliance is a large one to miss. To detect a smaller but perhaps still important effect on compliance (for example, 15%), a study would have to include many more subjects (almost three times as many) to achieve the same probability of detection. Alternatively, if the sample size remained at 50 in each group under study, the probability of detecting a 15% difference would slip to less than 60%. For those readers rendered cold by statistics this procedure may be viewed as a simple quality control mechanism to purge false results (or nonresults in this situation). On the other hand, stricter reviewers might contend that a β level of 0.05 should have been employed to equalize the risk of α and β errors. I would suggest, however, that it is more difficult to get negative results published and that the β error is probably the less serious of the two types of error anyway. In any event, both camps can have their way, as enough data are provided in this chapter and in the bibliography to permit application of either set of standards or no standards at all; those articles eliminated from the no correlation column in this chapter's tables have been retained in those which accompany the bibliography in Appendix I.

THE PRESENT STATE OF KNOWLEDGE

Features of the Disease

Table 4.1 displays the results of studies which assessed the relation between one or more features of the disease and patient compliance, and which met the standards of statistical significance and sample size set out above. As a first estimate of the relative lack of importance of disease factors, it is immediately apparent that less than half of the reports found any significant correlations, and that for these only a few factors showed consistency among the studies. Disease factors are thus relatively unimportant as determinants of compliance.

A few exceptions to this generalization merit comment. Of eight studies which found a correlation between the diagnosis and compliance, five dealt with psychiatric patients (7, 15, 92, 424, 528). These reports indicate that patients with schizophrenia, paranoid features, and personality disorders are less compliant than other psychiatric patients and, perhaps because of these subgroups, psychiatric patients in general are less compliant than patients with nonpsychiatric diagnoses.

Studies of disease severity have for the most part found no correlation with compliance. Six of 13 found an association, but even these are inconsistent. For example, one study (342) found that heavier smokers were more likely to be successful at quitting, whereas two others (269, 280) found just the opposite.

Counter to common wisdom, not a single study has found that increasing severity of symptoms encourages compliance. On the contrary, four investigations discovered that the more symptoms patients report, the lower their compliance. The conditions studied here included rheumatoid arthritis (277), anxiety neurosis (315), alcoholism (19), and general medical complaints (260). Three other studies, dealing with otitis media and pharyngitis in children (95), medical care utilization among Social Security recipients (321), and alcoholism (233) failed to find any relationship between symptom severity and compliance. On the other hand, the degree of disability produced by a disease does appear to influence compliance in a positive direction (138, 235, 240). Whether this is a reflection of the severity of the disease or, alternatively, simply the result of the increased supervision which often accompanies increasing disability was not examined directly, but the prior findings on disease severity and the findings on level of supervision which appear later in this chapter strongly support the latter explanation.

TABLE 4.1. Features of the disease

Feature	Association with compliance		
	Positive	*Negative*	*No association*
Diagnosis	Associations found:	7, 15, 27, 92, 260, 424, 444, 528	15, 95, 135, 192, 221, 223, 256, 272, 302, 312, 377
Severity	240*, 342	57, 65, 269, 280	95, 128, 221, 264, 272, 327, 437*
Symptoms		19, 260*, 277, 315	95, 233*, 321
Degree of disability	138, 235, 240*	19	256
Duration			7*, 17*, 121, 192*, 256, 269, 272, 342, 376, 441
Previous bouts	33		95, 127, 235, 327, 486, 487
Recency of last attack			235
Previous hospitalization	200, 377	315	223, 235, 330, 408, 536
Length of stay in hospital		414	330, 377, 428
Positive family history	235		200
Clinical improvement		192*	340, 341
Concurrent conditions			258, 414

*Compliance with appointments only.
Note: Numbers within the table refer to citations in the annotated bibliography in Appendix I.

Previous experience with a disease, including its duration and prior hospitalization for it, do not appear to influence compliance. However, both the physician's rating of disease prognosis (315) and a positive family history (235) are associated with higher compliance.

Clinical improvement was followed by lower compliance among depressed outpatients (192), but bore no relationship to compliance among children on short-term antibiotics for otitis media (340, 341). The latter observations are difficult to evaluate, however, as "feeling better or well" is one of the commonest reasons given by patients for defaulting (12, 82, 124, 220, 224, 236, 274, 302, 420, 424, 425, 499, 513). It is important to point out that the reasons for noncompliance given by patients cited above must not be taken at face value as discriminating features, since they are uncontrolled and subjective observations (thus they are not recorded in Table 4.1). For example, feeling better or well might be just as common among compliers as noncompliers but the symptomatic state of compliers was not reported in these studies. Furthermore, even among noncompliant patients, reasons offered often seem contradictory: "feeling worse" (425, 499), "lack of improvement" (124, 192), and "sickness" (220, 240, 424) have also been offered as explanations for low compliance.

Finally, concurrent illnesses in the same patient have not been found to influence compliance (258, 414) although the presence of concurrent illness in the family has been offered by patients as a reason for missing appointments (7, 17, 565).

In summary, disease features are not important determinants of compliance with the following exceptions: (1) psychiatric patients, particularly those with schizophrenia, paranoia, or personality disorders, tend to be low compliers; (2) increasing symptoms may be accompanied by decreasing compliance; and (3) increased disability may be associated with increased compliance. Since none of these factors offers much of an opportunity for the detection or improvement of compliance, future research in this area must have a relatively low priority.

Features of the Referral Process

Patients may be referred from screening projects to their regular sources of medical care or from one clinician or service to another. Although several studies examined patient characteristics related to attendance at referral appointments, very few evaluated the process of referral itself (see Table 4.2). The most important and best documented finding is that the longer the elapsed time between referral and the actual referral appointment, the lower the likelihood that the appointment will be kept (169, 194, 243). Finnerty and his co-workers (169) demonstrated that this timing can be critical. They found that among hypertensives the 50% attendance rate for referral appointments after a one to two week wait could be increased to 95% by reducing the waiting time to one or two days.

TABLE 4.2. Features of the referral process and clinical setting

	Association with compliance		
	Positive	Negative	No association
The referral:			
Time between screening and referral appointment		169*, 194*, 243*	
Source of referral	Association found: 240*		
Method of referral	Association found: 520*		
Specificity of referral	243*		
The clinic:			
Waiting time		7*, 186	
Method of scheduling	Association found: 434		
Time of day for appointment		243*	184*, 243*, 341*, 375*, 453*
Time since last appointment			184*, 375*, 453*
Day of week of appointment	Association found: 453*		184*, 260*
Distance to clinic	224*		240*, 243*, 260*, 327*
Having to leave work for visit	17*		260*
Weather			220*
Assignment of specific therapist	7*		
Patient load of therapist			260*
Mobile facilities	450*		
Particular clinic	Association found: 481*		
Type of visit	Association found: 224*		275*

*Compliance with appointments only.
Note: Numbers in the table refer to citations in the annotated bibliography in Appendix I.

In another referral study, Hertroijs (240) found that leprosy patients diagnosed through a screening program have a higher rate of default from care than do those who were self-referred or referred from other sources of care. This study may have important implications for screening programs in general and should be replicated for other disorders. Wilber and Barrow (520) have found that in hypertension screening, letter referrals were more successful than phone calls or direct referrals by indigenous workers at the time of screening. Finally, Hoenig and Ragg (243) have found that patients referred to a psychiatric outpatient department were more likely to attend if referred to a specific physician rather than just the clinic.

Further research into the effect of the referral process on compliance should have high priority, since the findings presented here suggest that rather simple logistical changes can substantially improve compliance with follow-up appointments.

Features of the Clinical Setting

As with the referral process, scant attention has been directed to the effect upon compliance of the mechanics of setting appointments and arranging clinics, despite the apparent importance of these variables and the ease with which many of them can be manipulated.

Two studies examined the effect of waiting time. Alpert (7) determined that 29% of patients with low attendance had reported waits of over four hours at visits previously attended, whereas only 16% of regular attenders made this complaint. Geersten et al. (186) found that noncompliers more frequently complained about long waiting times than did compliers. More objective evidence of the effect of appointment scheduling and waiting on attendance is provided in a very important study by Rockart and Hofmann (434). In a hospital outpatient setting they found that, when all patients were scheduled at the same time and seen on a first-come, first-served basis, mean waiting time was 85 minutes and the no-show rate was 27%. Aside from the level of nonattendance, they also observed that patients tended to arrive late and their physicians even later! It was observed that those patients wise enough to arrive late under the "block-unassigned" scheduling experienced a shorter wait. When all patients were scheduled for the same time but assigned to specific physicians the mean waiting time was reduced to 57 minutes and the no-show rate to 22%; the patients tended to arrive on time and the physicians were much less tardy. Finally, they found that providing patients with individual appointment times, though not with specific physicians, diminished the mean waiting time to 33 minutes and no-shows to 13%; both patients and physicians arrived early (no clinic offered individual appointment times with specific physicians). There have been several other studies of the finer points of clinic scheduling. The time of day did not influence appointment keeping in five studies (184, 243, 341,

375, 453), although one found lower attendance for women in the afternoon (243). Surprisingly, most studies failed to find a relation between the time since the last appointment and the likelihood of keeping the next one (184, 375, 453), though one study found that more frequent appointments were associated with lower attendance (260). The day of week (184, 260, 453) and the distance to the clinic (224, 240, 243, 260, 327) are unimportant, and the rest of the factors in Table 4.2 are either understudied or unimportant.

The recommendations for future research made above for the referral process apply doubly for the clinical setting: this is an important aspect of compliance that deserves much more attention. Since there is a relationship between attendance and compliance with the prescribed treatment (61, 198, 366, 428), it is not merely a matter of getting the patient and the doctor together. Furthermore, inconvenience at the clinic undoubtedly may lead patients to drop out of treatment entirely; this possibility urgently requires documentation.

Features of the Regimen

Although the method of referral and the clinical setting are important in bringing and keeping patients under medical care, improving the efficiency and convenience of these processes will not necessarily improve compliance with the treatment regimen itself (449). Various features of the prescribed treatment have a more immediate and direct impact on compliance (Table 4.3).

Alternative Treatments.

Alternative treatments are available for a number of conditions. Although some investigators have reported differential compliance rates for these alternatives, other investigators disagree. Ireland (265) found intramuscular streptomycin much more acceptable than PAS and somewhat more acceptable than INH, but McInnis (345) found no difference in compliance between INH and PAS. Ley et al. (310) found similar error rates between psychiatric patients taking tranquilizers and those taking antidepressants; however, Rickels et al. (427) reported that neurotics dropped out of treatment more frequently if they were prescribed fluphenazine than if they were prescribed chlordiazepoxide; and Willcox et al. (523) found lower compliance with chlorpromazine than with imipramine among depressed patients. One controlled clinical trial reported more dropouts among depressed patients on imipramine than among those on placebo (405), but four other drug trials failed to detect compliance differences between placebos and active drugs including penicillin (158), chlorpromazine (246), meprobamate (315), and chlorpromazine, meprobamate, or phenobarbital (355).

There is little disagreement, however, when the alternative is a parenteral formulation. If patient attendance can be ensured or outreach follow-up services

TABLE 4.3. Features of the therapeutic regimen

	Association with compliance*		
	Positive	*Negative*	*No association*
Type of treatment			
-for the same condition	Associations found: 23, 265, 266, 272, 405, 427, 523		95, 124, 158, 192, 223, 246, 310, 315, 345, 355, 414
-for different conditions	Associations found:		395
-parenteral treatments	106, 159, 160, 255, 273, 387	103, 236, 258	
Duration of therapy		42, 95, 192*, 202, 245, 246, 265, 348, 433, 436, 489, 524*	133, 137, 342
No. of drugs/treatments	455	65, 102, 127, 174, 236, 258, 302, 331, 376, 395, 513	
Frequency of dosing		65, 185	312, 345, 395
Dosage	377		
Side effects		377, 425	302, 523
Cost	105	7*, 65, 236	312
Health insurance	7*		
Safety lock containers		300	
Pharmacy dispensing		340, 341	

*Compliance with appointments only.
Note: Numbers within the table refer to citations in the annotated bibliography in Appendix I.

provided, compliance problems can be obviated by the simple expedient of injecting or infusing the medication under direct supervision. Logistically, this is usually only practical if the medication can be provided in a long-acting form. When such circumstances exist, this maneuver has met with uniform success as the following studies indicate. Injectable penicillin for acute streptococcal pharyngitis (106) and for rheumatic fever prophylaxis (159, 160) has been found both acceptable to patients and more successful than oral regimens in achieving favorable clinical outcomes. Long-acting phenothiazines for schizophrenia have dramatically reduced hospital readmission rates (273). Twice weekly intramuscular streptomycin injections for tuberculosis have produced similar benefits (255, 387). Along these same lines, intrauterine contraceptive devices have been associated with much better continuation rates than oral medication (23, 436, 463, 469, 489). The distressingly poor compliance of diabetics with self-injected insulin (511) attests to the fact that the important factor in this method of administration is not parenteral formulation alone. It is not known whether prolonged duration of action would promote compliance with self administered medications, enteral or parenteral; but, as suggested by Desmond Fitzgerald at the first McMaster Workshop/Symposium (661), prolonged action would at least make feasible medical staff supervision of drug utilization.

Classes of Medications.

In general, it may be said that alternative oral medications for the same condition do not produce substantial differences in compliance. This does not appear to be true with different treatments for different problems, however. Closson and Kikugawa (103) found only 17% compliance with antacids. They observed progressively higher levels of compliance for tranquilizers (40%), antituberculous drugs, sedatives, mydriatics, and estrogens (42%), analgesics (50%), antihypertensive agents (61%), diuretics (72%), insulin and antidiabetic drugs (78%), and cardiac drugs (89%). Hemminki and Keikkila (236) reported that compliance with "proper" drugs such as cardiac and diabetic agents was 85% although the rate was 42% with drugs for symptomatic relief such as antihistamines, spasmolytics, and plain psychotropics. Hulka et al. (258) also found higher compliance with cardiac and diabetic drug regimens than with other drug classes. Only Parkin et al. (395) failed to find differences among various drug classes ten days to one month following hospital discharge; unfortunately, they did not itemize the drugs studied.

The reasons for the substantial differences in compliance with different classes of medications observed in most studies are not at all clear. We know that the diagnosis per se has little influence on compliance, save perhaps for psychiatric disorders. We also know that different oral medications for the same condition have similar compliance characteristics. How, then, can one explain the variations in rates of compliance with medications among different conditions?

To start, one could speculate that there are important differences in such factors as the level of supervision for different conditions (see Chapter 8). Second, patients' perceptions may vary substantially by condition (see Chapter 6). Third, it is likely that medications for different conditions are much less similar than alternative medications for the same condition. The latter is the obvious implication in including this information under the title "Classes of Medications," but there is no satisfying explanation for the observations in this section. We would benefit from more extensive and thorough investigation of this important topic and no doubt from more perceptive interpretation!

Duration of Treatment.

The duration of treatment has an unequivocal effect on compliance: adherence to treatment decreases with time (42, 95, 192, 202, 245, 246, 265, 348, 433, 436, 489, 524). Only three reports failed to find such a correlation. One of these was cross-sectional rather than longitudinal (137), one dealt with dialysis patients dependent on medical staff (133), and the third demonstrated a nearly significant trend in the expected direction, based on self-reported compliance (342).

Complexity.

Similarly, the number of medications or treatments prescribed has an important effect on compliance: the more treatments prescribed, the lower the compliance rate (65, 102, 127, 174, 236, 258, 302, 331, 376, 395, 513). The report of Schwartz and her co-workers (455) was exceptional in that it found more errors committed by those who had been prescribed two or three medications than among those prescribed four to nine medications.

The influence of the number of times per day that medications are to be taken is not nearly so clear. Gatley (185) and Brand et al. (65) both found a fairly steep decline in compliance as the frequency of dosing increased from once a day to four times per day. However, McInnis (345), Lima et al. (312), and Parkin et al. (395) failed to find any correlation between compliance and the number of daily doses. Thus, although advertisements frequently claim that reducing the frequency of dosing will improve compliance, these claims should be ignored until this matter is clarified.

Dose Effects.

The dose of medication (as distinguished from the frequency of dosing) has received little attention. One study reported that hospitalized schizophrenics on a self-administration program were more compliant with higher doses of medication, but the dose range studied was narrow (377). Glick (192) reported the rather confusing observation that depressed patients receiving intermediate doses of phenylzine or tranylcypromine dropped out of treatment less frequently than patients on either low or high doses.

Side Effects.

One of the most common claims made by clinicians and echoed by drug manufacturers in their advertising is that side effects cause noncompliance. Rickels et al. (425) and Nelson et al. (377) cite data in support of this for psychiatric patients. However, the bulk of the available evidence undercuts this popular notion. Two controlled studies found no difference in the frequency of side effects between compliers and noncompliers (302, 523). In studies in which patients have been asked for their reasons for noncompliance (23, 82, 124, 192, 236, 240, 274, 291, 302, 425, 489, 499, 513) side effects have generally fallen far down the list, being mentioned by only 5%-10%. Not only are side effects infrequent for many medications but patients' complaints may not even be related to the drugs they are taking. For example, in the Veterans Administration antihypertensive drug trial (646) only 7% of patients in the actively treated group complained of symptoms which might have been attributed to their drugs; in the placebo group the frequency and even the distribution of complaints was similar, with the single exception that orthostatic complaints were less common. Even when side effects are present it cannot be assumed that noncompliance will result. Willcox et al. (523) found substantially different side effect rates for imipramine and chlorpromazine but no correlation between reported side effects and compliance.

Cost.

The cost of treatment has not been carefully evaluated for its effect on treatment adherence. Studies do not generally distinguish between the cost of the treatment or clinic visit and the actual cost to the patient. No account has been taken of lost wages, transportation, babysitting costs, and other expenses incurred by the patient in, for example, purchasing special diets. The effect of cost is not necessarily self-evident either. Cody and Robinson (105) were surprised to find that providing prescriptions at a nominal cost to psychiatric outpatients resulted in a significant increase in hospital admissions compared with admissions among patients receiving drugs at regular cost. Lima et al. (312) found no difference in compliance with a ten-day antibiotic regimen when they compared groups who paid for their medications with those who received them free of charge. However, cost is no doubt an important barrier to compliance for many patients, as has been demonstrated convincingly in three investigations (7, 65, 236). In keeping with these results, Alpert (7) found that patients who failed to keep their appointments were twice as likely to be without health insurance as those who kept their appointments.

TABLE 4.4. Important factors in compliance

	Effect on compliance
The disease	
1. Mental illness, especially schizophrenia, paranoia, and personality disorders	Negative
2. Symptoms	Negative
3. Disability	Positive
The referral process	
1. Time from referral to appointment	Negative
The clinic	
1. Waiting time	Negative
2. Individual appointment times	Positive
The treatment	
1. Parenteral drug administration	Positive
2. Duration of treatment	Negative
3. Number of medications/treatments prescribed	Negative
4. Cost	Negative
5. Safety containers	Negative
6. Erring and errant pharmacists	Negative

Dispensing.

Two investigations of problems related to dispensing medications have produced interesting results. The first, a controlled study comparing safety lock pill containers with regular containers, demonstrated significantly lower consumption of medication associated with the lock (300). Thus, it appears that safety lock containers thwart adults as well as children. Furthermore, many patients who did comply reported that they had removed the safety lock container tops and left them off between doses. Second, revealing studies by Mattar et al. (340, 341) found that community pharmacists dispensed less medication than was ordered on 15% of all prescriptions for a ten-day course of antibiotics for children with otitis media.

SUMMARY AND PRIORITIES FOR FUTURE RESEARCH

Table 4.4 summarizes the important factors this review found to be related to compliance. Some of these, such as the disease factors, can be regarded only as markers that indicate an increased probability of noncompliance. Other factors, such as the parenteral administration of medication, duration of treatment, and the number of medications or treatments prescribed, provide at the present time only limited opportunity for improving compliance. On the other hand, parenteral treatment, and as a corollary, prolonged action treatments, offer the exciting possibility of eliminating compliance as a problem for those few conditions for which such treatments now exist and in the future for any conditions for which safe preparations can be developed. The factors of time between referral and appointments and waiting time at appointments offer immediate possibilities for improving attendance.

Further research is required to determine the true impact of cost on compliance, with particular attention being accorded not only the amount the patient pays out of pocket for medications and visits but also the time lost from work, payments for babysitters, transportation, and the like. The single study on safety lock pill containers should be replicated and, if verified, should lead to changes in the routine dispensing of safety lock containers. Finally, further scrutiny of the amount of medication dispensed by pharmacists should be undertaken with a view to remedial action.

The major motivation for reviewing factors found to be associated with compliance is the hope that we might identify potential strategies for improving compliance. This chapter has identified several hopeful avenues to this end. It is clear, however, that very little can be taken for granted in this field: witness the negative effect of reducing cost in the study by Cody and Robinson (105). Proposals for improving compliance must be based on carefully conducted and methodologically sound, controlled clinical trials, and this important work must be given high priority in future research into health care.

5

Patient-Clinician Interactions and Compliance

Barbara S. Hulka

The interaction between patients and physicians is without doubt important to compliance. Unfortunately, however, it is extremely difficult to assess the nature of this interaction and to measure its components. As a result, any review of the topic has two major limitations: lack of a clear concept of what is meant by patient-clinician interaction and by compliance. I shall address the latter term first, since, in the context of this paper, the issue of compliance can be more readily resolved.

Compliance usually refers to the extent to which patients follow the instructions—proscriptions and prescriptions—of their physicians or other providers. The concern is generally with *noncompliance*, and the term often implies a pejorative affect toward patients, who are presumed to be at fault. However, certain authors (256, 825), whom I would regard as enlightened, suggest that the physician and his style of communicating with the patient may alter the patient's ability and inclination to comply.

Another factor mitigating the patient's ability to comply is the regimen itself. Therapeutic regimens frequently involve a variety of components, some of which necessitate changes in lifestyle (modifying eating, drinking, or activity levels), whereas others entail the taking of medications. Most authors (127) agree that the former are more difficult for the patient to comply with than the latter. Changes in lifestyle are also more difficult to measure in a valid, quantitative fashion. Therefore, compliance in this report will focus on medication-taking behavior and the types and amount of error which may occur. Having thus reduced the scope of compliance behaviors to be discussed in this chapter, the more difficult task of defining the patient-clinician interaction remains.

Two aspects of the interaction will be pursued. The first of these is the perspective which is frequently labeled the *doctor-patient relationship* (130, 670, 741, 866). Although the term is bandied about by many and is assumed to be important in the delivery of medical services, remarkably little is known about it. What is it; what are its components; how are they to be defined and measured? Without doubt, there is hardly a phrase in all the health services literature about which so much is said yet so little is known. The research reported here attempts to bite off a few bits of this multidimensional pie and to define, measure, and quantify them. Clearly, the effort is preliminary, but it does represent a move from the arena of global euphemisms to relatively constricted components amenable to scientific inquiry.

The second aspect of the patient-clinician interaction under scrutiny in this chapter is that subset of activities pertaining to the drug prescription and prescribing process itself. Although not so readily evident as a component of the interaction, the medication regimen as initiated by the physician and consummated by the patient should be quite directly related to medication-taking behaviors. For this reason, the medication regimen itself is implicated as part of the patient-clinician interaction.

With this background, then, let us pursue a study which my colleagues and I undertook to illustrate these aspects of the patient-clinician interaction.

METHODS

Setting

The study was undertaken in Fort Wayne, Indiana, a city of almost 200,000 people including contiguous urbanized townships. Primary medical care was provided by physicians in private practice supplemented by active emergency rooms in three voluntary hospitals. The organizational patterns of practice included solo practitioners, two- or three-man associations, and two loosely organized multispecialty groups.

Participants

Physicians.

A stratified random sampling procedure was used to select physician participants for the study. The sampling frame was composed of all internists and family physicians listed in the Fort Wayne-Allen County Medical Society Directory. The sampling unit was the individual practitioner or the group of practitioners, depending on the type of practice in which the physician was engaged. A table of random numbers was used to sequence physicians and practices in the order in which they would be asked to participate. Sixty-eight percent of the physicians contacted participated fully in the study.

Patients.

Patients with either congestive heart failure or diabetes mellitus were the subjects for the study, since these conditions are seen frequently in the offices of primary care physicians and they usually require the continued use of one or more medications for their control. Adult onset diabetics with disease duration of ten years or less were eligible. Congestive heart failure patients between the ages of fifty and seventy-five were admissible; almost all cases were due to either arteriosclerotic or hypertensive heart disease.

Patients were enrolled in the study at the time of an office visit to a participating physician. Patient enrollment from each practice continued over a four-month period. A member of the physician's office staff introduced the study to each eligible patient, and a patient participation rate of 84% was achieved.

Measures of the Doctor-Patient Relationship

Communication between Physician and Patient.

Separate measures of the physician's success in communicating instructions and information were devised for diabetic patients and for those with congestive heart failure. For each condition the physician was asked about a series of topics that had been identified as pertinent to the specific disease process and the patient's management of his condition. The physician indicated whether or not each patient had been instructed or informed in each area. The patient was subsequently presented with a corresponding series of questions to determine whether or not the information had been transmitted.

A communication score was devised to measure the proportion of information retained by the patient compared with the total amount provided by the physician. Communication scores ranged from 0 to 1, with higher scores indicating a better level of communication (257, 866).

Physician Awareness of Patient Concerns.

In developing a scale to measure physician awareness of patient concerns, specific issues which might cause anxiety to the patient were defined for each condition. These included concerns about the disease process and its symptoms, difficulty with maintaining a diet or therapeutic regimen, and loss of ability to maintain usual role functions and to care for oneself.

Each questionnaire contained 18 to 20 items in the form of graphic rating scales with 20 response locations representing a continuum from the most negative to the most positive affect. Several items were devised to tap each substantive area.

Physicians and patients completed identical versions of this questionnaire, but the instructions to each group differed. The patient was requested to express his or her own attitudes when responding to each item. In contrast, the physician was instructed to respond in terms of his or her perceptions of the individual patient's attitudes. In other words, the physician was asked to predict each patient's responses.

The score for this questionnaire was based on the mean of the absolute differences on all items for each doctor-patient pair. Since the distribution of patients' responses to each item could affect the magnitude of the doctor-patient differences, the final score was adjusted to eliminate the effect of the particular response locations chosen by the patient. The awareness score for each doctor-patient pair was a proportion which represented the fractional reduction in maximum doctor-patient differences associated with the physician's ability to predict his patient's concerns. Therefore, the larger the proportion the greater the physician's awareness (865, 866, 871).

Patient Satisfaction.

The satisfaction scale was designed to measure attitudes toward three distinct aspects of medical care: professional competence, personal qualities of the physician, and the cost and convenience of care. Thus, within the total scale there exist three distinct component scales.

The Thurstone Equal Appearing Interval Technique was used in developing the satisfaction scale. This was subsequently modified to a Likert Format of five response alternatives. In conjunction with the format change, the scoring method was also modified to incorporate both the item scale values derived from the Thurstone approach and the specific weightings determined by the response alternative selected by the patient. Reliability testing by the split half method provided correlations ranging from .68 to .86 for the three component scales. Patient scores were computed such that negative values represented negative attitudes and positive values indicated positive attitudes (867, 868, 869, 872).

Data Collection

Within two weeks of enrollment at the doctor's office, the patient was visited at home by a nurse-interviewer. At that time, the patient was asked to display current medications, indicate the function of each, repeat the scheduling recommendation of the physician, and indicate whether or not he or she was taking the drug as directed. In addition, the patient completed the attitude/concern questionnaire and also responded to the communication questions. The satisfaction questionnaire was administered at a second home visit about six months later.

Since drug names were infrequently recorded on the bottle, the pharmacy name and address and prescription number were transcribed from each container. A subsequent check of prescriptions at the pharmacy provided the name and schedule for each medication presented by the patient. Of the 76 pharmacies used by patients in the study, only one pharmacy refused to provide the information requested.

From the patient's medical record in the physician's office, the nurse-interviewer abstracted data on medications prescribed and not discontinued during the year prior to the home visit. These drug data were submitted to the physician for review and modification. Drugs for which dosage or schedule were unavailable were called to the physician's attention so that he could supplement the medical record data with his own knowledge of the patient's current medication. Thus, any inaccuracies or omissions in the record could be corrected, giving as complete a picture as possible of prescription drugs the physician believed his patient to be taking.

In addition to reviewing medications, the physician also completed the communication questionnaire for each participating patient and the questionnaire to measure physician awareness of patient concerns.

Computation of Drug Error Rates

Since data were collected from doctor-patient pairs, comparison could be made of drugs consumed by patients with drugs prescribed by their doctors, as well as drug schedules recommended by physicians with the patient's perception of the recommended schedule. In addition, the patient's verbal statement of whether or not he or she was taking each drug as prescribed was noted. With this data set, it was possible to formulate four distinctive types of medication errors for each doctor-patient pair:

1) *omission rate* = proportion of drugs prescribed by the physician that the patient was *not* taking;
2) *commission rate* = proportion of drugs the patient *was* taking of which the physician was unaware;
3) *scheduling misconception rate* = proportion of prescribed drugs taken by the patient for which the patient did *not* know the correct schedule;
4) *scheduling noncompliance* = proportion of prescribed drugs taken by the patient for which the patient knew the correct schedule but did *not* take as prescribed.

Scheduling was defined in terms of frequency of consumption per 24 hours and number of units (pills, spoonfuls, etc.) to be taken each time.

For each error rate a score was computed for each doctor-patient pair. Each score was a proportion ranging from 0 to 1. The lower the score, the smaller the error; the larger the proportion, the greater the error. The mathematical properties of these error rates have been discussed previously (258).

RESULTS

Study Group

Forty-six physicians contributed 357 patients to the study. Among these physicians, 33 were in family practice and 13 were internists. Each physician category was approximately equally divided between solo and group practitioners.

Of the patients, 234 were diabetics and 123 had congestive heart failure. These diagnoses were not mutually exclusive, since several heart failure patients also had diabetes and some diabetics had cardiac conditions (but not congestive heart failure). The mean age of the diabetics was 53 as compared to 63 for congestive heart failure patients. Approximately 55% of both patient groups were women. Fifty-eight percent of diabetics were high school graduates, compared to 42% of heart failure patients; more than two-thirds of both patient groups represented the middle or working classes.

Drug Error Rates

On average, both diabetic and congestive failure patients were omitting 18% of drugs prescribed, *and* taking 19% more drugs than their physicians realized, *and* making scheduling errors on about 17% of drugs. When all types of medication-taking errors were combined, the average total error for all doctor-patient pairs was 58%. Scheduling noncompliance has not been analyzed further since the mean error rate was low (about 3%), and it exhibited only minor variability.

Patient Profile and Medication Errors

Possible associations among patient characteristics, their diseases, and drug error rates are important for at least two reasons. First, if relationships do exist, these variables must be controlled for in the subsequent analysis of patient-clinician interaction and compliance. Secondly, if characteristics of patients and their diseases are associated with drug error rates, a descriptive profile could be developed which would be useful to clinicians in predicting patients at high risk for making drug errors.

Patient characteristics can be summarily reviewed, since their association with drug error rates was minimal. The characteristics analyzed included age, sex, marital status, education, current activity, number of people in household, and social class (Hollingshead two-factor index based on occupation and education). Using analysis of variance for comparing the means of two or more populations, there were no statistically significant associations ($P \leqslant .05$) between any of these variables and the drug error rates.

Several measures of disease severity were available. Duration of disease and number of other concurrent diseases might be expected to influence the medical status of the patient. Neither factor, however, was associated with drug errors.

For heart failure patients, there were two additional measures of disease severity: the New York Heart Association classification of functional impairment and the number of prior hospitalizations for congestive heart failure. Neither variable was associated with drug error rates.

A rather consistent pattern appeared among the diabetic patients, when the insulin-dependent were compared with those using oral agents or diet alone.

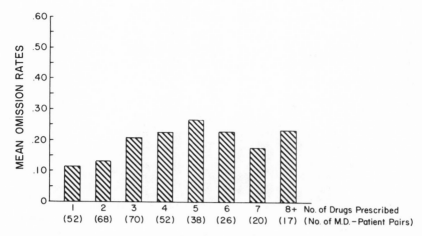

FIGURE 5.1.   Mean omission rates by number of drugs prescribed.

Patients requiring insulin had higher drug error rates than those not requiring insulin. However, the association was based on a small number of insulin-dependent patients (23) and was statistically significant for scheduling misconceptions only.

Patient-Clinician Interaction and Medication Errors

Two types of interactions were reviewed; those pertaining to the medication regimen and those identified as components of the doctor-patient relationship.

Medication Regimen.

1.   Number of drugs involved between doctor-patient pair. The number of drugs consumed by patients ranged from 0 to 14, and prescribing patterns showed a similar variation. A very likely hypothesis would suggest that the proportion of errors would increase as the number of drugs involved between the doctor-patient pair increased. Figures 5.1 through 5.3 were prepared to test this hypothesis. In each figure, a different mean error rate is shown in relation to the number of drugs involved.

Figures 5.1 and 5.2 represent the drug omission rates and drug commission rates, respectively. Errors of omission and commission increase with an increasing number of drugs involved. The Spearman rank order correlation coefficient based on a one-tailed test for a positive trend is significant at the .05 level for both rates.

Figure 5.3 presents the scheduling misconception rates that indicate lack of communication between physician and patient on medication dose and/or fre-

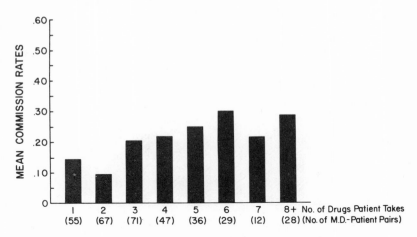

FIGURE 5.2.   Mean commission rates by number of drugs consumed.

quency. Although these rates peak at .23 with four drugs involved, the association between error rates and number of drugs involved is not statistically significant.

In summary then, errors of omission and commission increased with increasing number of drugs, whereas scheduling misconceptions did not demonstrate that association.

2. Knowledge of drug function. Another feature of the drug regimen concerned whether or not the patient knew the function of each medication he was taking. One might expect that the greater the proportion of drugs for which the patient knew the function the less likely he would be to make errors.

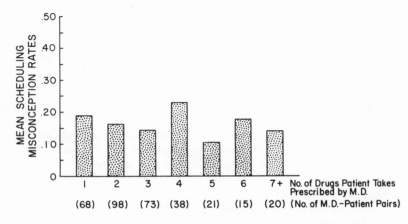

FIGURE 5.3.   Mean scheduling misconception rates by number of drugs both prescribed and consumed.

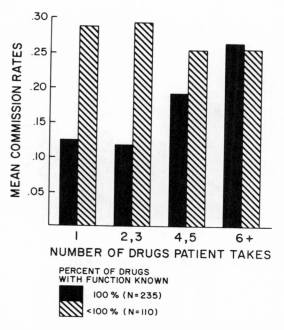

FIGURE 5.4. Commission rates by percentage of drugs with function known and number of drugs patient takes.

Drugs were assigned to the "function known" category if the patient displayed a reasonable knowledge of their function. For example, if a diuretic was taken "to get rid of water" or digitalis was taken "for the heart," these were considered acceptable responses. Only when the stated function was inconsistent with known pharmacologic and clinical properties or the patient denied knowledge of the function was the response categorized as incorrect. Overall, patients were reasonably knowledgeable about drug function; 69% of patients knew the function of all drugs they were taking.

Graphic presentations correlating drug error rates with knowledge of drug function, controlling for number of drugs involved, are shown in Figures 5.4 and 5.5. In both figures, there are two categories of function knowledge: function known for 100% of drugs and function known for less than 100%. Figure 5.4 shows that mean commission rates are high among those patients who did not know the function of all their drugs, irrespective of the number of drugs being taken. With the exception of patients taking six or more drugs, commission rates are higher for patients who did not know the function all their medication than for those who did. This association reaches statistical significance $(P < .005)$ only for the two to three drug category.

A similar finding for scheduling misconception rates is shown in Figure 5.5. The scheduling misconception rates are higher for patients who did not know

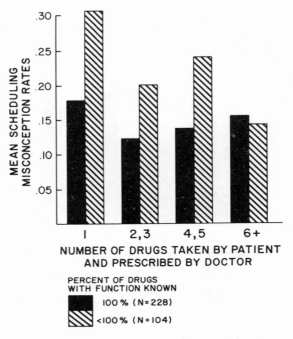

FIGURE 5.5. Scheduling misconception rates by percentage of drugs with function known and number of drugs both prescribed and consumed.

the function of all their drugs than for patients with 100% function knowledge. This association is consistent for each category of number of drugs except six or more. Statistical significance is reached at the .05 level for the two to three and four to five drug categories.

Omission rates were not associated with the percentage of drugs for which the function was known.

3. Complexity of medication schedule. The hypothesis was made that increased complexity is associated with increased error. The percentage of drugs scheduled once a day was selected as a measure of scheduling complexity, assuming that it is easier to remember the schedule for medications taken only once a day than for those scheduled more frequently.

Figures 5.6 and 5.7 illustrate this point. Mean commission rates for patients taking one to four drugs are shown in Figure 5.6. The percentage of drugs scheduled once a day has been divided into 100% and less than 100%; that is, patients for whom all drugs were scheduled once a day are compared with patients for whom some or all drugs were scheduled more than once a day. In general, commission errors are lower when all drugs are scheduled once a day, although this association is not statistically significant.

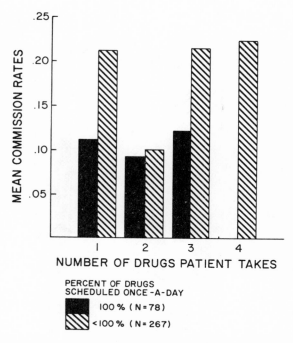

FIGURE 5.6. Commission rates by percentage of drugs scheduled once a day and number of drugs patient takes.

Scheduling misconceptions appear in Figure 5.7, where at each level of number of drugs involved, the error rate is lower when all drugs are scheduled once a day. This association is significant ($P < .05$) when the number of drugs being taken is one, two, or three. In both Figures 5.6 and 5.7, the number of drugs is limited to four, since almost no patients taking more than four drugs had 100% of them scheduled once a day.

Doctor-Patient Relationship.

The elusive phenomenon of the doctor-patient relationship has numerous components, three of which were defined and measured in this study. These have been labeled communication between physician and patient, physician awareness of patient concerns, and patient satisfaction.

1. Communication. The distribution of communication scores was reviewed separately for diabetic and congestive heart failure patients, then the relationship between these scores and the drug error rates was analyzed. No association was found for the diabetic patients, whereas the pattern for congestive heart failure patients was clear.

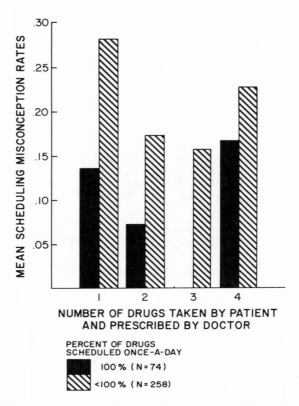

FIGURE 5.7. Scheduling misconception rates by percentage of drugs scheduled once a day and number of drugs both prescribed and consumed.

Communication scores were grouped in tertiles, and the mean drug error rates were computed for each of the three levels of communication. The graphed results for congestive heart failure patients are shown in Figure 5.8. For each of the three drug error rates, a pattern of increased error with decreased level of communication is evident. The differences are significant at P values less than .001 for omissions and P values between .05 and .10 for commissions and scheduling misconceptions.

Among diabetic patients, no association was found between overall communication and drug errors, although a very high correlation was found between specific communication items and the relevant behaviors. For example, if the patient knew the correct name of his hypoglycemic medication, he almost always had the correct medication on hand; if the name were unknown or in error, he was less likely to have the correct medicine. The same observation pertained to other aspects of therapeutic behavior such as urine testing for glucose or carrying diabetic identification. When patients were informed about what was

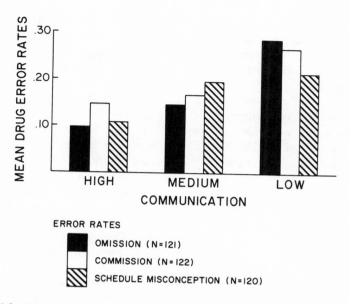

FIGURE 5.8. Mean drug error rates by level of communication between physician and patient: congestive heart failure patients.

expected of them, their behaviors conformed to that expectation more than 85% of the time. The major problem was communication; a third or more of the patients were unaware of what was expected of them in specific instructional areas.

2. Patient satisfaction. For congestive failure patients, increased satisfaction with professional competence and personal qualities of physicians appeared to relate in a linear fashion to decreased error; however, the association did not reach statistical significance and, in the interest of parsimony, no data are presented. That this relationship should exist is consistent with the findings of others (870).

3. Physician awareness of patient concerns. Physician awareness scores demonstrated no association with drug error rates among the entire set of patients nor in either of the disease subgroups.

IMPLICATIONS AND APPLICATIONS

Regimen

The intent of this chapter has been to identify modifiable features of the patient-clinician interaction which are correlated with medication-taking error. Certain characteristics of the medication regimen bear a significant relationship to the types and amount of error observed. The number of drugs involved for each doctor-patient pair is clearly associated with errors of omission and commission. The more drugs the doctor prescribes, the more the patient omits; the more drugs the patient takes, the greater the number about which the physician is uninformed.

This simple information should have important applications to both medical practice and patient performance. Reduce the number of drugs prescribed and consumed to the minimum number consistent with the therapeutic goals. This objective may even provide the rationale for the use of "combination" medications, those containing more than one active pharmacologic agent, although there is little experimental evidence on this matter (see Chapters 8 and 9).

The finding that increased frequency of scheduling medication is associated with an increased rate of scheduling misconceptions by the patient is hardly surprising. Scheduling misconceptions can be reduced by simplifying the medication schedule a patient is expected to follow. Choosing the simplest regimen compatible with the patient's daily habits or life events should reduce the amount of error.

Furthermore, when a patient shows a poor response to medication, the physician should consider first what drugs have been taken and how, rather than just adding more of the same or a different drug (331, 612).

Knowledge of drug function, as opposed to no knowledge or incorrect knowledge, was associated with decreased errors of commission and scheduling misconception. Error rates of both types were reduced when functional knowledge was reasonable for all drugs being taken. Review of the drug delivery system to identify critical points where the patient's learning can be reinforced is in order. Opportunities to enhance functional knowledge start with the physician at the time of initial prescribing. Functional knowledge can be reinforced by the pharmacist at the time the prescription is filled, and such reinforcement should be continued by the physician or other provider at follow-up visits (341). Follow-up visits can be more effective if medication is physically present so that both physician and patient can clearly visualize which drugs are being taken and for what purpose.

Communication

Among patients with congestive heart failure, communication of instructions and information was inversely associated with drug error rates: the better the communication, the lower the errors. Explaining the treatment, the disease, and the consequences of each is an important responsibility of the clinician. How can this best be done? As proposed by Lawrence Green in Chapter 10, an additional provider, trained in communication skills, may increase the transmission of necessary information. Others recommend a written format which may be elaborated on to the point of a detailed patient package insert. One format recently proposed by Griffith (864) displayed an information sheet prepared individually for each of the 500 most commonly prescribed drugs. The sheet contained information on instructions and directions for use, precautions, possible side effects, effect on activities of daily living, storage, refills, overdose, and treatment.

Other Aspects of the Patient-Clinician Interaction

Several reports in the literature suggest that we have not adequately defined the most relevant aspects of the patient-clinician interaction, particularly the role of the clinician in effecting compliance (130, 670, 741, 820, 825). Compliance has been shown to be better in private practice than in clinic settings; and within a private practice, patients are more compliant when their regular physician, rather than another member of the group or an unknown physician, does the prescribing (95).

Patients are more likely to take their medications if the prescribing physician believes in the efficacy and importance of those medications (774), but how the physician can express this conviction most effectively is more difficult to assess. In addition, fewer errors occur when patients' expectations from a visit are met and when patients are well satisfied with care (870).

Thus, investigative pathways are open for better conceptualization and definition of various facets of the patient-clinician interaction and for the design of more precise methods of measurement and analysis.

6

Patient Perceptions and Compliance: Recent Studies of the Health Belief Model

Marshall H. Becker, Lois A. Maiman, John P. Kirscht, Don P. Haefner, Robert H. Drachman, D. Wayne Taylor

INTRODUCTION: *Marshall H. Becker*

During the early 1950s, a group of social psychologists* working at the United States Public Health Service developed a theoretical framework for explaining the likelihood of an individual's undertaking a recommended preventive health action, for example, obtaining immunizations and participating in screening programs for early detection of asymptomatic disease (881). Since its initial evaluation in a screening program to detect tuberculosis (878), this formulation has been the subject of substantial direct study and has recently been the focus of considerable attention and research by behavioral scientists and health education specialists (32, 792, 882).

Usually termed the *Health Belief Model* (HBM), this theory, as illustrated in Figure 6.1, is based on the decision-making concepts of valence (or attractiveness of the goal to the individual) and subjective probability (or personal estimate of likelihood of goal attainment). The theory argues that whether or not an individual will undertake a recommended health action is dependent upon that individual's perceptions of: (1) level of personal *susceptibility* to the particular illness or condition; (2) degree of *severity* of the consequences (organic and/or social) which might result from contracting the condition; (3) the health action's potential *benefits* or efficacy in preventing or reducing susceptibility and/or severity; (4) physical, psychological, financial, and other *barriers* or costs related

---

*Drs. Godfrey M. Hochbaum, S. Stephen Kegeles, Howard Leventhal, and Irwin M. Rosenstock.

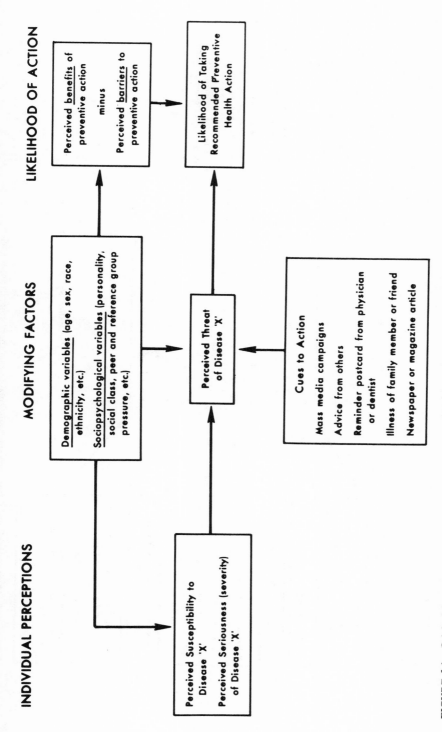

FIGURE 6.1. Original formulation of the health belief model.

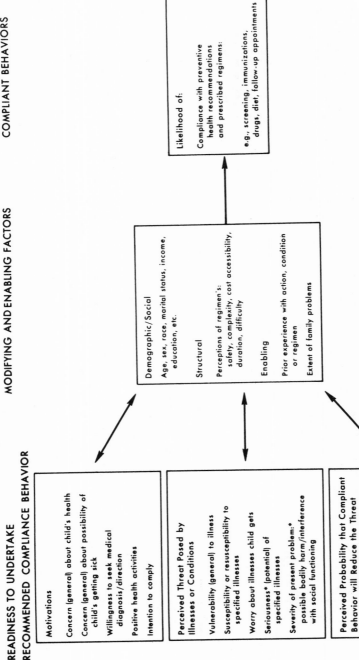

READINESS TO UNDERTAKE
RECOMMENDED COMPLIANCE BEHAVIOR

Motivations

Concern (general) about child's health

Concern (general) about possibility of
child's getting sick

Willingness to seek medical
diagnosis/direction

Positive health activities

Intention to comply

**Perceived Threat Posed by
Illnesses or Conditions**

Vulnerability (general) to illness

Susceptibility or resusceptibility to
specified illnesses

Worry about illnesses child gets

Seriousness* (potential) of
specified illnesses

Severity of present problem:*
possible bodily harm/interference
with social functioning

**Perceived Probability that Compliant
Behavior will Reduce the Threat**

Faith in doctors and medical care

Perceptions of the proposed regimen's
efficacy to prevent, delay, or cure
the problem

Feelings of control over problem

MODIFYING AND ENABLING FACTORS

Demographic/Social

Age, sex, race, marital status, income,
education, etc.

Structural

Perceptions of regimen's:
safety, complexity, cost accessibility,
duration, difficulty

Enabling

Prior experience with action, condition
or regimen

Extent of family problems

*At motivating but not inhibiting levels.

COMPLIANT BEHAVIORS

Likelihood of:

Compliance with preventive
health recommendations
and prescribed regimens:

e.g., screening, immunizations,
drugs, diet, follow-up appointments

FIGURE 6.2. Hypothesized model for predicting and explaining mothers' compliance behaviors.

to initiating or continuing the advocated behavior. The HBM also stipulates that a *cue to action* or stimulus must occur to trigger the appropriate behavior by making the individual consciously aware of his feelings about the health threat. Such cues can be either internal (for example, perception of symptoms) or external (such as mass media campaigns, interpersonal interactions) (874). Although it is assumed that various sociodemographic and structural factors can influence the individual's health beliefs and perceptions, these variables are not viewed as directly causal to compliance.

The original HBM, which was directed towards an individual's desire to avoid a specific disease threat, has since been revised (875), as shown in Figure 6.2, for pediatric compliance, to include: (1) *general health motivations*, based on measures of health concerns, practices, and beliefs about prevention that are seen as relatively nonspecific and stable across situations; (2) *resusceptibility* to illnesses previously contracted (including the condition under study); (3) *general faith* in physicians and medical care; and (4) *characteristics of the doctor-patient relationship* which might enhance or impair compliance. The interested reader is referred to more complete descriptions of the model in the earlier edition of this book (794) and elsewhere (215, 603, 604, 879, 880).

However, prospective investigations generally have not found correlations between health beliefs at the beginning of a course of therapy and subsequent compliance as strong as correlations between health beliefs and concurrent compliance. This may suggest that the relationship between health beliefs and compliance is at least partly bidirectional, with health beliefs becoming congruent with actual compliance as well as the reverse of this. The two studies which follow explore these possibilities in the areas of obesity and hypertension. Other illuminating reports of recent vintage have appeared in a variety of publications (36, 873) and as dissertations (876, 877).

A TEST OF THE HEALTH BELIEF MODEL IN OBESITY*:
Marshall H. Becker, Lois A. Maiman,
John P. Kirscht, Don P. Haefner, Robert H. Drachman

INTRODUCTION

Juvenile obesity is widely recognized as a major health problem (898), particularly because of its suggested association with severe adult obesity (902). Unfortunately, the literature on patient compliance with various treatments for obesity reveals results that are "remarkably similar and remarkably poor" (486).

*This investigation was supported by Grants HL5P17, HL14207, and HL18045 from the National Heart and Lung Institute, and 5K04 HD 00061 from the National Institute of Child Health and Human Development. An earlier report of this study appeared in the *Journal of Health and Social Behavior* 18: 348-366, 1977.

Attempts to characterize the obese adolescent psychologically have been disappointing (885, 887, 888), and interventions based on physiological, psychological, and group methods yield rates of compliance generally ranging from 0% to 28% (889, 904, 905). The only consistent finding is that both patients and physicians are pessimistic about the possibility of successful weight reduction (897). This perceived lack of success may be due in part to research approaches that tend to ignore fundamental attitudes and subjective perceptions about health and obesity.

Dietary adherence is somewhat unusual in the class of health behaviors: (1) the threat posed to health is not immediate but rather future oriented and linked to other conditions; (2) appropriate action may be undertaken for other than health reasons (e.g., body image, social acceptance); and (3) even when identified as a health problem, obesity may not be regarded by many persons as an "illness" in the usual sense of the term. These factors therefore create a new situation in which concepts of the Health Belief Model may be extended and tested.

For groups such as children, the elderly, and many of the disabled, the relevant health beliefs and attitudes of "responsible others" are often the primary determinants of the degree to which the dependent patient follows the treatment program (604). This control over the child's health behaviors has been documented for actions such as obtaining immunizations (500) and dental care (886, 893), taking medication (34), and utilizing a variety of health services (883).

Beyond direct control, researchers have emphasized the influence of mothers' health beliefs on the attitudes and behaviors of their children. For example, Zborowski (906) linked mothers' overprotectiveness to children's perceptions of health-threatening situations, and Mechanic (900) found that the child's attention to symptoms was related to the mother's interest in health matters. Perhaps most important to the present study is Litman's finding (896) that the mother's influence was the primary determinant of the child's food habits and attitudes; he notes (page 505) that "the most persistent theme running through our three generation study was the rather pervasive role played by the wife-mother in the health and health care of the family." For these reasons, this study focuses on the mother's health motives and perceptions as predictors of her child's weight loss.

Methods

The study was conducted in the large ambulatory pediatric clinic at a major teaching hospital. From July 1973 to July 1975 mothers of children newly identified by clinic physicians as obese were referred to the clinic dietitian for instruction and a weight reduction plan, then invited to participate in a project to learn more about individuals' health opinions and concerns. Only persons claiming to be responsible for the child's daily care, and for bringing the child to the clinic when necessary, were included in the study.

The 182 eligible mothers were interviewed for approximately one hour concerning their beliefs, concerns, and motives relative to health in general and to obesity in particular (the interview items were designed specifically to operationalize dimensions of the HBM).

Subjects were then randomly assigned either to one of two levels of a motive-arousing intervention or to a control group (no intervention). The two experimental treatments were: (1) a "high fear" message and booklet concerning obesity and its possible unfavorable consequences; or (2) a "low fear" message and booklet with similar (but less threatening) information.*

Although the literature on threat appeals is somewhat ambivalent (899), the evidence favors using threat as an adjunct to recommendations about health (895), particularly at the beginning of a regimen (884). It does not appear that arousing fear necessarily leads to belief or behavior change in the direction intended, but rather that people seek to resolve the fear, and that threats interact with other individual dispositions such as the amount of initial concern and coping ability (890). To the extent that a threat presents a personally relevant danger and is coupled with modes for coping with that danger, it provides useful information, especially to those with lower levels of concern (895). As a strategy, threat offers a possible way to tailor messages to the intended audience (901). There are several reports of effective use of health threats (293, 894, 903), as well as prior attempts to employ threat in modifying health beliefs (215, 413, 891).

Data on weight change were obtained by the dietitian every two weeks for two months (i.e., four visits). Upon initial assessment, the children were, of course, overweight to varying extents; therefore, differing amounts of weight reduction were prescribed for each child. To achieve standardization across patients, the study's major dependent variable is the ratio of weight change between visits to weight on initial visit.

To create another, more general measure of the mother's compliance behaviors, a ratio of long-term clinic appointment keeping (excluding those with the dietitian) was calculated for each child (where available; N = 145) by dividing appointments kept by appointments made during a standard twelve-month period.

A number of HBM dimensions were represented by multiple questionnaire items. In order to obtain more reliable measures, the items relating to a given dimension were combined into an index. Three steps were used in assessing the

---

*Length of these items precludes their publication; however, all study materials are available from the authors upon request.

adequacy of an index: first, the items included had to possess some face validity relative to that dimension; second, inter-relationships among items were examined, and items (or an item) that did not yield at least modest associations were excluded; and third, internal consistency of the index was assessed by calculating a consistency coefficient (892). Indexes retained in the analysis yielded coefficients of .47 to .96; those with lower degrees of internal consistency were dropped. In general, indexes reflecting general concern about child's health, perceived threat of illness, and perceived negative health consequences of obesity yielded the highest consistency, whereas items tapping specific benefits of the diet and barriers to following the diet did less well in terms of coherence.

Personal characteristics such as age and education were measured with single questions. One index was created, however, that combined items on personal health status, educational level, income, and number of children in the home. This combination was intended to reflect personal problems. However, because of a low degree of index reliability, single item measures of problem circumstances were used in the analyses.

Results

Sixty-two percent of the 184 study subjects completed all phases of the trial. Detailed statistical analyses suggested that the attrition of the study group probably had little influence on the findings.

General Health Motivations.

The interview began with an appraisal of the degree to which the mother was concerned about the child's general health, both alone and in comparison to health concerns for her other children. As the data in Table 6.1 indicate, these items were strong predictors of weight loss, as was the mother's concern about the possibility of her child's getting sick. When these items are combined, the resulting index also yields correlations which are high, but which run somewhat below the level of the single question on child's general health.

To tap another dimension of health concern, mothers were asked to what extent they agreed or disagreed with the statement "If you wait long enough, children will get over most any illness," and to indicate whether, when their child seems a little sick, they "usually take him/her to a doctor right away or wait a day or two." Neither measure was predictive, perhaps because the questions reminded the mother of her child's mild and/or acute illnesses, experiences quite dissimilar to the present condition of obesity and need to diet.

A third aspect of mother's motivation is more covertly assessed, and is based on her report of whether or not she gives her child vitamins regularly, buys special foods "to improve or protect the family's health," makes certain the

TABLE 6.1. Correlations (gammas) between general health motivation and compliance variables

Motivation variables	Weight change on follow-up visit (FUV)				Clinic appointment-keeping ratio
	First FUV	Second FUV	Third FUV	Fourth FUV	
Concern about: Child's health	.541*	.330*	.326*	.252*	.140†
compared with her other children	.354*	.229*	.113	.068	−.017
Chance of illness	.502*	.319*	.332	.200†	.110
Concern index	.514*	.307*	.315	.209†	.133†
Children get well without M.D.'s help	−.041	.027	.015	.028	.088
Take to M.D. versus wait	−.110	.097	−.019	.162	−.043
Special health practices index	.332*	.408*	.281*	.241†	−.005
Concern about own health index	.184†	.128	.077	.111	.100
Chance keep child on diet	.527*	.428*	.418*	.341*	.089

*P ≤ .01.
†P ≤ .05.

child gets sufficient exercise and rest, and so forth. Engaging in these special health practices is shown to be associated with compliance, although not with clinic appointment keeping.

Although concern about the child's health appears to influence dietary compliance, mothers' personal health worries (in general, and about the chance of getting sick) were poor predictors of weight loss. Clearly, in this context, concerns for the child are more salient and relevant.

Finally, to obtain an indirect measure of intent, each mother was requested to estimate the likelihood that she would be able to keep the child on the prescribed diet. (Davis [128] found that 44% of the noncompliant patients he surveyed admitted that they had never intended to comply; see also Alpert [7].) Of the general health motivation items, this variable produced the best overall correlations with weight change.

With the exception of general concern about the child's health, the motivation measures were not significantly associated with clinic appointment keeping. This outcome may have resulted because the general-level items were not predictive of weight loss or of appointment keeping, and also because the remaining variables were diet specific and therefore unlikely to be predictive of an unrelated activity.

Perceived susceptibility.

As concern about the child's health was predictive of compliance, so also was the mother's perception of how easily her child gets sick. As the correlations in Table 6.2 show, the latter measure was more consistently correlated with weight loss across the follow-up visits, and it was a better predictor of appointment keeping.

Mothers were also asked to rate the likelihood of their child ever developing each of eight illnesses or conditions. Results obtained for the four items involving possible heart and circulatory threats reveal substantial associations with weight loss, and all but rheumatic fever were significantly related to appointment keeping as well. (The other four illnesses were anemia, pneumonia, asthma, and mumps; these correlations were also substantial, varying between .410 and .177.) Combining the eight illnesses yielded correlations with weight loss that are significant but somewhat weaker than those obtained for most of the individual items. However, an "index of general susceptibility" comprising both the general and specific vulnerability measures produced the highest correlations both for weight at the first follow-up visit and for appointment keeping.

A mother's conjectures about her child's probable future health behaviors (whether general or specific to weight and smoking) were not meaningfully linked to either of the dependent variables. These findings may reflect the subjects' differential appraisals of their childrens' present habits and desires, together with the realization that, although they could exert great control over the

TABLE 6.2. Correlations (gammas) between perceived susceptibility and compliance variables

Susceptibility variables	Weight change on follow-up visit (FUV)				Clinic appointment-keeping ratio
	First FUV	Second FUV	Third FUV	Fourth FUV	
How easily child gets sick	.491*	.433*	.422*	.348*	.185†
Chance child could get:					
Index of 8 illnesses	.298*	.280*	.274*	.229*	.088
Strep throat	.440*	.261*	.329*	.324*	.218†
Rheumatic fever	.433*	.292*	.300*	.291*	.105
Heart trouble	.251*	.190*	.210†	.235†	.149†
Hardening of arteries	.353*	.218*	.263*	.273*	.213†
General susceptibility index	.504*	.334*	.360*	.308*	.254*
Chance child will:					
Be overweight	.086	-.052	-.038	-.011	.075
Smoke	.033	-.033	.049	-.006	-.083
Take good care of health	.001	.129	-.024	.043	.088

*P ≤ .01.
†P ≤ .05.

child's diet and other health actions, this would not be the case when he or she became an adult.

Perceived Severity.

It is evident from the correlations in Table 6.3 that more compliant mothers had heightened perceptions of the potential seriousness of their children's illnesses.

Measures of "perceived severity" were constructed to parallel those employed for vulnerability. First, the interview attempted to determine how worried the mother was about the child's illnesses.

Although these correlations are significant, they are lower in comparison to the equivalent measure of general susceptibility. The absence of association with appointment keeping might be explained by reasoning that some mothers who keep follow-up appointments perceive such medical care interactions as efficacious in reducing the severity of the child's usual illnesses.

Next, using the earlier list of eight conditions, the subject was asked, "If your child were to get (each illness), how worried do you think you would be?" The best compliers are clearly mothers who were strongly aroused by the thought of what some illnesses could do to the child. In this instance, the correlations (including the illness index) run well above those obtained for susceptibility; in addition, these items are significantly related to appointment keeping. The overall score for general severity was a good predictor of weight loss.

Although employed successfully as a predictor in other studies of patient compliance, no association was found between the dependent variables and respondent's report of how much the child's usual illnesses "keep her from doing the things she needs to do." Further analysis also showed that this variable did not cluster with the other, straightforward severity items. Again, the explanation may depend upon perception of obesity as something other than an illness; moreover, a child's obesity probably would not actually interfere with the mother's usual activities, at least not in the same way as a typical acute illness. One might then conclude that it would be more appropriate to examine the mother's perception of how much the weight problem disrupts the *child's* normal activities (e.g., interactions with peers, eating/feeding, participation in athletics). The strong correlations for that dimension, as shown in Table 6.3, support this alternative interpretation of the "social severity" concept.

The remaining severity variables involve perceptions of threats specific to obesity. Worry about the child being overweight and the extent of agreement with the statement "being overweight could cause serious illness" were both substantially correlated with compliance (the latter was also associated with appointment keeping). The severity of overweight index (composed of "interference with child's activities" and the mother's worries about the child's obesity

TABLE 6.3. Correlations (gammas) between perceived severity and compliance variables

| Severity variables | Weight change on follow-up visit (FUV) | | | | Clinic appointment-keeping ratio |
	First FUV	Second FUV	Third FUV	Fourth FUV	
Worry about child's illnesses	.487*	.355*	.339*	.303*	.053
Worry if child got:					
Index of 8 illnesses	.452*	.247†	.304*	.234†	.120†
Strep throat	.506*	.303*	.337*	.249†	.224†
Rheumatic fever	.595*	.431*	.349*	.343*	.187†
Heart trouble	.640*	.401*	.351*	.370*	.217†
Hardening of arteries	.614*	.452*	.408*	.375*	.204†
General severity index	.525*	.351*	.326*	.278*	.097
Child's illnesses interfere	.049	.030	.051	−.043	.001
Overweight interferes with child's activities	.489*	.292*	.377*	.330*	.106
Worry about child's overweight	.419*	.300	.265*	.212†	.071
Overweight cause serious illness	.448*	.279*	.281*	.311*	.162†
Severity of overweight index	.556*	.348*	.358*	.298*	.066

*P≤.01.
†P ≤ .05.

generally and about possible sequelae specifically) produced the strongest correlations for the first and second follow-up visits, but the "interference" item alone was more powerful at the third and fourth visits.

It is of interest to note, in comparing the obesity-specific and general severity indexes, that the former was a better predictor of weight loss, whereas the latter was more accurate for forecasting appointment keeping.

Perceived Benefits.

The first three variables in Table 6.4 were meant to illustrate the HBM dimension concerned with the subjects' faith in medical information and care. None of these items are significantly related to weight loss; this may reflect a mix of current increased sophistication on the part of mothers concerning what they think they know about caring for their children's health (including nutritional knowledge), and a view of obesity as something relatively unrelated to illnesses and remedies. The "sophistication" argument receives some support from the substantial negative correlation between the helpfulness of information from the dietitian and appointment keeping (better appointment compliers perceived the diet information as less necessary). Nonetheless, subjects who did not feel that their children seemed "to get the kinds of illnesses that doctors can't do much for" were more likely to have kept their general clinic appointments, probably because this variable operates at the more abstract level of perceived ability of the clinic to help the sick child.

The remaining items in Table 6.4 represent different aspects of repondents' feelings of control over obesity and its consequences. Subjects were first asked what things a person can do to keep from having heart trouble, and those who mentioned *diet*-related actions (e.g., lose weight, avoid cholesterol) were significantly better compliers for the first two follow-up visits (although this motive seems to decline in importance by the third visit). Finally, mothers who disagreed with the statement "there isn't much anyone can do about how much he weighs," and who attributed the child's overweight to circumstances over which they do have control, were found to achieve better weight loss. (None of the "control over weight" variables predicted appointment keeping.)

Perceived Barriers.

Table 6.5 presents the study results concerning the effects of possible barriers to compliance. To determine perceived safety of the diet, the interview assessed respondent's strength of agreement or disagreement with the phrase "sometimes I worry that going on a diet can cause health problems." Although at first this question does not predict weight loss, the correlations climb to significant levels by the third follow-up visit, suggesting that those who originally felt more secure about the diet's safety were more likely to stay with it over time. This variable

TABLE 6.4. Correlations (gammas) between perceived benefits and compliance variables

Benefit variables	Weight change on follow-up visit (FUV)				Clinic appointment-keeping ratio
	First FUV	Second FUV	Third FUV	Fourth FUV	
Child gets illnesses M.D.s can't help	−.034	.063	.111	.175	.215*
Old remedies sometimes better	.023	.054	.008	.000	.049
How helpful was information from dietitian	−.079	.015	−.062	.045	−.253*
Things that might prevent heart disease	.353†	.268*	.145	−.061	.052
Control over weight	.420†	.344*	.320*	.337*	.088
Overweight attributed to self versus fate	.263*	.303*	.454*	.367*	.026

*P ≤ .05.
†P ≤ .01.

TABLE 6.5. Correlations (gammas) between perceived barriers and compliance variables.

| Barrier variables | Weight change on follow-up visit (FUV) | | | | Clinic appointment-keeping ratio |
	First FUV	Second FUV	Third FUV	Fourth FUV	
Safety of diet	−.032	.130	.199*	.212*	.223†
How difficult to affect weight	−.131	−.092	.055	.160	.001
Child on a diet before	.005	.025	−.070	.217*	−.033
Ease of diet compared to others	.147	.131	.297*	.325*	.162
Family problems	.182*	.201*	.087	.033	.030
Easy versus difficult get through day	.197*	.307*	.300*	.066	−.118
No reason to miss appointment	.014	.243*	.233*	.227*	.268*

*P ⩽ .05.
†P ⩽ .01.

may also provide another indirect measure of the subject's confidence in prescribed advice, since it also was found to be correlated with appointment keeping.

Mothers were then asked, "How difficult would you say it will be for you to
do something to help this overweight problem?" Their responses were not
associated with the dependent variables. This failure to predict may derive from
the respondents' general difficulty in making future-oriented appraisals, from a
wait-and-see attitude toward a regimen with which they did not yet have experience, or perhaps because the perceived ease or difficulty of the diet had little
bearing upon ultimate compliance. The last speculation is supported in part by
data from another part of the research. At the first follow-up visit, subjects
were asked to estimate how much the child minded being on the diet, and the
degree to which the diet was difficult to follow, was hard to plan, was hard to
prepare, necessitated preparing separate meals, was expensive, caused the family
to give up favorite foods, and caused problems with eating out. None of these
possible problems was significantly correlated with weight loss.

Whether or not the child had ever been on a diet was not significantly associated with weight loss until the fourth follow-up visit. Perhaps recollection of
how things had gone before utlimately provided extra motivation to continue
in the face of temporary problems or setbacks. Additional evidence for this
possibility comes from analyses which revealed that the dropout rates between
follow-up visits were lower for mothers of children with prior diet experience
than for the remaining subjects. Further, among the experienced mothers, those
who found the present diet easier began to obtain significantly better weight
loss by the third follow-up visit.

Because circumstances in the home might interfere with compliance, the
mother's perceptions of the frequency with which the family was troubled by
problems, and of whether she found it relatively easy or difficult to get through
the day were evaluated. Both variables showed a somewhat curvilinear relationship to weight loss, starting with significant levels at the first follow-up visit,
peaking at the second follow-up visit, and declining to nonsignificance by the
last visit. Thus, having fewer difficulties at home appeared to enable better
compliance during the first month of the diet, but declined in influence as the
regimen continued.

The last item in Table 6.5 is based on responses to the open-ended question,
"Sometimes mothers can't bring the child back to the clinic for the next appointment. What are some of the things that might make *you* miss an appointment for your child at the clinic?" Because many mothers said "nothing would"
or "I don't miss appointments," a special analysis was performed in which
subjects were coded into two categories of this independent variable: no reason
given, and any reason given. Correlations between this "no excuse" dimension
and weight loss were found to be significant after the first follow-up visit, and,
as would be expected, were most highly associated with appointment keeping.

Sociodemographic Variables.

The large number of nonsignificant correlations shown in Table 6.6 reflect the usual situation in attempts to use sociodemographic variables to predict patient compliance. Only "age of child" and "mother's marital status" were significantly associated with weight loss (no sociodemographic item predicted appointment keeping). Mothers of older children were better compliers; and since correlations for the mother's own age were not significant, the effect appears to be due solely to the child's age. The direction of the findings is somewhat surprising, since an older child might be expected to exert more detrimental control over the regimen (e.g., snacks, eating away from home), and to be able to object more successfully to the rigors of the diet. That the reverse was in fact true suggests that the older child was using the extra control to adhere to the diet, perhaps because he or she experienced peer pressures related to the social desirability of losing weight.

Two kinds of analyses were conducted to assure that the age of the child was not a source of spuriousness in the HBM-compliance association. First, Pearson correlations were calculated between the child's age and the mother's score on each of 14 health belief indexes; only one significant association (with "index of susceptibility to specified illnesses") was obtained (.16). Second, weight loss at the first and fourth follow-up visits was regressed on age of child; multiple regression was then performed on the weight change and belief variables using the age-removed residuals from the previous regression. The resulting betas were almost the same as those obtained by simply regressing weight change on beliefs, and the multiple correlations declined only slightly (from .648 to .618 for the first follow-up visit, and from .463 to .454 for the fourth follow-up visit).

The influence of marital status (ordered, for the gamma, as married, widowed, divorced, separated, never married) may derive both from the helpfulness of having the spouse present to exert influence, and from the relationship of this variable to the "family problems" dimension discussed earlier (gramma= .271).

The Intervention.

As described earlier, post-interview subjects were randomly assigned to: (1) receive a "high fear" message and booklet about obesity; (2) receive a similar, but lower threat, communication and booklet; or (3) no intervention at all (the control group). Analysis of variance assured that no significant differences existed among treatment groups on the initial amount of overweight (i.e., that random assignment was effective).

Figure 6.3 displays the cumulative percentage of initial weight gained or lost by the treatment and control groups at each follow-up visit. The experimental conditions were significantly associated with weight change at each visit. Although, in the aggregate, the controls actually gained weight at first, children of

TABLE 6.6. Correlations (gammas) between demographic factors and compliance variables

Demographic factors	Weight change on follow-up visit (FUV)				Clinic appointment-keeping ratio
	First FUV	Second FUV	Third FUV	Fourth FUV	
Age of child	.111	.206*	.211*	.221*	.100
Age of mother	.119	.120	.146	.114	.060
Sex of child	.049	.053	.003	.221	.213
Race of child	.267	.390	.520	.503	−.093
Number of siblings	.055	−.028	−.011	.032	.137
Mother's martial status	.108	.270*	.443†	.329*	.088
Mother's education	.120	.003	−.064	−.118	−.038
Number of people in home	.049	−.020	.015	.018	.030
Family income	.147	.002	.047	.037	.013

*P ≤ .05.
†P ≤ .01.

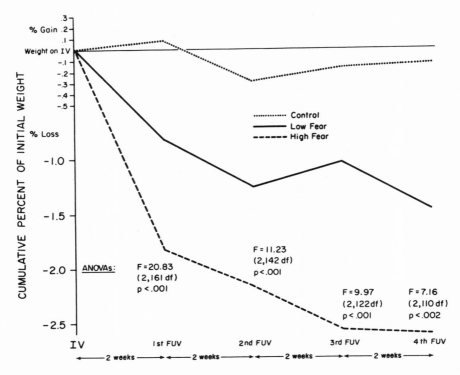

FIGURE 6.3. Cumulative percentage weight change from initial visit, by treatment group.

subjects in both of the experimental groups had lost considerable weight by the first follow-up visit. Across the four follow-up visits, the high fear intervention had the most consistent long-term effect (although its influence appears eventually to have declined). The low fear group lost ground slightly between the second and third follow-up visits, but subsequently exhibitied another substantial drop in weight. Finally, except for the second two-week period, the control group always evidenced weight gains between follow-up visits. Expressed in correlational terms, gammas between communication groups (ordered high, low, control) and weight change (ranked from loss to gain) across the four follow-up visits were: .594, .438, .447, .444, respectively (all significant). There was, of course, no association between communication group and prior appointment keeping.

Discussion

Based on this study's findings, the HBM appears to be useful in explaining and predicting a mother's adherence to a diet regimen prescribed for her child,

DEMOGRAPHIC VARIABLES

Age of child
Mother's marital status

THREAT VARIABLES

Susceptibility:

BENEFITS

MOTIVATION VARIABLES

Concern about:

  Child's health *
  Chance child get sick
  Index *
  Special health practices
  index
  Chance keep child on diet

How easily child gets sick *
Index of 8 illnesses
  (those related to heart) *
General susceptibility index *

Severity:

Worry about illnesses child gets
Index of 8 illnesses *
  (those related to heart) *
General severity index

Worry about child's overweight
Overweight can cause serious illness *
Overweight interferes
Severity of overweight index
Child's concern about own weight

MD can help illnesses
  (App't.-keeping only)
Diet-related activity might
  prevent heart disease
Control over weight
Overweight attributed to
  self versus fate

BARRIERS

Safety of diet*
Prior experience/relative ease
Family problems/getting through
  day
No reason to miss clinic
  appointments*

* = Also predicted clinic appointment - keeping

FIGURE 6.4. Reduced list of variables found to be predictive of weight loss.

as well as in forecasting the likelihood that she will keep general clinic follow-up appointments made for the child. At both a general level and at a level relating specifically to obesity and dieting, variables significantly associated with a child's weight change were found in each major category of the model. These results are summarized in Figure 6.4. Perceptions related to health motives, to threat (i.e., to susceptibility and severity, whether general or weight-specific), and to benefits of and barriers to the diet, show positive relationships to weight loss, while appointment keeping was modestly associated mainly with the more general motivation and threat measures. Except for "age of child" and "mother's marital status," subjects' personal characteristics were unrelated to the dependent variables.

Although the correlations often decline in magnitude by the fourth follow-up visit, they usually remain significant. This attenuation implies that health beliefs may be most important initially; but, with time and concurrent experience with the diet and weight-change outcomes, other variables may become important as well. The changing correlations are not explained by changes over time in characteristics of the study population. The first and second halves of the group (i.e., early and late study entrants) were compared on sociodemographic characteristics (e.g., age of child, education, marital status), and no significant differences were observed. In terms of dropouts, another set of analyses compared belief scores and weight loss at first follow-up visit for two groups: mothers who remained in the study across all four follow-up visits, and mothers who dropped out of the study at any time after the first follow-up visit. It was found that: (1) belief-belief and belief-behavior correlation patterns were virtually identical for both groups; and (2) multiple regressions using beliefs to predict weight loss at the first follow-up visit were quite similar (multiple correlation = .68 for those who remained, .56 for dropouts). Furthermore, there were no significant differences in demographic variables among dropouts after each follow-up visit.

Several checks were made to test the possibility that "objectively" severe obesity produced both high scores on HBM variables and greater weight loss (such a possible source of spuriousness would not affect the experimental outcomes, since treatment groups did not differ significantly in initial amount of overweight). Using the ratio of actual weight to ideal weight at the start of treatment as the measure of severity of overweight, gammas were calculated between this construct and weight loss at each follow-up visit; *none* was statistically significant (.023, .031, .040, and -.005 for visits one through four respectively), demonstrating that more extreme initial overweight was not associated with greater weight reduction. Another series of correlations between actual versus ideal weight and each of several belief indexes were also nonsignificant (gammas ranged from -.08 for "index of general susceptibility" to .11 for "index of general severity"). Thus, the degree of initial overweight does not appear to enhance perceptions of threat along HBM dimensions.

To evaluate the whole HBM (i.e., combination of beliefs *across* belief dimensions) as a predictor of compliance, multiple regression analyses were performed in which the weight change measures were regressed against belief indexes and items. (The latter were selected to represent the critical HBM elements, and were put into the regression in an order from general measures to more weight-specific items.) Table 6.7 presents the analyses for the basic HBM dimensions, showing substantial multiple Rs from this combination for each follow-up visit and for appointment keeping, levels well above the zero-order correlations obtained by any single study item or index. Together, the nine items account for approximately 49% of the variance in weight change on the first follow-up visit and 17% of the variance in appointment keeping.

A somewhat different combination of measures was also evaluated, based only on indexes (and, thus, reducing the number of elements in the regression as well as introducing additional dimensions). The entire set of general health indexes (relating to the mother's beliefs about the child's health) were combined into one general health threat measure. A single index of beliefs about the diet was also constructed, and an index of overweight as a health problem was included. Results, shown in Table 6.8, indicate multiple Rs quite similar to those obtained by the first combination (the Rs are slightly higher for follow-up visits two through four, but slightly lower for the first follow-up visit and for appointment keeping). Thus, only six index measures can still account for a significant proportion of the variance in the dependent variables. These findings also suggest that: (1) measures of general beliefs concerning the child's vulnerability to health problems are most important in weight loss during earlier follow-up periods, whereas weight-specific measures are relatively more important later;

TABLE 6.7. Multiple regression 1, with weight change and appointment keeping regressed on major HBM belief indexes and items

Belief indexes and items (in order)	(c)*	Weight change on follow-up visit (FUV) (betas)				Clinic appointment keeping ratio (betas)
		First FUV	Second FUV	Third FUV	Fourth FUV	
General concern about child's health	(.77)	.10	.15†	.07	.02	.17
Special health practices	(.86)	-.08	-.26†	-.13	-.09	.08
General susceptibility	(.91)	.25†	.13	.11	.14	.23†
General severity	(.96)	.08	.03	.03	-.04	-.11
No reason to miss appointment	(item)	.04	.16†	.22†	.12†	.20†
Chance keep child on diet	(item)	.31†	.25†	.23†	.24†	.10
Severity of overweight	(.85)	.11	.03	.13	.11	-.06
Control over weight	(item)	.09	.03	.16†	.11†	-.05
Safety of diet	(item)	-.12	-.02	.03	.05	.20†
Multiple R =		.702	.596	.566	.465	.414
R^2 =		.493	.355	.320	.216	.171

*Internal consistency coefficient for index.
†$P \leq .05$.

TABLE 6.8. Multiple regression 2, with weight change and appointment keeping regressed on combined belief indexes

Belief indexes (in order)	(c)*	Weight change on follow-up visit (FUV) (betas)				Clinic appointment keeping ratio (betas)
		First FUV	Second FUV	Third FUV	Fourth FUV	
General health threat	(.92)	.43†	.32†	.24	.02	.48†
Medical benefits	(.87)	−.10	−.12	−.21†	−.15	−.14
Concern about own health	(.55)	−.12	−.05	−.14	−.10	−.07
Special health practices	(.86)	−.12	−.29†	−.16†	−.15	.13
Severity of overweight	(.85)	.17	.12	.22	.35†	−.22
Overall efficacy of diet	(.48)	.14†	.21†	.18†	.25†	−.00
Multiple R =		.641	.606	.591	.514	.342
R^2		.411	.367	.349	.264	.117

*Internal consistency coefficient for index.

†$P \leqslant .05$.

(2) although it is surprising that beliefs concerning the efficacy of medical care generally are negatively related to weight loss, this finding reinforces the notion that weight is seen as a problem that must be dealt with outside the medical care system; (3) a mother's concern with her own problems may interfere with her dealing with the child's day-to-day health problem; (4) the influence of perceived benefits from the diet appears consistently; and (5) only the general health threat measures prove to be a significant predictor of appointment keeping.

The analyses, therefore, indicate that signficant predictions about weight loss can be made just by knowing about the mother's general health concerns and her threat perceptions regarding the child. Specific concerns and feelings about weight and about the diet, however, enhance predictive accuracy and seem to become increasingly important over time.

The experimental conditions were specifically associated with weight change, and the influence of that association on the belief analyses remains to be explored.

Using the experimental groups as a dummy variable, the multiple regressions were redone, with the group variable entered first. An example of the outcome is provided in Table 6.9. As expected, treatment group was a significant predictor of weight change at each follow-up visit. However, the belief variables were *also* accurate predictors of weight change, and at approximately the same levels as before. Another approach used analysis of variance on experimental groups and weight loss within aggregates of subjects who were all high (or low) on relevant health beliefs. This approach confirmed the significant independent effects of beliefs and of the fear-arousal intervention.

Finally, evidence was obtained for an effect of the intervention combined with health beliefs. Table 6.10 permits examination of mean weight loss at each follow-up visit, classified *jointly* by experimental group and by high versus low splits on a health threat combined index. "Highs" fared better than "lows" in general, and high fear treatments accomplished more than low fear ones which, in turn, were better than controls; however, the differences for controls were consistently much greater than those found for either fear group. Also, the experimental treatments show the greatest difference for subjects with the lowest levels of health threat beliefs.

In summary, the data lend further support for a model of individual health-related behavior based on valence of goal and subjective probability of goal attainment, and incorporating estimates of health motives, disease threat, and benefits of action. Whether taken singly or in combination, these dimensions were shown to account for substantial amounts of the variance in this study's measures of dietary compliance and appointment keeping. Further, although the HBM itself suggests no particular strategy for altering beliefs, the fear-arousal intervention tested in the study had a marked effect on compliance behavior. It is suggested that the HBM be employed as a basis for additional

TABLE 6.9. Multiple regression 3, with weight change regressed on belief indexes and experimental group as dummy variable

Belief Indexes (in order)	(c)*	Weight change on follow-up visit (FUV) (betas)			
		First FUV	Second FUV	Third FUV	Fourth FUV
Experimental group	(—)	.25†	.20†	.18†	.17
General concern for child's health	(.77)	.21†	.20†	.17	.05
General susceptibility	(.91)	.30†	.20†	.27†	.29†
Medical benefits	(.87)	-.06	-.05	-.14	-.06
Concern about own health	(.55)	-.15†	-.11	-.16†	-.12
View of diet	(.51)	-.05	.04	.05	.06
Diet benefits	(.47)	.19†	.15	.08	.09
Multiple R =		.666	.545	.567	.486
R² =		.444	.297	.321	.236

*Internal consistency coefficient for index.
†P ≤ .05.

TABLE 6.10. Mean weight change at each FUV, by both treatment group and level of health threat

Health threat		Treatment group			Visit
		High fear	Low fear	Control	
High		1.93	1.27	.61	FUV 1
Low		1.64	.49	−.44	
	Difference	.29	.78	1.05	
High		2.14	1.23	1.32	FUV 2
Low		2.13	1.28	−.34	
	Difference	.01	−.05	1.66	
High		2.79	.82	1.25	FUV 3
Low		2.14	1.16	−.42	
	Difference	.65	−.34	1.67	
High		2.45	1.12	1.13	FUV 4
Low		2.84	1.71	−.44	
	Difference	−.39	−.59	1.57	

research on other patient behaviors, in different settings, with different socio-demographic populations, and using experimental designs to test the relative value of other interventions aimed at modifying the model's belief dimensions and subsequent health behaviors.

A TEST OF THE HEALTH BELIEF MODEL
IN HYPERTENSION: *D. Wayne Taylor*

A sizable body of published data now exists (see Table 5 in the annotated bibliography in Appendix I) that shows positive correlations between patients' compliance and their "health beliefs" as described by Marshall Becker at the beginning of this chapter. Three important implications have been drawn from these data. First, the data have been interpreted as indicating that a patient's compliance is largely determined or caused by his health beliefs. Second, the implication has been drawn that physicians might be able to identify noncompliant patients by inquring into their patients' perceptions of their illness and treatment regimen. Finally, it has been speculated that compliance might be improved by strategies designed to modify health beliefs and perceptions.

Although the majority of studies have found support for the Health Belief Model (HBM), there are several studies which disagree (see Table 5 in Appendix I and Chapter 15 on nursing and compliance). Furthermore, investigations of the HBM which have been performed to date have all been subexperimental in design. Such studies can detect correlations between health beliefs and compliance but fall short of establishing that these links are of a causal nature. Thus, it is unclear whether (1) health beliefs of an appropriate sort cause people to behave in a compliant fashion, or (2) compliant behavior causes people to hold certain health beliefs (to reduce cognitive dissonance, for example), or (3) unknown factors cause both high compliance and appropriate health beliefs. A convincing demonstration that health beliefs are responsible for compliance would require a randomized controlled trial in which health beliefs were modified (for example, by an educational process) and corresponding changes in compliance resulted. While we await the performance of such an experiment we must be content with less convincing correlational evidence.

We can and must, however, make a distinction between two types of correlational data. First, most health belief studies have measured health beliefs at the same point in time, and sometimes after, the assessment of compliance. Correlations from such studies can determine whether compliance and verbally expressed attitudes and perceptions are consistent with each other, but they do not permit conclusions regarding cause and effect. A second and more convincing type of correlational study involves the measurement of health beliefs at some point prior to the assessment of compliance. Data from these investigations has the advantage of showing whether health beliefs precede compliance, thus providing a stronger indication of causality. It is obvious that the inferential advantages of such prospective studies is lost if the study begins at some point after the initiation of treatment or if the patients have had prior experience with the treatment (from a previous bout of illness). For if this were the case, it could be argued that health beliefs and compliance had already been set by other unknown factors or by a process of rationalization, and that the analysis merely reflected a stable situation in which both health beliefs and compliance behavior remained consistent with each other. A convincing correlational test of the HBM would therefore require individuals prescribed the therapeutic regimen for the first time among whom health beliefs were measured before the initiation of the regimen and then compared with subsequent compliance. We have conducted such a test within a hypertension detection and treatment program in which various strategies were tested for their ability to improve compliance.

Methods

The experimental part of this research has been reported elsewhere (228, 449). The features of the study which relate to the test of the health belief model are described below.

Patients were enrolled in the trial following blood pressure screening of a random two-thirds sample of steelworkers employed at a foundry in Hamilton,

Ontario, Canada. After excluding men who were taking prescribed medication of any kind or who had been treated for hypertension previously, 245 men remained with sustained hypertension (DBP $\geq$ 95 mm Hg) on their most recent company medical examination and on two subsequent blood pressure checks made by trained technicians. Although 230 of these men agreed to participate in the study and although we ensured that all of these men kept a referral visit to a physician, only 153 were started on treatment and physicians discontinued treatment on 25 men before the end of the twelve-month trial. This report is thus for the 128 men who were started and continued on antihypertensive therapy by a physician over a twelve-month period.

Patient perceptions of personal susceptibility to developing hypertension, the seriousness of hypertension, the benefits of treatment, attitudes toward drug taking, and the dependency implications of illness were assessed in a standardized interview which also included questions on medical history, symptomatology, and family and social relationships. This interview was first conducted during the blood pressure screening phase, before a diagnosis of hypertension had been made, and was repeated six months after patients were referred to physicians for therapy. The various questions used to assess each health belief were coded and summed to create five health belief scales: susceptibility, seriousness, benefits of treatment, drug attitudes, and perception of the dependency implications of illness. To assure that the questions selected for a particular scale were in fact homogeneous with respect to the belief being measured, correlations were computed between each item and the total score obtained by summing all other items in that scale. Only items for which these correlations were statistically significant (P < .05), at both the screening and six-month interviews, were retained in the health belief scales.

Compliance with the prescribed drug regimen was assessed six and twelve months after the initiation of treatment by unobtrusive pill counts conducted during home visits after the patient had left the room to produce a urine specimen and also by asking the patient in a nonthreatening manner to estimate how often, on average, he missed taking his medication. Pill counts were compared to physician and pharmacy records of pills prescribed and dispensed. The results of pill counts and subjective measures of compliance were expressed as the percentage of the prescribed medication which was taken by the patient.

In addition to the test of the causal hypothesis implied by the health belief model, i.e., whether pretreatment health beliefs influence subsequent patient compliance, the study design permitted an examination of four other questions. First, study of the relationship between health beliefs and compliance, both measured six months after the initiation of therapy, permitted assessment of whether the consistency between health beliefs and compliance seen in cross-sectional studies could be demonstrated here. Second, an examination of the correlation between six-month health beliefs and 12-month compliance allowed us to ascertain whether health beliefs measured after the initiation of therapy

TABLE 6.11. Correlations between pre-treatment health beliefs and compliance

Pre-treatment beliefs	Six-month compliance		Twelve-month compliance	
	Pill count	Self-report	Pill count	Self-report
Susceptibility	.01	−.03	−.02	−.02
Seriousness	−.01	−.01	.10	.05
Benefits	.07	.08	.08	.12
Drug safety	.15*	.12	.05	.03
Social dependency	.23†	.18*	.21†	.21†

*P < .05.
†P < .01.

could predict future compliance. Third, a multiple regression analysis in which compliance served as the dependent variable for the combined set of health belief model scales assessed the extent to which a holistic consideration of health beliefs improved upon correlations observed for individual components of the model. Finally, since some authors have implied that physicians might identify noncompliant patients better by inquiring into health beliefs, we examined partial correlations between patient compliance and health beliefs, controlling for patients' verbal reports of their compliance. These partial correlations indicated whether an inquiry into health beliefs was likely to provide more information than could be gained by the simpler and more direct approach of asking patients to estimate their own level of compliance. In the above analyses both parametric and nonparametric correlations were computed; since the results were extremely close, only Pearson product moment correlations are reported.

Results

As a test of the hypothesized causal link between health beliefs and compliance, pretreatment health beliefs were correlated with both six- and twelve-month pill counts and with self-reported measures of compliance. Of the five scales examined, only the one that assessed attitudes towards the dependency implications of illness, showed significant correlations with compliance at six and twelve months (Table 6.11). Patients who felt that illness did not imply a state of dependency on others were more likely to comply than those who believed that illness entailed dependency. (A positive attitude toward the safety of drug taking also reached statistical significance, but this was for only one of the four prospective measures of compliance.)

In contrast to the general failure of pretreatment beliefs to predict subsequent compliance, three of the four health belief model scales assessed six months after the beginning of treatment showed significant correlations with six-

TABLE 6.12. Correlations between six-month health beliefs and compliance

Six-month beliefs	Six-month compliance		Twelve-month compliance	
	Pill count	Self-report	Pill count	Self-report
Seriousness	.17*	.19*	.27†	.20*
Benefits	.02	−.02	.08	.12
Drug safety	.16*	.16*	.32†	.23†
Social dependency	.20*	.19*	.23†	.21†
Multiple R = .26	.25		.39	.30
R^2 = .07	.06		.15	.09

*P < .05.
†P < .01.

and twelve-month compliance as shown in Table 6.12. Although pretreatment perceptions of drug safety and the seriousness of hypertension were not significantly correlated with six- and twelve-month compliance, these same perceptions measured at six months were significantly correlated with both concurrent (six-month) and subsequent (twelve-month) compliance. Six-month perceptions of the dependency implications of illness continued to show significant correlations with compliance, and six-month perceptions of the health benefits of anti-hypertensive therapy remained unrelated to compliance. A subject's perception of his personal susceptibility to developing hypertension obviously could be made only before the diagnosis of hypertension and therefore was not assessed at six months.

In order to determine the explanatory power of the health belief model scales when considered together, a multiple regression analysis was performed between six-month health beliefs and six- and twelve-month compliance. The multiple correlation coefficient, R, and the proportion of variance in compliance explained by the combined set of beliefs, R^2, are shown at the bottom of Table 6.12. The best result achieved was an R of .39 between six-month health beliefs and the 12-month pill count measure of compliance indicating that six-month beliefs accounted for only 15% of the variance in the subsequent objective measure of compliance.

Finally, in order to determine whether an assessment of health beliefs would add significantly to the identification of a compliance problem, beyond that which could be learned by simply asking the patient to estimate his own compliance, partial correlations were computed between each of the six-month beliefs and the six-month pill count measure of compliance, controlling for patients' verbal reports of their compliance. A correlation of .72 was found between the subjective report and pill count measures of compliance, indicating that the patients' subjective reports could explain 52% of the variance in the objective

TABLE 6.13. Partial correlations between pill count compliance and health beliefs, controlling for self-reported compliance

Six month beliefs	Six-month compliance by pill counts	
	Simple R	Partial R
Seriousness	.17*	.06
Benefits	.02	.05
Drug safety	.16*	.07
Social dependency	.20*	.09

*$P < .05$.

pill count measure of compliance. As shown in Table 6.13, all partial correlations between six-month health beliefs and compliance were near zero, indicating that an inquiry into patients' health beliefs could not explain any additional variance in the pill count measure of compliance.

Discussion and Conclusions

Health beliefs related to hypertension and its treatment that were assessed before the initiation of drug treatment for hypertension did not predict compliance six and twelve months later. However, health beliefs expressed six months after the initiation of treatment were found to be consistent with compliance measured at the same point in time and also predictive of subsequent (twelve-month) compliance. These results support the hypothesis that health beliefs, instead of preceding and determining compliance behavior, develop along with compliance behavior as a result of experience with treatment gained by patients in the early weeks or months of therapy. If this is indeed the case, attempts to improve compliance by trying to modify health beliefs should not prove successful.

The scale which measured beliefs regarding the dependency implications of illness was the only one which showed significant correlations between the pretreatment state and subsequent compliance, and thus is a possible exception to the above conclusion. It may justly be argued, however, that this observation lends support only to the health "locus of control" model for explaining compliance, since beliefs regarding the dependency implications of illness have never been formalized as an element of the "barriers to compliance" component of the HBM, as it was utilized here.

Our results also indicate that a general inquiry into health beliefs at the beginning of treatment is not helpful in the identification of patients who will encounter future compliance problems. If one waits until patients have gained some experience with the treatment regimen before measuring health beliefs, our results reveal that the health belief scales do show significant correlations with compliance, and together explain 15% of the variance in compliance. However, the simple procedure of asking the patient to estimate his own compliance fared much better, explaining 52% of the variance in compliance. In addition, the partial correlations between health beliefs and the pill count measure of compliance were all near zero when controlling for patients' subjective reports of compliance, indicating that after asking the patient to estimate his own compliance an inquiry into health beliefs did not provide further useful information in the identification of patients with compliance problems.

This report should not be misconstrued as suggesting that health attitudes and beliefs of patients are never the cause of low compliance, nor that they can be ignored in the practice of medicine, for the focus of this chapter is much narrower. What these data do suggest is that in the practical business of attempting to identify noncompliant patients and to predict compliance over the next few months of therapy, a routine inquiry into health beliefs is not likely to be of much help.

It must be pointed out that the particular setting in which these results were obtained raises some questions about their generalization. Is it possible that these results are peculiar to the treatment of hypertension and other asymptomatic conditions in which the objective of treatment is the prevention of disease for which the patient is at increased risk, rather than the cure of immediate sickness? If so, the health belief model might still be of practical use in the latter situation. We might also wonder whether these results are peculiar to the type of patients involved, and whether health beliefs might be more salient and important determinants of compliance for others, such as mothers caring for their children or pilots for their eyesight, than for hypertensive steelworkers beginning a long-term course of therapy for the eventual prevention of stroke, kidney damage, and premature death. It is also possible that patients with a more extensive history of prior and coexistent illness (recall that we excluded subjects who were taking any form of prescribed medication at the beginning of the study) have built up a more extensive set of beliefs and perceptions regarding disease and its treatment which may strongly influence their response to a new diagnosis and prescription.

The present study has been valuable in identifying a particular setting in which the health belief model has not been useful in explaining compliance behavior. Whether or not this failure is due to the above or other reasons, it is clear that future investigations should attempt to distinguish those patient groups and clinical situations in which the health belief model can be of practical use in dealing with the problem of noncompliance as opposed to those where it offers little help.

III
STRATEGIES FOR IMPROVING COMPLIANCE

7

Ethical Issues in Compliance

Albert R. Jonsen

It is a pleasure to address the "ethical issues in compliance." The pleasure arises not because the issues are particularly pleasant—indeed, they are often particularly aggravating—but because, unlike most of the issues we medical ethicists are called to address, compliance is a familiar everyday sort of ethical problem. Withdrawing life support mechanisms, fetal experimentation, decisions about Down's babies with duodenal atresia—these are dramatic, intense issues, the stuff of which Marcus Welby episodes and evening television news are made. Compliance will probably never achieve a high Neilson rating or even a headline (although, in some respects, it ought to).

Indeed, compliance is less of an ethical issue than it is an issue of homiletics. The latter is a subject with which few physicians are acquainted. It is defined as "the art of preaching, of giving sermons intended to edify a congregation on some practical matter." As I read through the literature on compliance, I am struck by how much it resembles, save for the statistics and controlled trials, the problems faced by the minister charged with leading his parishioners to the godly life. For centuries, the pastor explained over and over the orderly steps, the daily activities which, if faithfully followed, would bring his flock to "happiness in this life and eternal bliss in the next." While perhaps devoting an occasional sermon to horrendous sins such as tyranny or treason, he would almost always attend to the more habitual sins of anger, gluttony, and lust, for it is in the routine of life, not in its rare and dramatic moments, that virtue is won. And, sad to say, the faithful pastor saw his exhortations go unheeded as his charges wandered from the straight path into the neighborhood tavern or the neighbor's bed. He preached compliance with a salvific regimen and was often disappointed.

The literature on compliance tells us a message which our good minister would recognize. He would agree with Barbara Korsch, even without reading her data, that, "lack of warmth, friendliness, failure to take into account patients' concerns and expectations . . . lack of clearcut explanation . . . and using medical jargon . . . contribute significantly to patient dissatisfaction" (907). He would recognize his own flock in the descriptions of patients' noncompliance behavior: they are careless, forgetful, too busy, noncomprehending, and nonbelieving. He would in humility confess he saw himself in the profile of the physician: poor at explanation, failing to sympathize, failing to motivate, too lofty in tone and phrase. He would conclude, after reading through Sackett and Haynes's book (794), that, alas, compliance posed very much the same problem as piety: even the best intentions become quickly ensnared in the flaws of the human condition. And, unlike our good pastor, physicians cannot invoke divine grace to heal those flaws.

The comparison between compliance and piety may sound facetious, but it is drawn to make a point about the nature of compliance studies. Students of compliance would like to have their problems clearcut and their data hard. Yet, they are unlikely ever to be satisifed with the questions and answers that constitute the compliance problem. Those who would like definitive criteria to recognize the nonconformer will be frustrated by Hulka and co-workers' conclusion that, "neither characteristics of patients nor severity of disease were influential in determining the extent of medication errors" (256). It is rather that irrational and unpredictable reality, known to the theologians as "fallen human nature," that is influential. Those who look for the precise dimension of the problem will be discouraged by Gillum and Barsky's summation: "Factors most consistently related to noncompliance are: (1) psychological factors; (2) environmental and social factors; (3) characteristics of the therapeutic regimen; and (4) properties of the patient-physician interaction" (670). Or, in words more familiar to the theologian, the "universe unredeemed" explains noncompliance. Why do people knowingly neglect to do what is in their best interest? Any answer you seek will lead you away from the familiar evidences of the clinical world into the mysterious territory of the theologian and his favorite problem: the freedom of the will.

The point, then, of my apparently facetious simile that compliance is like piety, is this: when the epidemiologists move from their familiar tasks of recording the incidence and prevalence of dengue fever or schistosomiasis to the new endeavor of explaining why and how hypertensives exhibiting "type A" behavior fail to take their hydrochlorothiazide, they move from the scientific and statistical to the ethical and almost to the theological. The mysteries of the latter disciplines are not solved by even the best observation and the most sophisticated statistics.

My simile has a second, less didactic point. It can serve as an organizing theme for the rest of this essay. Piety has two sides: the fundamental truths on which it rests and the fundamental problems with the observance of those truths that, in the language of theology, are called temptations and, if yielded to, sins. The ethics of the compliance problem can be viewed in a similar way. There are some fundamental truths that define the ethics of compliance and some fundamental problems. In the remainder of this sermon, I will expose the dogma and the possible delinquencies from it.

Fundamental Truths of the Ethics of Compliance

The term *ethics* can be understood in two ways. First, it can refer to the quality of behavior expected from a person (a professional) in the ordinary course of his activities. In this ordinary course, what are the accepted standards from which departure is blameworthy? The second meaning of ethics refers to the problem of the right action in a "crisis," when the ordinary course of activities is disrupted, the accepted standards seem inapplicable, and the problem at issue is ill defined. In passing, it should be noted that, in current medical ethics, so much attention is paid to ethics in the second sense, that the fundamental truths of the patient-physician relationship are sadly neglected.

The fundamental truths of the ethics of compliance are well stated in Fink's definition of the *consensual regimen*: "a negotiated mutual contract in which both provider and client can be said to have given 'informed consent,' which is practical in terms of the current set of health problems and resources, 'no-fault' attitudes toward noncompliant behavior, and mutual responsibility for outcome" (658). This is the ideal for the patient-physician relationship in which compliance behavior is expected. It states an ethical ideal of freedom, mutual understanding, and mutual responsibility. It also suggests a practical ideal: within such a relationship compliance should be mutually satisfactory.

In addition to the relationship of mutual responsibility, the conditions proposed by Sackett for the ethical nature of compliance must be present: the diagnosis must be correct and the therapy must do more good than harm. Sackett also notes that not only must there be mutual responsibility of patient and physician in the prescription of medication and in its taking but also, "the patient must be an informed, willing partner in execution of any maneuver designed to alter compliance behavior" (795). These definitions and conditions state the fundamental and ethical truths of compliance behavior. They are the expected standards of behavior in the ordinary course of caring for patients. To say they are "ethical" in this sense does not mean, of course, that they are easily achieved or are commonly practiced. It means, rather, that they are the uncontroverted standards toward which patient and practitioner must strive. Should they depart from these standards without some reasonable justification, blame could be rightly attributed.

In the light of these fundamental truths, at least four problems appear. These are the temptations of compliance behavior; yielding to them results in the sins of compliance behavior. These problems are the "crises" in which application of the fundamental truths is difficult. We shall list them as four questions: (1) What ought to be done when a patient is persistently noncompliant? (2) What are the ethical limits of efforts to improve compliance? (3) Can compliance behavior be studied in ways which are both scientifically rigorous and ethically appropriate? (4) To what extent is the provider responsible for noncompliance?

The following sections will touch briefly on these four problems. Each deserves discussion more ample than space allows, but the definition of the problem, some considerations which ought to be elements in its solution, and a statement of the definitive failure to solve it must suffice.

Treatment of the Noncompliant Patient

Patients are sometimes persistently noncompliant. Some make hearty efforts and collapse early; others half-heartedly drag along; still others will obdurately refuse, in an explicit or implicit manner, even to start. In addition, suppose that such patients cannot or will not go elsewhere and cannot leave care without serious detriment to themselves. It can be asked whether the attending physician has a moral responsibility to continue to care for such patients. (The legal responsibilities are relatively clear.)

There are several elements to be considered in answering this problem. First, it is rash to suppose that noncompliance of this sort equals the refusal of treatment which would absolve the physician of further responsibility. Noncompliance may instead represent needs in the patient deeper than any that medication can satisfy. The ethics of medical care, it should be remembered, rest on ambiguous and not always compatible imperatives; the physician's responsibility to care derives from the patient's request for care and, on the other hand, derives from the patient's need for help, even when not explicitly requested. The first imperative establishes a kind of "contract," called in the law fiduciary, in which the patient contracts for services by entrusting himself or herself to the physician's care. The second inperative arises from something deeper in the patient than the free ability to contract; it arises from the state of desperate need, which may be inarticulate. Physicians are often torn between these two imperatives, recognizing a need even in the face of refusal. In the matter of noncompliance, it seems that the second imperative should rule. An explicit refusal has not been uttered; indeed, the repeated return of the patient belies any presumption of refusal. Thus, it seems that the physician, no matter how frustrated, retains ethical responsibility for the patient.

Still, how can this responsibility be fulfilled? First, an examination of conscience is indicated: Does the physician rightly understand and appreciate the patient's motives, life setting, and comprehension? Does the physician properly evaluate his or her own skills and strategies? If, after such an examination of conscience (whose items are abundantly found in books and articles on compliance), no answer is found, the next ethical question must be asked: Is it time to shift from a "curing" to a "caring" mode of treatment? Physicians seem to find it difficult to make this shift. They are trained in the use of medicines and have them at hand; they are often quite unskilled in the more subtle "medicine" of support for which there exists no physical armamentarium. Indeed, the ethical physician will often feel guilt that nothing is being done for the patient, although the persistently noncompliant patient may respond better to faithful, supporting care than to diuretics. It should be noted, however, that such care has its own ethical limits. A physician's time and medical resources are limited; others have more tangible needs. It is not unethical, in such circumstances, for physicans to determine that their diagnostic and therapeutic skills can be employed better elsewhere.

Of course, there are more ethical and less ethical ways of terminating the relationship. A serious attempt to wean the patient from dependence, an honest proposal that the patient may be more satisfied with someone else, even an offer to help in finding that someone, are ethically preferable to the abrupt termination.

The sin of abandonment occurs when there is a unilateral termination of responsibility for a patient by a provider of last resort (who can find the time and resources) while there remains any hope of benefit in the relationship itself. Many physicians feel that they are wasting their time in such relationships, but they have chosen to join a profession that advertises itself as offering more than medicine.

Ethical Limits of Compliance Improvement

The second critical problem for the ethics of compliance lies in ways in which compliance behavior is improved. There are two basic patient-directed strategies for improving compliance, education and behavioral modification. These strategies have inner ethical constraints: education should be truthful and behavior modification should be noncoercive. However, it may be felt that the goal of attaining health is so important that it justifies some distortion of truth or some application of coercion, such as fear. Thus, a physician wishing a hypertensive patient to adhere to guanethidine conceals the possibility of impotence; another physician exaggerates the possibility of strokes or promises more than the medication can deliver. It is, of course, no secret that misinformation or fear of punishment can prompt persons to do what they would not otherwise do.

The elements of an answer to this problem are complex. First, as a matter of principle, it should be maintained that the object of information, presented in whatever manner, is insight; and the object of training, however automatized, is freedom. All strategies aimed at improving compliance must provide the patient with insight into his or her own situation and self, as well as with the ability of doing otherwise than conforming when he or she judges it best. Within this principle, however, certain considerations seem reasonable. First, health should not be considered a unique or singular goal. It should be, for patient and physician alike, one element within the overall goal of attaining a human, free, and dignified manner of life. The drive to obtain health should not compromise other valid human goals. Secondly, information can be conveyed in ways that match the needs of time, situation, and "right to know," yet still be truthful within the whole picture. Persons are sometimes not ready to hear a truth and will, if it is forced upon them, refuse, repress, or fail to comprehend. Such a truth, which will not be incorporated into comprehension and decision, is useless. Still, any strategy for unfolding the truth must aim at the ultimate revelation of the whole picture and the ultimate opportunity for the patient to decide for himself or herself. The physician who judges that the truth should be imparted in this way must scrupulously examine personal motives and the reasons for so doing. Similarly, the emotions of fear or shame are not evil in themselves, for attitudes are evil only in their effect upon ultimately free decisions. Indeed (as our pastor will acknowledge), they are emotions which can be salutary. Once again the use of these emotions, which have a long history in the rhetoric of persuasion, must contribute to, rather than overwhelm, free decision. The sin or failure in the ethics of training is *coercion*, the application of physical or psychological pressure to the extent that the patient's own deliberation about his or her situation is impaired. The sin in the ethics of information is the *lie*, the concealment of those facts that will lead a person away from a decision which, even though it may not be "in his interests" as others define it, is a decision which is truly his or her own.

Ethical Constraints on Research

The problem of deception brings us directly to the "crisis" of carrying out research on compliance within ethical constraints. It is obvious that, unless research is done on compliance behavior, important information about the efficacy of therapeutic regimens will be lacking. This will lead to inappropriate prescription and waste of medical resources as well as to waste of patient time and money. It leads ultimately to poor medical care and persistent illness which might otherwise be cured. However, much of the compliance research must employ protocols which are ethically problematic. Studies of compliance apparently must rely on deception in order to obtain the information they seek. Obtaining informed consent about the compliance study would appear to vitiate the study since, once patients know their compliance with the regimen is under investigation, they will comply. Researchers are forced to ask whether it is ethical to withhold information which, if given, would vitiate the study.

Several considerations make up the elements of an answer. First, within the context of any therapeutic regimen under study, any withholding of information which might be suspected to compromise the known therapeutic values of the regimen is clearly unethical. Second, the risks and benefits of compliance-improving strategies should be assessed separately from the risks and benefits of the therapeutic regimen itself, and the information about them provided to the patient in such a way that the patient can make a separate judgment about them. Finally, information about procedures which are harmless or involve only minimal risk need not be provided in specific terms (for example, a randomization between two drugs considered equally effective but given in two forms about which questions may be legitimately asked). However, the general information that a clinical trail involving randomization, will take place should be provided. Any concealing of information should be considered "sinful deception" if it involves withholding substantive matters which one could presume might materially influence the decision of the patient to be treated, or not treated, or to be treated in a certain way.

The Ethics of Physician Responsibility

The last ethical problem is perhaps the most serious, since it touches the qualification of the provider. Questioning the virtue of the preacher is not, in itself, a refutation of the truth of his message; but medical care is not, in this respect, like theology. The deficient provider of medical care causes damage which is palpable (and liable). The virtue requisite in the physician is knowledge, that is, the possession of correct information; skill, the competence to apply the information to particular situations; and (often neglected) the will to educate and motivate patients and to supervise them closely. Three serious sins can be attributed to the physician. The first is carelessness, the blameworthy failure to have the proper information about drugs and procedures, about the patient and the patient's social setting. The careless physician will fail to take reasonable efforts to educate and motivate. The second sin is irrationality, the prescription of medications that are not appropriate for the illness and are thus inefficacious or harmful, either in themselves or insofar as they keep the patient from the more appropriate drug. It would be monstrous for physicians to pride themselves on achieving high compliance to an ineffective or harmful regimen. Third, the authoritarianism to which physicians are often tempted can be a serious sin. Compliance, it seems, is best achieved in a partnership of understanding. The authoritarian physician, giving orders without preparing patients for their acceptance or supporting them in their observance, can undermine compliance. Of course, firmness and, for some patients, benevolent paternalism may be quite effective but, even then, an eventual partnership should be the goal.

It is within this context that I wish to add my comment to the many comments on the suitability of the word *compliance*. The word has often been criticized for being too authoritarian in tone or too condescending (although a review of its meanings in the *Oxford English Dictionary* will reveal many quite fitting ones). When better words are being offered, I would suggest *complacence* which in its etymological origins means being pleased together: both physician and patient are satisfied with their interaction. However, I fear its current connotation of smug self-satisfaction would but compound misunderstanding. I wish to criticize compliance because it suggests the ethical "blooper" of blaming the victim. To refer to the problem as compliance is to pose it as a problem of the behavior of patients and, consequently, to seek its causes in the patient. In so doing, the sins of the careless, irrational, authoritarian physician are visited on the heads of his patients. Those who study and write about compliance know physician behavior is crucial but, by naming their problem after patient behavior, they skew the picture. Perhaps the best text with which we can close this sermon on the ethics of compliance is "physician heal thyself!"

8

Strategies to Improve Compliance with Referrals, Appointments, and Prescribed Medical Regimens

R. Brian Haynes

INTRODUCTION

Preceding chapters have documented the magnitude of noncompliance, described the methods and problems of measuring it, and explored its nature. Although these explorations have uncovered many useful ways in which noncompliance might be avoided or remedied, it is clear that our understanding of the problem remains limited. It is also worth remarking that knowledge of the phenomenon does not necessarily impart solutions, no matter how attractive certain avenues of approach may appear. Conversely (and happily) it should also be noted that improvements in compliance need not await rational analysis, since much of medical and other health care is founded on empirical methods for dealing with poorly understood processes.

Nonetheless, we have also been cautioned that from an ethical perspective we must not proceed without constant concern for the possibly harmful consequences of our attempts to increase compliance, regardless of whether they are based on theoretical or empirical grounds. Negative effects from compliance strategies could arise in two ways. First, increased adherence to a prescribed treatment could result in an increase in dose-related side effects. Second, the strategies, inasmuch as they interfere with an individual's usual method of handling health problems, might themselves cause psychological or social damage. In our own work, for example, we have found that labeling people as hypertensive is associated with a substantial increase in work absenteeism (908), although this effect is least among those who were compliant with treatment. It remains to be seen, however, if improving compliance among those who are not adhering to treatment improves their work activities or other dimensions of their social or emotional function. Surely this should be explored in future compliance investigations. At a minimum we must aspire to improve adherence only with those treatments or actions for which we have reasonable evidence of efficacy, and we must maintain constant vigilance for any harmful results of our interventions, however well intentioned.

With these issues fixed in mind, this chapter and the succeeding ones address strategies for improving poor compliance. The problem will be tackled from many angles. This chapter will synthesize what has already been accomplished in improving compliance with referrals, appointments, and prescribed treatments for people with medically defined illnesses. Subsequent chapters will consider individual strategies in greater detail and will tend to look more to the future than to the past. The focus will then switch to the most difficult problems of all: the addictions of smoking and alcohol abuse. Finally, we will consider the role of the key personnel who carry out compliance interventions and the organization of the health services that facilitate their actions. We will also take a highly practical look at implementing worthwhile strategies in busy clinical settings. Throughout, the authors have attempted to keep their contributions as practical as possible, that is, to show us how we can implement effective strategies for improving compliance in our own clinical or other health care settings, as well as to warn us of strategies which are not yet ready for general use despite their apparent success in the rarefied atmosphere of research.

METHODS OF REVIEW

Except where stated, only studies with clearly defined control groups or control periods of observation are included, and in each instance sufficient data must have been included to permit statistical analysis. In practice this means that the investigators were obliged to provide both the number of individuals studied and the rates of compliance in the groups which were contrasted.

Reports which met these "entry criteria" were analysed in the following way. Methodologic merit was assessed according to the standards outlined in the annotated bibliography (Appendix I), with particular note being made of whether randomization had been used in the evaluation. To permit comparison with strategies studied in other investigations, the impact of a given intervention was assessed simply by subtracting the proportion of compliant individuals in the control group from the proportion in the intervention group. This method has important advantages. First, it can be applied to most studies directly or through interpretation of the data they provide. Second, it provides a simple and immediate measure of absolute effect. For example, if a strategy increases the proportion of compliers from 40% to 75%, that means that for every one hundred patients to whom it is applied thirty-five additional patients will be provided with the opportunity to benefit from their prescribed therapy. Finally, it permits the construction of other indexes such as the percentage of potential improvement that was actually achieved. However, there are some disadvantages to this method as well. First, different studies employed different standards to define a compliant patient, and this can create problems in comparisons. For example, in our own work with hypertensives (228, 449), we defined adequate compliance as the consumption of at least 80% of prescribed medication. There is biological merit in this definition, as it was only at or above this level that compliance correlated with blood pressure reduction. On the other hand, studies by Gordis among children receiving rheumatic fever prophylaxis (673), have shown that only about one-third of the medication usually prescribed need be consumed to begin to demonstrate protection. Thus, a low absolute level of compliance may be partially protective in one regimen but worthless in another. To the extent that the definition of "good" compliance either fails to reflect therapeutic benefit or varies markedly from one regimen to another, the value of the comparisons between investigations will suffer. This problem is mitigated by assessing findings within studies rather than among them, and once again reinforces the appropriateness of insisting on appropriate control groups or control periods in each study.

A second difficulty created by the method of comparison utilized here is that some investigators reported actual compliance rates rather than the proportions of patients judged compliant. This means that the denominator for compliance rates is the number of treatment units prescribed (for example, pills) rather than the number of "compliant" patients. This makes comparisons across studies difficult although, of course, assessment of the strategy within the study is still revealing. The moral of the foregoing discussion is simply that comparisons across studies must be made with considerable caution. The important factors in judging the value of a compliance-improving strategy are whether it worked at all and the extent to which its usefulness has been demonstrated in different settings.

A final point before proceeding with the results of this analysis: all strategies that produced changes in compliance which failed to reach traditional levels of statistical significance have been reported here as if they had no effect. Accordingly, some worthwhile strategies will fail to receive credit because they were tested among too small a group of patients. This danger of the "type II" or β error was judged to be less important than that of the "type I" or α error of according undue credit to a worthless strategy merely because of random fluctuations in compliance between the experimental and control groups compared.

RESULTS OF THE REVIEW

Improving Referral Rates

Referrals can be made either within the medical care system (between various clinicians) or from outside the system, as from a screening program. As D. L. Sackett and J.C. Snow pointed out in Chapter 2, compliance with referral appointments can be distressingly low. Loss of the individual at this initial step is pathetic: the fight against his disease is given up without a single battle.

TABLE 8.1. Interventions to improve referral and appointment keeping

Citation	Clinic	Strategy	Methods rating*	Compliance (%)		Effect on outcome**
				Control	ΔC†	
	Referrals for:					
193	Glaucoma	Patient education	14(r)	76	+13	
241	Adolescent psychiatry	Preintake counseling	12	60	+30	
242	Psychiatry	Preintake counseling	18(r)		+20	+
172	Hypertension	Special referral clerk	13(r)	63	+21	n.s.
520	Hypertension	Letter to patient	9	45	+14	
	Appointments for:					
109	Cardiology	Mailed reminders	9	66	+8	
352	Pediatrics	Mailed reminders	7	69	+14	
461	Pediatrics	Telephone reminders	9(r)	56	+22	
	Pediatrics	Mailed reminders	9(r)	56	+17	

*Methods rating: see bibliography; (r): randomized trial.
†ΔC: change in compliance; percent of patients compliant in control group substracted from percent compliant in intervention group.
**Effect on outcome: + means improvement (P < .05) in intervention group; n.s. means no significant change.

Studies which have evaluated strategies to improve referral appointment keeping are displayed in Table 8.1. Strategies such as patient education (193), preintake counseling (241, 242), special referral clerks to remind patients and help them overcome scheduling and transport difficulties (172), and simple letters to patients (520) have met with substantial success. It would therefore appear that those making referrals have a choice of maneuvers and could use the one which is easiest and most economical to execute in their setting.

In the earlier assessment of the determinants of compliance (Chapter 4) it was documented that the interval between referral and the actual appointment is critical. While the effect of reducing the referral time has not been rigorously assessed, one study (169) did report a substantial improvement in referral appointment keeping when these appointments were scheduled only one or two days in advance rather than one to two weeks. When an appointment cannot be arranged this promptly, a call, letter, or reminder card sent to the patient one to two days in advance of the scheduled appointment will probably suffice.

It is useful to consider for a moment the extreme importance of determining the end result of compliance strategies, no matter where they are applied along the path from disease detection to cure. It profits neither the patient nor the medical care system to detect and link a patient to further assessment or care if the treatment offered is not ultimately accepted. Unfortunately, all too few "compliance studies" investigate what happens to the patients they influence. For example, of the five studies just reviewed, only two determined treatment outcomes. It is obvious to us all that bringing patients into the health care system may not result in health benefits. This is well documented by the study of Fletcher and co-workers (520) who found no difference in the proportion of patients with controlled blood pressures five months following referral, despite a substantial increase in the proportion of paitents successfully linked to a source of care. On the other hand, providing patients referred to psychiatric services with information on what to expect and how to gain the most from therapy did improve both their attendance and their cooperation at therapy sessions (242). It is this type of information that is needed before practical implementation of such procedures.

Improving Appointment Keeping

As was the case for referrals, various types of reminders (see Table 8.1) have been successful in increasing the attendance rates of those already under care. In general, simple post cards are easiest and are the least expensive method. Telephone calls are perhaps slightly more successful if contact can be made, as found by Shepard and Moseley (461), but contact rates in this study were only 75% even after as many as three attempts. This study also provided enough information to permit a crude estimate of the cost of telephone calls and mailed cards. The cost of preventing a single broken appointment was $1.20 when post cards were used and $1.85 when telephone calls were made. On the other hand, the direct cost to the clinic for a broken appointment (including scheduling the appointment, retrieving the records, reviewing the notes, and contacting the patient as necessary) was estimated at $1.12. Thus, preventing appointment breaking is not necessarily profitable. However, the cost figures failed to include physician time wasted or revenue lost from broken appointments, items which would be of importance in many settings.

The appropriateness of reminders obviously depends on the importance of the visit and the likelihood of nonattendance. It can be recommended here that, if the clinic attendance rate is less than 85% (regarded as an optimum by some for routine follow-up care) and if follow-up is important, a postal reminder card, mailed so that is arrives one to two days in advance of the scheduled appointment, is the best method in terms of both cost and convenience.

If the clinic has a chronically low attendance rate, however, findings from the review of determinants in Chapter 4 suggest that clinic reorganization, designed to reduce waiting time and to provide specific as opposed to block appointment times, will be successful; however, these manipulations admittedly lack experimental validation. Whatever the short-term effects of sending appointment reminders, they cannot be expected to result in high compliance with appointment keeping if clinic visits are inconvenient and time consuming for patients.

Finally, the strategies for improving compliance with treatments reviewed below can also be expected to improve attendance.

Improving Adherence to Short-term Treatments

Table 8.2 provides the results of four controlled studies of ways to improve treatment compliance for ten-day courses of antibiotics for various infections. All of the studies reported significant improvements in compliance. Strategies used included verbal and written instruction (106, 460), instructions plus take-home pill calendars (136, 314), various special forms of pill packaging designed to aid memory (314), and intramuscular injections (106). Three other studies, also reporting successful results, are cited in the table. Fink and his co-workers (165, 166) reported that a nurse acting as a "Family Health Management Specialist" greatly improved compliance with short-term pediatric regimens and was as successful at this as a doctor acting in the same role (166). The final study found that pill containers with timed-alarm buzzers improved the accurate consumption of placebos by volunteers (16).

Three of the reports offered internal comparisons of strategies. Colcher and Bass (106) found penicillin in urine samples nine days after the start of therapy in 58% of patients in a control group, in 80% of a group that received instructions emphasizing the need for a full ten-day course, and in 87% of patients given an intramuscular injection. Both of the latter groups were significantly

TABLE 8.2. Interventions to improve compliance with short-term treatments

Citation	Condition	Strategy	Methods rating*	Compliance (%) Control	ΔC†
106	Streptococcal pharyngitis	Instruction by therapist	14(r)	58	+22
		Intramuscular injection	14(r)	58	+29
460	Acute infections	Written instructions	14	63	+22
314	Acute infections	Calendar & instruction	13(r)	28	+9.5
		Unit doses & instruction	13(r)	28	+33.9
		"Strep-Pak"	13(r)	28	+60.5
136	Otitis media	Pharmacy instruction + pill calendar	10	8.5	+41.5
166	Acute pediatric	Special attention —by doctor	9	65	+25
		—by nurse	9	65	+25
165	Acute pediatric	"Family Health Management Specialist"	11(r)	18	+51
16	Volunteers	Special pill containers: self-stop alarm	10	84	+5
		patient-stop alarm	10	84	+13

*Methods rating: see bibliography; (r): randomized trial.
†ΔC: change in compliance (difference in proportion of patients found compliant in intervention group and control group).

more compliant than the control and experienced significant reductions in treatment failures and relapses; the two experimental methods did not differ significantly from each other for either compliance or outcome. Linkewich et al. (314) observed incremental increases in compliance when the following strategies were added to usual dispensing practices: a pill calendar plus instruction; unit-dose strips of pills; and finally, a commercial reminder package of pills (Wyeth QID-Strep-Pak®). All of the intervention groups were significantly more compliant than the control (a condition for the entry of their findings on the table), and the last group had statistically significantly higher compliance than the rest. Azrin and Powell (16) found that an alarm signal that the subject was required to turn off was associated with significantly better compliance than one which turned off automatically after a few seconds.

As for attendance, there are several simple methods of improving short-term treatment compliance. In terms of ease and economy there seems little point in using intramuscular injections, special pill containers (with or without alarm devices), or extended role nurses when equal effectiveness can be attained with simple, direct instructions from the physician or pharmacist, augmented by a brief written statement or calendar. We are indebted to Colcher and Bass (106) for vertifying the improvement in outcome which follows such minimal efforts. My firm recommendation is that, in every institution, the therapists and pharmacists get together to decide who will carry out this task. It would do no harm if both instructed the patient, but, in lieu of accord between the groups, the onus is clearly on the therapist.

Improving Adherence to Long-term Treatment.

The light shed by the above investigations does little to illuminate the dark corner of chronic compliance problems. Instructions and simple reminders at best produce only transient benefit and at worst are a considerable waste of the effort, time, and good intentions of all the health care personnel who are dedicated to the proposition that sweet reason should prevail, that the patient who has been "educated" ipso facto will take on the responsibility for administering his own care. As we shall soon see, this is not the case. Compliance with long-term treatments can be improved in certain circumstances, but the effort required is intensive, often clumsy, and must be maintained as long as compliance is required.

"Patient Education" and Disease Instruction.

Table 8.3 shows the results of six vigorous attempts to educate patients about their disease and its management. The methods included programmed instruction (148, 449), lectures and demonstrations (61, 86, 493), and personal instruction and counseling (229). Although these measures substantially increased patients' knowledge about their conditions, none of them improved either compliance or therapeutic outcomes.

Medication Counseling.

Table 8.3 reports the effect of efforts by pharmacists (101, 107, 419) and nurses (331) to provide patients with clear and unequivocal instructions about their medications, so that there would be no grounds for them to fail to know what was expected of them and how they could accomplish it; in Blackwell's terms (Chapter 9), comprehension was assured. Only one of these studies reported an improvement in compliance. In this investigation (107), one of the authors phoned patients at home about two weeks following hospital discharge and asked them to count their remaining pillls. "Perfect" compliance, which included both the correct amount and the appropriate timing of medication, was reported by 92% of patients who had received a pharmacy consultation just prior to hospital discharge, by 88% of patients who had had a consultation plus a two-day period of in-hospital self-administration of medications, and by only 24% of the control group patients. The authors provided little information about the types of disease or the types or duration of medications involved, though most patients appeared to have chronic medical complaints. The use of a standard of "perfect" compliance and the gathering of compliance information over the telephone give rise for concern about the validity of the results. Taken at face value, however, it appears that compliance was improved by pharmacy consultation over the short term of the study. None of the other three studies found improved compliance in either the short term (101, 331) or longer term (419). The latter study is interesting in that it reveals what an arbitrary standard of "good" compliance can do to results. Rehder and co-workers (419) assigned hypertensive patients to one of four groups: a control group that simply received their medications in regular safety cap pill bottles; a group that received pharmacy counseling about drugs and hypertension; a group that received a special bubble package pill container with four separate slots per day for pills; and a final group which received both counseling and the special pill container. By pill counts, performed on returned containers (only about half the patients returned with their containers), 48% of patients in the control group had taken at least 95% of their prescribed medication, whereas in the other three groups the proportions of compliant patients were 60%, 90%, and 92%, respectively. Thus, the results were statistically significantly better in all three intervention groups, and the last two groups were significantly more compliant than the one which received counseling alone. However, when the measure of compliance was the percentage of pills consumed (rather than the proportion of patients taking at least 95% of prescribed medication), the control group had taken 87% and the others 90%, 95%, and 98%, respectively. Although this trend paralleled the former analysis, the differences were not statistically significant, nor were they

TABLE 8.3. Interventions to improve compliance with long-term treatments

Intervention modality	Citation	Condition	Strategy description	Follow-up	Methods rating	Compliance (%) Control	ΔC†	Δ outcome**
Disease instruction	148	Diabetes	Programmed instruction	3 mo.	9			no
	61	Diabetes	Lectures & demonstrations	6 mo.	13			no
	86	Hypertension	Lectures	8 wk.	9		nil	no
	449	Hypertension	Programmed learning	6 mo.	18(r)		nil	no
	493	Diabetes; hypertension	Lectures	4 visits	13(r)		nil	
	229	Tuberculosis	Instruction & counseling	2 wk.	18		nil	
Medication instruction	107	General medical	Pharmacy discharge consultation	14 d.	8		+68	
	101	General	Pharmacy instructions	2-47 d.	10	24	nil	
	331	Chronic medical	Nurse drug counseling	1 wk.	6		nil	
	419	Hypertension	Pharmacy counseling	3 mo.	12		nil	no
Special pill container	419	Hypertension	"Bubble package" container	3 mo.	12		nil	no
	147	Hypertension	"Compliance-Pak"	1 visit	12(r)		nil	
	300	General	Child-resistant containers	3-23 d.	9		negative	
Free medication	57	Pregnancy	Free iron from clinic	2 mo.	15(r)		nil	
				9 mo	11(r)			relapses+19%

Study	Condition	Intervention	Duration	Methods rating*		ΔC†	Δoutcome**
Extended supervision							
118	Tuberculosis	Isolation order	>6 mo.	7	90	+7	improved
117	Tuberculosis	Outreach clinics & home retrieval	variable	10	74	+21	improved
512	Tuberculosis	Home visits to dropouts	>1 yr.	10	34	+15	improved
521	Hypertension	Home visits by nurse	2 yr.	12	50	+36	improved
348	Hypertension	Monitoring by pharmacist	5 mo.	8	17	+62	improved
201	Well-baby care	Continuous, comprehensive care	1 yr.	9(r)		nil	no charge
Behavior modification							
228	Hypertension	Home b.p. self-monitoring, tailoring treatment to habits, positive reinforcement	6 mo.	18(r)	43	+22	improved
Serum drug monitoring							
324	Epilepsy	DPH levels & feedback	3 mo.	12(r)	30	+38	improved
462	Epilepsy	Ethosuximide levels & feedback	6 mo.	14	76	+14	improved
189	Epilepsy	DPH levels & feedback	30 wk.	12			
145	Asthma	Theophylline levels		11	9	+31	improved
213	Cardiac	Digoxin levels & feedback	16 wk.	12	52	+30	improved
Injections							
273	Schizophrenia	Fluphenazine	2 yr.	7			improved
160	Rheumatic fever	Benzathine penicillin	3 yr.	13(r)	49	+51	improved
159	Rheumatic fever	Benzathine penicillin	4 yr.	12(r)	31	+58	improved

*Methods rating: see bibliography; (r): randomized trial.

†ΔC: change in compliance due to intervention.

**Δoutcome: "improved" means statistically significant benefit in intervention group.

clinically meaningful, since blood pressures were not correlated with these differences in compliance. Thus, this study shows that the selection of cutoff points to separate compliers from noncompliers can result in overenthusiastic conclusions about the benefits of compliance-improving strategies. We are indebted to these authors for providing information both on individual compliance rates and on proportions of patients judged compliant by other criteria. Other investigators would do well to follow their example.

Special Pill Containers.

Three studies which met our review criteria for inclusion examined the compliance effect of various types of pill containers. We have previously discussed the results of Rehder et al. (419): a bubble package pill container was associated with a statistically significant increase in the proportion of hypertensive patients meeting a 95% standard for "good compliance" and effected a small increase in the proportion of pills consumed. No systematic change in blood pressure was observed. In a six-month follow-up period, during which patients were encouraged to fill their own containers, 54% chose to do so; compliance was not assessed during this period. Eshelman and Fitzloff (147) evaluated the effect of a commercial Compliance Pak® on compliance with once-a-day chlorthalidone among patients with hypertension. Compliance was assessed by two methods, thin layer chromatography of urine and pill counts on returned pill containers. Despite telephone calls to remind patients to return their unused pills, follow-up was incomplete for 33%. The two methods of assessing compliance among the remaining patients were in disagreement; the urinary measure found 93% of patients using the "Pak" to be compliant, statistically significantly higher than the 69% compliance rate among controls who used regular containers. The pill count, however, revealed that 63% of the patients in the intervention group were taking 80%-109% of their prescribed medication, versus 61% in the control group. Which result was correct? Unless patients in the intervention group had access to pills other than those contained in their "Paks," or the timing of their pill taking or urinary assessment differed from that of controls, it appears that the pill count is closer to the truth and that the device was not helpful. If the chromatographic method of assessing chlorthalidone used in this study is similar to the one which we attempted to develop for use in our hypertension-compliance investigations, then the interpretation of its results is rendered difficult because of the very long halflife of chlorthalidone and the great individual variability in its metabolism. It is of further interest that when subjects receiving the "Pak" were asked whether it aided memory, opinion was divided equally and was not correlated with either urine or pill scores. In fact, one patient admitted removing all the pills from the "Pak" and putting them into a regular container.

The final evaluation of pill containers (300) was an attempt not to improve compliance but rather to assess the possible negative influence of child-resistant pill containers. Unfortunately, as noted earlier in the discussion of the determinants of compliance (Chapter 4), the effect was indeed negative, with statistically significantly lower compliance among those receiving safety capped containers. Moreover, in many homes the intended purposes of the caps was thwarted by leaving them permanently off the bottles. If the results of this study are replicable, the implications are clear. At the very least, patients' ability to remove these safety caps should be determined by their pharmacists at the point of dispensing, and special arrangments made for those who have difficulty doing so. A second implication is equally important. Studies evaluating special devices to enhance compliance should include a control group which receives nonsafety cap containers.

Barry Blackwell will also discuss pill containers in Chapter 9; for my part, although they appear about as useful as other methods for short-term treatments, I am not impressed with their use for long-term therapy.

Free Medication.

As reviewed in Chapter 4, the cost of treatment is possibly a deterrent to compliance. However, this conclusion lacks rigorous validation and, indeed, two studies which reduced the cost of medication disproved this eminently sensible theory. Bonnar et al. (57) found no difference in the frequency of stools positive for iron when comparing antenatal patients who received free medication with those who received a regular prescription to be paid for out-of-pocket. Even more disturbing, Cody and Robinson (105) found that hospital readmissions increased by 19% among schizophrenic outpatients who received their medications at a nominal cost compared to a randomly allocated control group who had to purchase their medications at usual cost. The savings to the intervention group were substantial, for the monthly price of their prescriptions was reduced from a high of $40 before the study to a flat rate of $1. Compliance was not assessed directly in this study, but relapse is a well-documented consequence of noncompliance in schizophrenia (245, 246) and such an outcome measure is in any event more important than compliance.

The results of the latter investigation seem extraordinary because, at the very least, one would not expect compliance to decrease when medication costs were substantially reduced. Reducing the cost of medication should, therefore, be tested in other settings before abandoning it as a compliance strategy. On the other hand, the option of providing medications free or at a minimal cost will not be available in many settings, particularly at the primary care level, so that even if future studies were to reveal compliance advantages, the potential for applying this strategy would be limited.

Extended Supervision.

The discouraging results of tests of educational methods, special pill containers, and reduced cost of treatment may be contrasted with the success achieved by the strategies discussed in this and succeeding sections. Table 8.3 displays the results of six studies in which extended supervision was the key or major element. It must be stressed that the classification of this strategy is admittedly arbitrary, as it is difficult to isolate the nonspecific effect of supervision from other components in these studies. Extended *supervision* entails increasing the frequency of clinic visits, adding home visits, establishing outreach clinics, adding an extra member to the medical team to monitor achievement of the therapeutic goal, or, ultimately, hospitalizing noncompliant patients. Unfortunately, in all the studies cited here, some additional activity usually transpired during the added supervision, and more often than not this activity could be classified under the rubric "patient education" or "counseling." To those who would argue that these, rather than extended supervision, are the active elements it should be pointed out that the patient education studies we have already reviewed (in which lectures, demonstrations, and teaching programs were tested in isolation) showed no long-term benefits. It is thus my conclusion that, with one exception, the studies of extended supervision reviewed here demonstrated worthwhile effects, regardless of any ancillary activities that took place.

In Curry's study (118) of tuberculous veterans, patients who had been absent without leave on previous or current hospital admissions were served with an isolation order. Violation of this isolation order, which required cooperation with prescribed treatment (including hospitalization) until regular discharge, resulted in an alternative of up to six months in jail or two years probation. "A.W.O.L." rates diminished from 10.4% of all admissions to 3.2%, and patients were noted to be much more cooperative when jail was the alternative. Legal sanctions such as this are drastic measures which only society can place in the hands of physicians. Their existence is a matter which is best left to law courts and lawmakers, who have properly decided that their use be limited to those diseases which pose an immediate and substantial risk to others as well as to the victims themselves. Thus, measures designed to improve compliance but that also restrict the patient's freedom of choice or activity are not advocated here. On the other hand, a period of voluntary hospitalization with supervised administration of medication can be very helpful in distinguishing problems of therapeutic efficacy from those of compliance. Such strategies are especially useful for the many conditions such as hypertension for which direct measures of compliance are generally unavailable. If compliance is established as the problem, then successful treatment in hospital at least permits less intensively supervised programs to start off on a firm footing.

A good example of an ambulatory program with extended supervision is reported in a second study by Curry (117) in which a major clinic for the treatment of tuberculosis was decentralized to provide services in communities with a high prevalence of the disease. These outreach clinics were staffed with "patient-oriented district teams" which included a public health nurse who telephoned or visited patients who had missed appointments. The percentage of broken appointments decreased from 26% to 5% with the introduction of these clinics and to 4% with the further implementation of home visits by nurses. In another study of tuberculous outpatients, Watts (512) reported that simple bookkeeping procedures which kept track of those who broke appointments and the use of two home visitors to retrieve dropouts resulted in a substantial improvement in follow-up at the Mulago Hospital in Uganda. Both this study and Curry's first study also examined treatment outcomes and demonstrated statistically signficant improvements with implementation of their programs.

Multifaceted strategies were employed in two studies which attempted to improve compliance in hypertension. Wilber and Barrow (521) sent a public health nurse to visit 88 hypertensive patients, instruct them in the nature and care of high blood pressure, check their blood pressure, and emphasize the importance of taking medication regularly. The compliance levels and blood pressure readings of this group were then compared with those of a group of patients who had not accepted home visits; the proportions of patients under treatment and whose blood pressure was under good control before intervention were comparable in the two groups. However, only 50% of the nonvolunteer group were found to be on treatment at the end of a two-year follow-up period, and only 34% had achieved good blood pressure control, whereas in the volunteer group 86% were taking treatment and 80% were under good control. James McKenney, who elaborates on the role of pharmacists in compliance in Chapter 16, also has studied compliance among hypertensive outpatients. He and his co-workers (348) found that regular blood pressure monitoring, coupled with patient teaching and drug manipulation by a pharmacist (working in cooperation with treating physicians at a multispecialty neighborhood health center), resulted in substantial improvements in both compliance and blood pressure control during the intervention period. Both of these studies provided additional information which supports the theory that it is the increased supervision component which is the operative factor in the compliance improvements they observed. Postintervention follow-ups (of two years in the former study and six months in the latter) revealed a substantial fall back toward baseline compliance and concomitant rises in blood pressure in the intervention groups.

The final study in this group (201) reported on an experiment that provided increasing continuity and comprehensiveness of care to infants of primiparous adolescents in a low class neighborhood. The strategy for well-baby care included an educational program as well as public health nurse home visits when patients missed appointments. No improvement in compliance was observed for immunization or vaccination schedules (save for polio vaccine) or with well-baby visits, and there were no differences in morbidity and mortality over the year of observation. The strategy in this study seems to fit as well as any in the concept of increased supervision which has been illustrated here. The negative results obtained should thus serve as a warning that increased supervision will not work in all settings.

One of the important points that arises from the studies of the role of supervision is that the more specific the supervision the more effective and efficient the procedure. Thus, when attention can be directed specifically—through monitoring a biologic endpoint such as blood pressure that is closely related to compliance or, better still, through monitoring the consumption of the treatment, either by assessing drug levels in body fluids or by administering the treatment directly using parenteral formulations—the effect on compliance can be dramatic.

Behavior Modification.

Many of the most effective strategies for improving compliance informally use behavior modification principles. For example, verbal encouragement by the therapist is one of the more potent "reinforcers" that can be applied to ambulatory patients. In our own work (228), which will be described in more detail shortly, a formal behavior modification program was applied to noncompliant hypertensives. It included self-monitoring of both blood pressure and pill consumption by patients at home, coupled with tailoring medication taking to daily events of a reinforcing nature, plus providing monetary incentives and other forms of positive reinforcement for improved compliance and blood pressure control. The result was a 21% improvement in average compliance among members of the intervention group compared to a 1% fall in compliance among controls. Such programs may not be practical in routine clinical settings, but they do show that these principles can be applied successfully.

Serum Drug Monitoring.

Table 8.3 contains the results of five studies in which serum drug levels were monitored. Applied to the diphenylhydantoin (189, 324) or ethosuximide (462) treatment of epilepsy, theophylline treatment of asthma (145), and digoxin treatment of cardiac disorders (213), the results were uniformly encouraging. Two of the studies evaluated treatment outcome (189, 462), and both reported improvements.

Laboratory facilities are currently available in most centers for diphenylhydantoin and digoxin determinations and they should be used routinely for compliance monitoring.* Theophylline measurements are not generally available.

---

*Attention must be given to the timing of drawing specimens for these and other drugs in view of the profound differences in blood levels that occur as a function of time elapsed since the last dose.

There seems little reason why the same principle cannot be applied to any drug which gives steady state serum levels. However, the same results may not apply to many other drugs which have variable absorption or metabolism or which disappear rapidly from the bloodstream. It may also be true that qualitative tests, as opposed to the quantitative tests which were used in these studies, will not produce the same benefits. The theophylline study showed that the same results could be achieved using salivary levels, and there seems no inherent reason why determination in other body fluids such as urine and sweat could not be used in the same way. The ideal, from the practitioner's point of view, would be simple dip stick tests of saliva or urine to provide semiquantitative on-the-spot information to guide treatment and compliance decisions. We are a long way from achieving this for most drugs, but unless or until such a goal is realized, the routine monitoring and management of compliance problems in usual clinical settings will likely remain impractical or difficult. Table 11 in the annoted bibliography lists methods of drug level assessment tested or suggested for compliance studies.

Parenteral Administration of Treatment by Medical Staff.

When a drug has a suitable parenteral formulation which is long acting, supervised administration becomes feasible and compliance problems can be circumvented. Three studies illustrate the substantial advantages in compliance and treatment outcome which thereby accrue. In a two-year "mirror image" study of schizophrenics who were switched from oral phenothiazines to intramuscular fluphenazine, Johnson and Freeman (273) found a 26% reduction in the number of hospital admissions and a 52% reduction in the number of hospital days following the switch. In two studies of rheumatic fever prophylaxis (159, 160) groups of children receiving benzathine penicillin injections once a month had statistically significantly fewer relapses than control patients on oral medications.

Although parenteral forms are available for most drugs, their durations of action are so short that supervised administration becomes impractical on a routine basis. This lack of availability may be due more to pharmacologic prophesies of doom based on adverse reactions and on consequent drug manufacturer policy decisions than to technical problems, however (661). The benefits found in the studies just cited compel a reexamination of these issues with clinical pharmacologists and, in view of the benefits, an exploration of the extent to which concerns about toxicity may be overstated. At present, it appears that long-acting agents are routinely rejected by drug manufacturers as being commercially unattractive because of these frequently undocumented fears (661).

Coincidentally, and in keeping with previous comments on supervision, the favorable results with injected medications are more likely attributable to supervised administration than to the parenteral formulation itself. Compliance with self-injected insulin has been found appallingly low (511), whereas supervised oral medication consumption, such as occurs in hospitals and among day patients (223), results in substantially increased compliance. Thus, long-acting parenteral formulations may make supervised administration logistically feasible, obviating confinement of the patient to continuous institutional care or the need for daily clinic visits. Accordingly, there is no reason why equivalent results could not be attained with long-acting oral agents. In addition, although no properly controlled studies have been reviewed on this subject, reports on the continuance of contraception have shown improved results with intrauterine devices when compared with oral contraceptives and other forms of contraception (23, 436, 463, 469, 489). The IUD may be considered as a form of parenteral treatment. Its use also illustrates the ultimate in long-acting reversible treatments and demonstrates that if the duration of action of a treatment is longer than the usual period between clinic visits, the need for supervision can actually be diminished.

Application to Hypertension: A Model
for Compliance Problems in Chronic Disease Therapy.

Hypertension has been touted as the model disease for the study and solution of the problems of chronic medical therapy. It is highly prevalent, causes awesome morbidity and mortality, and has efficacious treatments although these treatments must be continued for the duration of the victim's life and, as we know, are all too often neglected by the victim. Actually, the preemptive claims of those interested in hypertension that it is *the* model for chronic treatment management problems are perhaps somewhat pretentious as there are other diseases which would serve (and have served) equally well, among them the psychoses and tuberculosis, not to mention smoking and alcoholism. Nevertheless, it serves well as a model and it seems opportune at the end of this review of tested strategies to illustrate many of the points made by considering, as a group, the available compliance studies for this one condition. This will also provide an opportunity for me to describe our own trial of compliance-improving strategies of which I can provide a firsthand account, thus switching from reviewer to reporter. This will be a somewhat more comfortable though perhaps less impartial role.

Table 8.3 provides the results of a number of unsuccessful attempts to improve the compliance of hypertensive patients. Since we have already discussed all of these studies I will be brief in summarizing them. Methods which utilized information exchange about the disease and its treatment as their main approach (86, 419, 449) were uniformly unsuccessful. Failures were noted for teaching patients to monitor their own blood pressure at home with clinic checks of the results (88) and for providing increased convenience of care at the work site (449). A special referral clerk (172) was able to improve the referral rate substantially, but the result five months later was no increase in the proportion of patients taking medication or achieving blood pressure control. Special pill containers also failed to improve compliance or blood pressure (147, 419). These studies include maneuvers in all of the strategy categories (except reduced cost of medication) that were found to be unsuccessful in our earlier review of chronic diseases.

In our own work (449), 5,400 male employees of a local steel mill were screened for untreated hypertension. Two hundred forty-five men met our criteria of sustained blood pressure elevation over three screening sessions, no therapy for at least the last six months, absence of surgically treatable secondary hypertension, and no daily medications. Two hundred thirty men (94%) agreed to participate in the study. For the initial six months, participants were randomly allocated to receive treatment either in the community (on their own time, from their regular family physicians) or at the plant (on company time, with full pay, and with treatment provided by the full-time plant physicians). The latter condition was termed "augmented convenience." A random half of each group also received an educational package in the form of a specially prepared slide-and tape show and take-home booklet with programed learning stops. An assistant helped those who received the program until they exhibited mastery of the material (defined as a score of at least 80% on a posttest). Periodic checks to assess retention of information were made. The material dealt with the nature and dangers of hypertension as well as the means and benefits of therapy. It spent a substantial amount of time teaching patients how to tailor their treatment to their daily routine to make remembering to take medication easier.

The results of the first intervention and treatment at the work site were as follows: Industrial physicians began 76% of patients on treatment whereas community physicians started only 49%. This result is hardly astonishing, since the industrial physicians had actually solicited the program because of their concern about untreated hypertension. At the end of six months, however, there were no statistically signficiant differences in treatment compliance or blood pressures between the two groups. This result was unexpected, particularly considering the larger proportion of patients on treatment at the work site. We do not have a verifiable reason for the lack of success. A partial explanation may be that although the group at the plant perhaps had increased access to care, this in no way led to increased convenience in adhering to the treatment, for the regimens prescribed by both industrial and community physicians were equivalent in numbers of drugs and frequency of administration.

Turning now to the effect of instruction, at the end of six months the intervention group displayed substantially greater knowledge about hypertension and its treatment with 85% exhibiting "mastery" of the material as opposed to 18% in the comparison group (P < .01). However, compliance rates and blood pressures were not significantly different for the two groups. We had anticipated this result and thus were not surprised by it. However, we had thought the teaching of specific ways in which to improve memory in pill taking might have some detectable impact. That it did not reinforces the conclusion that information exchange methods for patients do not alter compliance even if they are highly successful in transmitting relevant information, at least in situations in which treatment regimens are relatively simple to follow.

Turning to successful attempts, Table 8.3 provides the results of four worthwhile interventions. We have discussed all these but one. The studies of McKenney et al. (348) and Wilber and Barrow (521) utilized mixed strategies which included the active ingredient which has been labeled extended supervision including, in this case, monitoring of a biological endpoint closely related to compliance.

In a unique investigation which has not been citied in the review up to this point, Inui et al. (264) provided tutorials on hypertension, its therapy, and its relation to patient compliance for a group of interns, residents, and attending staff at a general medical clinic. The physicians were told to apply to hypertension the Health Belief Model which Marshall Becker and others have described in chapter 6. They were advised that, based on previous findings at the clinic, if patients had a diastolic blood pressure over 100 mm Hg, the probability of noncompliance was 90% and if the patient had a past history of hospitalization the probability of noncompliance was 96%. Physicians in a control group were merely told that some of their patients were to be observed. Compliance was assessed by pill count on two home visits to each patient at intervals separated by 60 days. Physicians in the experimental group found 61% of their patients to be taking over 75% of their prescribed medication, compared with only 32% of the patients in the control group. Blood pressures were controlled (diastolic pressure less than 100 mm Hg) in 69% of the intervention group's patients, compared with 36% of the control group's patients. Furthermore, blood pressure differences were found to be sustained some six months after the tutorials had been given. It should be noted that compliance with diet and appointments was not influenced. If the results of this study are replicable, then the implications for medical student and physician postgraduate education are clear.

The last study in this section is the second phase of our own investigation (228). As was outlined, hypertensive men assigned to treatment at work or in the community and allocated to receive or not receive an educational program were assessed six months after referral for treatment; these groups were found not to differ in compliance rates or blood pressure response. The six-month results were used to select all those patients who met the dual criteria of compliance rate less than 80% and diastolic blood pressure over 90 mm Hg. The 39 men who met these standards were randomly allocated either to continue with their usual care or to a behavior modification group. The latter group also continued to receive therapeutic management from their usual physicians. In addition they were taught to take and record their own blood pressure and pill consumption, their prescribed regimens were tailored in timing to their own particular daily routine and habits, and their blood pressure was checked about every two weeks. Blood pressure and compliance improvements were rewarded with praise and the award of $4.00 credit toward the purchase of their blood pressure cuff and stethoscope (no money actually changed hands). The program was carried out entirely by a high school graduate with no formal health care or psychology training. Compliance rates rose 21% in the intervention group and fell 1% in the control group based on an assessment by pill count at a home visit six months after the beginning of the program. Diastolic blood pressure dropped significantly in the intervention group although the magnitude of the drop was small (5.6 mm Hg) and was not significantly different from the 1.3 mm Hg drop in the control group. This aspect of the program was somewhat frustrating in that we felt it would be inappropriate for the program assistant to contact physicians to tell them to increase treatment when it appeared that the blood pressure goal of 90 mm Hg diastolic had not been reached despite the achievement of adequate compliance. Nevertheless, it remains to be tested whether tying changes in dosing and types of medication into such a compliance service will improve therapeutic response. It should be noted that individual components of this program have not been successful when tested in isolation in other studies. Thus, Carnahan and Nugent (88) found no benefit in home self-monitoring of blood pressure and Arnold Johnson and co-workers at McMaster University have found no benefit of this maneuver or of monthly blood pressure monitoring by home visitors (unpublished data).

No one has attempted to monitor drug levels in serum or urine among hypertensives, although laboratory methods for measuring propranolol (68), thiazides (319), alpha-methyldopa (319, 556, 630), and chlorthalidone (147) have been described or utilized for measuring compliance in descriptive studies. No acceptable long-acting hypotensive agents are currently available so that the strategy of supervised administration is not practical for hypertension at present.

CONCLUSIONS

The results of the studies reviewed here can be distilled into a small, select group of worthwhile compliance-improving strategies (Table 8.4).

When the problem is one of the referral of an individual from the community (as the result of screening) or referral of a patient from one service to another within the system, several methods will improve the rate of successful referral, among them letters to the patient, a referral clerk to remind and assist patients,

TABLE 8.4. Successful compliance-improving strategies

Compliance problem	Strategy
Referrals	Letter to patient Referral clerk Patient instruction (Short referral time)
Appointments	Mailed reminders Telephone reminders (Efficient clinic scheduling)
Acute medical regimens	Explicit verbal & written instruction Parenteral treatment Special pill packaging Pill calendars Extended-role nursing
Chronic medical regimens	Monitored drug levels Parenteral medications Increased supervision Behavior modification Physician instruction

and teaching the patient the reasons for and implications of referral and how best to benefit from treatment. Although not tested formally, it appears that reducing the referral time to one or two days or timing the reminders to arrive one or two days before the referral appointment will maximize success.

To improve attendance at scheduled appointments, mail and telephone reminders have produced at least short-term improvement; the former strategy is less expensive. In the long run, poor attendance may result from long waiting times at the clinic; although formal experimental validation is lacking, it appears that streamlining the clinic procedures would improve appointment keeping.

For short-term medical regimens, high compliance can be achieved by providing explicit verbal and written instructions with the medication. Alternatives (more complicated or less available but at least as effective) include parenteral treatment, special pill packages and calendars to inform and to remind patients, and extended-role nurses to supervise care and instruct patients.

Compliance with long-term medical regimens is more difficult to achieve, but improvements can be attained by a variety of methods. Depending on the clinical situation and therapy, the most efficient and effective of these are the monitoring of drug levels and the use of parenteral long-acting medications. A nonspecific and expensive way to improve compliance is to increase supervision, such as by increasing the frequency of appointments, providing home visits, or, if all else fails and the disorder warrants, hospitalizing the patient for a brief period. Formal behavior modification programs are not generally available, but their principles can and should be applied in routine clinical care. For example, by setting explicit goals for patients to achieve and rewarding each improvement by encouragement and praise, compliance can be substantially improved. In addition, tailoring the treatment to the patient's daily behaviors may also help to cue compliance. Finally, instructing therapists in the nature of the compliance problem and providing them with simple strategies for the detection and improvement of compliance may permit them to deal with the problem in their usual clinical settings, obviating the need for a compliance expert—yet another member of the already crowded medical care team.

RESEARCH PRIORITIES

Improving compliance with long-term disease regimens is not yet a simple matter. The need for immediate, direct measures of compliance is apparent. Since this information can be used to improve as well as monitor compliance, development, dissemination, and utilization of such methods should be pursued with vigor. The success achieved by parenteral treatments suggests that pharmacologists and drug manufacturers should be strongly encouraged to develop and test more of these formulations. In lieu of these, increased supervision with attention focused clearly on the achievement of the treatment goal seems a viable, though expensive, way to improve compliance. Tactics for maximizing the efficiency of this strategy should be explored. Finally, the effectiveness of teaching clinical personnel to recognize and manage compliance problems should be verified in several settings and for several conditions. If these teaching sessions prove successful, they should become an integral part of the curricula for training health professionals.

9

The Drug Regimen
and Treatment Compliance

Barry Blackwell

INTRODUCTION

The first annotated bibliography on patient compliance by Haynes and Sackett (693) reviewed some 200 variables reported in 246 papers. Table 9.1 shows a crude compilation from these data of the factors that affect compliance (614). The factor found most commonly to interfere with compliance was the complexity of the regimen.

Since this original observation, there have been a number of conceptual developments that concern this as part of compliance, including:

1. A clearer separation of the term *complexity* into two major components: the influence of frequency of dose and the effect of number of drugs prescribed daily (692).
2. An attempt to estimate the impact of each of these components on both comprehension (understanding the regimen) and various aspects of compliance (following the regimen).
3. Efforts to relate metabolic and pharmacologic considerations to simplification of drug regimens.

This paper will review the above factors with regard to the present state of knowledge, practical applications, and priorities for future research.

PRESENT STATE OF KNOWLEDGE

The various studies that concern the effect of multiple drugs are shown in Table 9.2, and those that deal with frequent dosing are listed in Table 9.3.

The quality of research represented in these papers is variable, extending from informally reported studies (909) to quite sophisticated recent research (258, 395). In particular, only a few studies have separated the effects of multiple medication from those of frequent dosage; the two factors are not independent variables since increasing the number of pills may also increase the number of

144

TABLE 9.1. Factors that affect adherence

Factors that increase adherence		Factors that decrease adherence	
Factor	Number of studies in favor	Factor	Number of studies in favor
Patient views disease as serious	7	Complexity of regimen	12
Family stability	7	Behavior change required of patient	4
Compliance with other aspects	5	Clinic waiting time	4
Patient satisfaction	1	Block versus individual booking	2
Close supervision by physician	4	Therapy painful	2
Private practice versus clinic	2	Psychological problems	2
Patient expectations met	2	Low frustration tolerance	2
Physician accepts patient	2	Nervous symptoms	2
Mother agrees with physician	2	Working mothers	2
Degree of disability	2		

SOURCE: From Blackwell 1976 (614).

occasions on which pills are to be taken. Some general conclusions that emerge from these combined data are shown in Table 9.4. For the purpose of the following discussion, a *dose* will be considered a single tablet, capsule, or equivalent of a given medication. This is distinguished from the *frequency of dosing*, which refers to the number of occasions each day on which the patient must take medication.

Frequency of Dose

Despite the recent emphasis on "once daily" regimens, there is no clear consensus linking frequent dosage with low compliance. The often cited study by Clinite and Kabat (102) involved only 30 patients, lacked statistical evaluation, and indicated that compliance was not consistently reduced until eight or more doses were prescribed daily. Porter's study in family practice (405) showed that dosage frequency was the second of nine factors in a regression analysis of items contributing to noncompliance with long-term treatment, but the 21% contribution was not statistically significant. The figures given by Ayd (909) are more impressive but consist of summary statements from unpublished data. He stated that 30% of patients on twice daily regimens failed to take over a quarter of their medication, compared with 70% who failed to do so on four times daily regimens. Table 9.5 shows the only published data that clearly support the belief that compliance is reduced by multiple daily dosage. The study

TABLE 9.2. Effect of multiple drugs in compliance

| | | | Effect of multiple drugs on | |
			Compliance	Comprehension
Reference	*Population*	*Drugs*	*Compliance*	*Comprehension*
Weintraub et al. (513)	Cardiovascular outpatients	Digitoxin & diuretics	Decreased if on ⩾ 2 drugs	Not related
Schwartz et al. (455)	Geriatric outpatients	Miscellaneous	Not distinguished* 2-3 decreased 4-9 no change	
Neely & Patrick (376)	Geriatric outpatients	Miscellaneous	Decreased if on ⩾ 3 drugs	Not studied
Malahy (331)	Medical outpatients	Miscellaneous	Decreased	Not related: level of education, labeling & instructions had no impact
Latiolais & Berry (302)	Specialty outpatient clinics	Miscellaneous	Decreased	Decreased
Clinite & Kabat (102)	V.A. outpatients	Miscellaneous	Decreased if on ⩾ 4 drugs	All patients were counseled before
Francis et al. (174)	Pediatrics	Miscellaneous	Decreased if on ⩾ 3 drugs	Not studied
Ayd (909)	Psychiatric & medical outpatients	Miscellaneous	Decreased if on ⩾ 3 drugs	Not studied
Curtis (120)	Home visits for chronic care	Miscellaneous	Decreased if on ⩾ 3 drugs	
Parkin et al. (395)	Medical outpatients	Miscellaneous	Decreased if on ⩾ 3 drugs	Decreased
Hulka et al. (258)	Diabetic & hypertensive outpatients	Miscellaneous	Decreased	Not affected

*See text.

TABLE 9.3. Effect of multiple dosage in compliance

			Effect of multiple dosage on	
Reference	Population	Drugs	Compliance	Comprehension
Clinite & Kabat (102)	V.A. outpatients	Miscellaneous	Decreased if on > 8 doses daily	
Parkin et al. (395)	Medical outpatients	Miscellaneous	No relationship	Not studied
Gatley (185)	Family practice outpatients	Miscellaneous	Decreased if on > 4 doses daily	Not studied
Hulka et al. (258)	Hypertensive and diabetic outpatients	Miscellaneous	Not changed	Not studied
Ayd (909)	Medical and psychiatric outpatients	Miscellaneous	Decreased if on > 2 doses daily	Increased errors
Porter (405)	Family practice outpatients	Miscellaneous	Not changed (nonsignificant trend)	Not studied

TABLE 9.4. Summary of reports on effects of multiple drugs and dosage on compliance*

	Negative	Doubtful	Positive
Multiple Drugs	10	1	0
Multiple Dosage	2	2	2

*The digits in the table are simple counts of the number of research reports reaching a given conclusion (e.g., 10 reports found that multiple drugs had a negative influence on compliance).

was conducted by a family practitioner in England (185); there are no supporting statistics, but the figures suggest that compliance is not substantially reduced until the dosing frequency increases to four times or more daily.

Number of Drugs Prescribed

As indicated in Table 9.4, the evidence suggesting that multiple drugs reduce compliance is quite consistent, with ten out of eleven studies indicating that this factor has an adverse influence on compliance. The quality of the studies listed in Table 9.2 is again variable, but is certainly more sophisticated than that directed towards frequency of dosage. A repeated finding in six of these studies was that compliance falls off sharply when the number of different medications reaches three or more daily. An isolated exception is the finding of Schwartz et al. (455) that for geriatric outpatients large numbers of medications (four or more) did not seem to add significantly to the base rate of poor compliance. Their explanation for this result was that patients for whom large numbers of medications were prescribed received special attention for their drug regimens, thus making the regimen truly a "way of life" and reducing the possibility of error.

Comprehension or Compliance?

There is an important artifact in the study of Schwartz et al. (455) that highlights the significance of more recent attempts to distinguish between the influence of complexity on comprehension and other aspects of compliance. These investigators collected information on several types of errors including omission, self-medication, incorrect dosage, improper timing, and inaccurate knowledge. In calculating the effect of the number of medications, these factors were combined into a composite error rate so that the highest rate of "noncompliance" occurred in those patients prescribed no medications at all! Inaccurate knowledge about drugs, the second most common source of error, accounted for 20% of all errors and occurred with 41% of the patients making errors. Table 9.2 indicates the quite variable attention paid to comprehension in studies of the effect of multiple drugs on compliance; a majority failed to make any distinction

TABLE 9.5. Effect of multiple dosage on compliance

	Number of daily doses				
	1 OD	1 BID	1 TID	1 QID	2 QID
Percentage compliance	67	50	44	22	25
Number of patients	3	6	32	37	8

SOURCE: From Gatley 1968 (185).

between comprehension (understanding the regimen) and compliance (following the regimen).

The study by Latiolais and Berry (302) illustrated that the degrees of comprehension and of compliance are related. They found that patients using medication correctly knew the names of their drugs and had been counseled by physicians significantly more often than those who made errors. Two other studies reported that compliance with multiple drugs was diminished even after written and verbal instructions were given at the time of prescription (102, 331).

Two recent studies reveal the difficulty involved in attempting to relate multiple prescribing to patient compliance. Hulka and her co-workers (258) utilized the novel methodology of matching physicians and patients in pairs, then studying the concordance between physician intention and patient behavior. Five separate components that contributed to a lack of concordance were defined and dealt with separately in relation to 357 patients treated by 46 physicians.

There was a distinct and statistically significant correlaton between the number of drugs prescribed by the physician and the failure to take them. In attempting to define this further, the authors distinguished between scheduling misconception (or noncomprehension) and scheduling noncompliance. Neither of these factors alone was statistically significantly related to the number of drugs taken. This apparent incongruity with the finding that total omission was related to the number of drugs was explained by the fact that comprehension and compliance were separated only for discrepancies between dosage and frequency of ingestion, but not for total pill taking behavior.

This separation of comprehension and compliance has been achieved best by Parkin et al. (395). One hundred thirty patients with acute medical conditions were followed after discharge from hospital. Forty-six (35%) did not understand their regimens. Of the remaining 84 patients, 20 (15% of the total) did not follow the instructions. Thus, in this investigation noncomprehension was a more powerful factor than noncompliance.

Table 9.6 illustrates how these factors interact with both the number of drugs prescribed and the frequency of dosing. It can be seen that the frequency of daily dosage had a relatively weak impact on comprehension, since the percentage of errors only increased when four or more daily doses were prescribed,

TABLE 9.6. Effects of multiple drugs and dosage on comprehension and compliance

| | | Percentage of errors | |
		Comprehension	Compliance
Daily drugs	1	7	7
	2	8	16
	3	19	44
	4	43	30
	P	.001	.025
Daily dosage	1	8	No relationship
	2	7	No relationship
	3	9	No relationship
	4	26	No relationship
	P	.025	N.S.

SOURCE: Adapted from Parkin et al. 1976 (395).

and dose frequency had no effect at all on errors due to compliance. In contrast, the number of drugs taken daily had a significant effect on errors due to both poor comprehension and poor compliance; the error rate clearly rose when three or more drugs were prescribed together. The finding that these two separate factors in the regimen may have different effects on comprehension and compliance has important practical implications that will be discussed later.

Metabolic and Pharmacologic Considerations

Metabolic and pharmacologic considerations have different significance with regard to the separate issues of frequency of dosing and multiple medications.

Frequency of Dose.

Historically, the most hallowed feature of drug administration is that it should take place frequently, every day at fixed intervals. The reasons behind this routine are obscure; there is no evidence to suggest that the ancient materia medica have shorter halflives than their modern synthetic substitutes. One explanation for frequent dosing may be that Galencial preparations were often pharmacologically inert and relied for their effect on the reminder that taking a pill provided of the reassuring presence of the prescriber. Nostrums do have dose-response and duration-of-effect curves; for example, the placebos used in analgesic research have a peak pain-reducing action that occurs one to three hours after administration.

Modern pharmacokinetic studies have revealed that dosage regimens can be estimated from information about drug metabolism. A basic assumption of these calculations is that drugs should be given as often as is necessary to ensure that a steady plasma level is obtained but that accumulation in the body does not occur. Achievement of this criterion depends on rates of absorption, metabolism, tissue storage, and excretion. Based on these factors, the dosing interval can be calculated by the product of a mathematical constant (1.443) and the known halflife of elimination of the drug. In practical terms, this means that any drug with a halflife over seventeen hours need be administered only once every twenty-four hours.

Many drugs—including major tranquilizers, antidepressants, antiparkinsonian agents, methadone, and antiepileptic drugs—once customarily given in divided doses are known to have halflives in this order and are now given once daily. Ayd (910) has carefully reviewed the many well controlled studies on central nervous system drugs that have demonstrated the efficacy and safety of once-daily regimens.

However, it is now becoming apparent that even quite rapidly metabolized drugs may be given less frequently and that it may be a mistake to equate therapeutic action with plasma levels. For instance, all six subjects given single doses of a ^{14}C labeled major tranquilizer showed very similar patterns of metabolism, including a halflife of nineteen hours; however, their physiological responses differed widely, and the degree and duration of sedation and changes in blood pressure varied considerably in relation to blood levels (sedation was much more closely correlated to blood level than was hypotension) (920).

This lack of an exact relationship between drug metabolism and therapeutic action is not surprising in light of the many factors that can influence the effects of drugs, including binding to receptors, storage in body tissues, and the influence of extraneous environmental factors in precipitating symptoms.

Two recent studies in the management of hypertension have given practical demonstrations of the possibility of less frequent dose schedules even for drugs with short plasma halflives. For instance, methyldopa has a plasma halflife of only one and one-half hours but the duration of its blood pressure lowering effect occurs from between four and twenty-four hours after dosing. Indeed, carefully controlled comparison of a once-daily bedtime methyldopa regimen with a three times daily schedule showed that both produced the same degree of blood pressure control, with the possibility of somewhat fewer side effects with the once-daily schedule (921). Similar conclusions were obtained in the study comparing the antihypertensive effects of the beta-blocking drug oxprenolol when given twice or three to four times daily (916). This drug has a serum halflife of only four hours, but it is apparently stored in body tissues and only slowly released back into the bloodstream. The implication of these findings is obvious: we can reduce the frequency of dosing for many medications without sacrificing their therapeutic activity. Unfortunately, as discussed earlier, the influence of this reduced dosing frequency on compliance is not at all apparent at present.

Multiple Drugs.

The fact that multiple drug use is related to poor compliance must be coupled with the observation that physicians very frequently prescribe more than one drug at the same time. Our recent survey of psychotropic drug use in five separate hospitals in the same city revealed that half the patients were receiving at least two drugs simultaneously (919). Indeed, many psychiatric patients are concurrently taking six or more drugs daily (909). The studies by Hulka et al. (258) found that patients with diabetes were taking up to twelve medications concurrently (mean 2.9), and those with congestive heart failure up to fourteen (mean 4.7).

The pharmacologic and metabolic arguments against polypharmacy are numerous, and consist of many practical demonstrations of the way in which one drug may alter the activity of another through inducing, blocking, or satiating enzyme systems, or by modifying the absorption or excretion of the other.

Appeals to the medical profession for rational prescribing practices produce remarkably little impact, and the attitudes that must underlie multiple prescribing are very poorly understood. The practice of "adding on" rather than substituting drugs or manipulating dosage may be deeply rooted in concerns such as avoiding the admission of failure to the patient or avoiding the criticism of another professional by discontinuing the treatment he had prescribed.

There are obviously times when more than one drug is necessary for effective treatment, and in such instances the use of a combination product might appear a logical compromise to improve compliance. Unfortunately, many of the existing combination products consist of illogical and ineffective ingredients. Because anxiety and pain are almost inevitable accompaniments of disease, many combinations are mixtures of analgesics or sedatives with more potent agents. The extent to which such combinations are used is surprising; over 300 million prescriptions are written each year in the USA for combination products, accounting for 20% of all drugs prescribed.

In 1971, the American Food and Drug Administration introduced legislation that required pharmaceutical manufacturers to prove the efficacy of all fixed combination prescription drugs marketed before 1962, and to show how each ingredient contributed to the claimed effects. This requirement has stimulated a spate of research, but few of the results have been positive in either a scientific or commercial sense. The only products to meet the requirements were the diuretic-reserpine combinations used in hypertension (914). At the same time, the legal and legislative delays in fully implementing these regulations account for the fact that a third of the 200 drugs most widely used five years after this legislation are combination products whose efficacy has yet to be proven.

The large commercial interest plus the scientific difficulties involved in demonstrating efficacy have led to the emergence of patient convenience and compliance as major arguments used to bolster the case for combination products.

Unfortunately, none of the newer studies showing efficacy of either combination products or once-daily regimens have investigated compliance as an independent measure of outcome. The reasons for this failure are methodologic in part and are discussed below.

PRACTICAL APPLICATIONS OF CURRENT KNOWLEDGE

The lack of a clear consensus in the compliance literature, coupled with the increasing complexity of the issues, contributes some skepticism and even cynicism about the significance of the compliance problem. As Charney states,

> If we look dispassionately at both sides of the "compliance-prescribance" axis, some sort of rough-and-ready natural law seems to be at work, balancing the interests of both the physician and the patient: The physician will be expected to prescribe with only approximate accuracy, and the patient will be expected to comply with only modest fidelity. Thus has mankind been able to survive bleeding, cupping, leeches, mustard plasters, turpentine stupes, and Panalba (622).

The scientific data relating the effects of frequent dosage and multiple medications do not yet reveal compelling conclusions. Nonetheless, practical applications of common sense solutions should not wait on 5% probability levels. With this in mind, it is useful to consider both the potential advantages and the disadvantages of attempts to simplify the treatment regimen.

Potential Advantages of Simplifying the Regimen

Improved Compliance.

In general, compliance can be improved by reducing medications to the minimum number necessary daily to produce the desired result, and by minimizing the frequency of pill taking. The first of these factors is the most powerful, but it runs contrary to established prescribing practices. The impending removal of many combination drugs from the market may exacerbate this problem; a survey conducted for the United States Pharmaceutical Manufacturers Association found that only 22% of physicians stated they would convert to single entity drugs if combinations were not available (918). Both a better understanding of the attitudes that underlie multiple prescribing and efforts to change physician behavior are required. Logical decision-making processes should be taught, among them the step care principles for the management of hypertension (913), and rational prescribing practices for psychotropic medication (912). A reduction in the complexity of a regime is likely to be most effective in improving compliance when it is coupled with educational efforts to increase comprehension.

Patient Convenience.

Less frequent medication can be fitted more easily into the patient's lifestyle, and can make it possible for the individual to avoid the inconvenience or embarrassment of public pill taking.

Patient Economy.

The cost of medication is reduced by giving larger milligram doses in single amounts. For instance, DiMascio (915) has calculated that the cost of 400 mg of thioridazine (Mellaril) daily is 54.4¢ when given in 25 mg tablets four times daily, but only 14.6¢ a day if a 200 mg tablet is given twice daily. This represents a saving of about $140 over one year. A similar point has been made by Moser and Wood (759) for the management of hypertension. Drugs such as propranolol or spironolactone are often given up to six times daily at a cost of up to $1.50, compared with a 15¢ single dose of a diuretic agent.

Staff Efficiency.

Ayd (909) has pointed out that less complex regimens can result in considerable saving of staff time plus a potential reduction in medication errors by those who dispense drugs.

Reduction in Drug Interactions.

The potential for metabolic and pharmacologic interaction is clearly reduced by providing the minimum number of medications.

Potential Disadvantages of Simplifying the Regimen

Losses of Efficacy.

The few studies comparing different dose frequencies all indicate that less frequent regimens are as effective as multiple dose regimens (914, 916, 917, 921). The fact that the prescribing of multiple drugs is often associated with the ordering of low doses provides indirect evidence that the more vigorous use of individual medications might be equally effective (919).

Increase in Side Effects.

The possibility that larger, less frequent doses of drugs may cause increased side effects is not well supported in the literature. The studies cited above report no difference in side effects among the regimens studied. There is even some evidence to the contrary when drugs are prescribed in the evening, since patients are not troubled during sleep by extrapyramidal or anticholinergic effects such as dry mouth or blurred vision (909). Drugs with sedative actions, given at night, may produce the additional benefit of obviating the cost and inconvenience of prescribing a hypnotic.

Caution should nonetheless be observed in some instances when large single doses of medication are used. For instance, elderly patients given large bedtime doses of antihypertensive or psychotropic medications could experience postural hypotension and fall on getting out of bed at night to visit the bathroom. Furthermore, it is possible that some of the cardiotoxic effects of tricyclic antidepressants are related to blood levels of the drug, and a case of sudden death has been reported in a six-year-old child given 300 mg of imipramine in a single dose at night for "school phobia" (911). Thus, large single daily dosages of drugs should be used with caution and discrimination, and their use should be coupled with careful clinical observation.

PRIORITIES FOR FUTURE RESEARCH

Recent research on drug regimens has revealed several issues and problems that require attention in future research.

Definition of Factors Influencing Compliance

The distinction between faulty comprehension and poor compliance is a valuable one, but there must be clearer definitions and a general agreement on terminology.The two most recent studies to shed light on this matter (258, 395) use a variety of descriptive terms such as *drug omission, scheduling noncompliance, noncomprehension,* and *noncompliance* that are overlapping and potentially confusing.

The distinction between these two dimensions, comprehension and compliance, is likely to be particularly useful in assessing the effectiveness of strategies designed to alter the separate components in specified patient populations (for example, comprehension in the elderly is likely to be a particular problem). As a result, the limitations of educational strategies will become more obvious, and attention can be addressed to the more complex issue of noncompliance in the face of comprehension.

Definitions of Compliance Related to Drug Class

Three recent studies indicate that class of drug may have an influence on compliance (103, 258, 395). The work by Hulka et al. (258) is particularly significant because it indicates that problems related to the regimen are more frequent in the less serious disease categories. Patients taking gastrointestinal drugs and tranquilizers make more scheduling errors than those with serious cardiac and diabetic conditions. It will be helpful if future studies continue to describe treatment populations carefully so that conclusions can be specific to particular regimens. This may be especially important in attempts to determine whether attention to education or motivation will be more successful for specific diseases, and in assessing the degree to which alterations in the regimen are able to affect either of these variables. There is a danger that too much attention may be paid to disease models like hypertension (where instruction has had little effect), with the risk that overgeneralized and unduly skeptical conclusions may be drawn about the inability to influence compliance.

Effect of the Regimen on Compliance

Despite all the attention paid to the regimen, the details of its effect on compliance remain inadequately studied. Part of the problem is related to a basic paradox in research strategy. Studies designed to compare the *efficacy* of different regimens (once daily versus multiple dosage) must make the two regimens identical in order to control for nonspecific effects; this is done by adding a placebo to the once-daily regimen, thereby equalizing the frequency of drug administration in the two regimens being compared. However, this manipulation makes it impossible to determine concurrently the effect of dosing frequency on compliance and the efficacy of the regimen. There is little doubt that the emphasis on proving the efficacy of different regimens, rather than on studying their influence on compliance, is related to the insistence of governmental drug regulating agencies that manufacturers divert their efforts in this direction.

A solution to this dilemma would be to conduct additional drug studies under naturalistic conditions without the addition of placebo, or to compare at least three treatment conditions in which the drug is given: once daily without placebo, once daily with placebo, and the multiple dosing schedule. There is an obvious possibility that although a once-daily schedule may increase compliance, it might reduce efficacy due to the absence of the placebo effect accompanying repeated administration. The relative importance of compliance and the placebo effect might also differ among drug categories and patient populations.

10

Educational Strategies to Improve Compliance with Therapeutic and Preventive Regimens: The Recent Evidence

Lawrence W. Green

INTRODUCTION

The purpose of this review is to examine recent developments in the research literature to find ways in which health education is or should be moving in order to maximize its contribution to health care.

This presentation is addressed to a multidisciplinary audience of practitioners and research specialists, so it begins with a redefinition of the scope and essential features in health education. It is immediately clear from this exercise that the assigned distinctions between "behavioral" and "educational" strategies (695) are artificial, unnecessary, and impossible to maintain in practice.

Some principles and methods of health education are then reviewed to critique their applicability in health care. Recommendations are offered for the improvement and extension of knowledge and for the practice of health education strategies. The state of the art is found still firmly anchored in behavioral science and learning theory but afloat on thin reeds of evidence in the health care system. In practice, the application of health education is casual, unsystematic, ritualistic, perfunctory, or neglected in most situations. In the third part of the review, applications to specific health behaviors and to specific populations through specific channels are summarized. The recent developments in

Preparation of this chapter was supported in part by grants 1R25HL17016 and T32H107180 from the National Institutes of Health and by contract SA-7974-75 from the Office of the Deputy Assistant Secretary for Planning and Evaluation/Health, United States Department of Health, Education and Welfare, to the Division of Health Education, Department of Health Services Administration, School of Hygiene and Public Health, The Johns Hopkins University, and the Health Services Research and Development Center, The Johns Hopkins Medical Institutions, Baltimore.

ambulatory chronic disease care have given considerable impetus to a strengthening of the scientific base of health education through a rapid expansion of experimental research.

PREVIOUS STRATEGIES AND PERSPECTIVES

The proper point of departure for this review is the excellent set of reviews presented in the predecessor to this book (794) by Brian Haynes, Victor Neufeld, Stanley Rosenberg, Ivan Barofsky, and Donald Fink. Haynes (695) summarized the methodologic and success ratings of 16 studies which tested what he characterized as *educational strategies*, "those attempts to improve compliance through the transmission of information about a disease and its treatment to patients" with or without a "motivational" appeal, with the intermediate objectives of affecting "patients' knowledge and attitudes" (page 70). He contrasted these with 20 behavioral studies of methods which "focus more directly upon the behaviors involved in compliance" and "include attempts (1) to reduce barriers to compliance . . . ; (2) to cue or stimulate compliance; and (3) to reward or reinforce compliance." By these definitions, Haynes found "that the behavioral and combined strategies may hold a substantial edge over educational [only] strategies in terms of improving both compliance and therapeutic outcomes." (page 74).

Neufeld (765) went on to examine the 16 "educational" studies in greater depth and found only one with a score of six or better on a scale of 0 to 10, based on five criteria from principles of learning, with each study rated 0, 1, or 2 for the adequacy with which its educational methods applied each of the five principles. He also found their research methodology seriously deficient and concluded that "a broader yet more precise definition of learning" (page 89) is needed, along with "greater collaboration in the design and execution of research into patient education" (page 91). This, he hoped, would reduce the triviality of interventions and outcomes studied and would strengthen the quality of the research designs and the educational programing. I have reached a similar conclusion in a review of other studies covering the same period (961).

If the studies reviewed by Haynes cast a dark shadow on the merit of "educational" strategies, then Rosenberg (789) more than compensated by reviewing the six most spectacular successes in the patient education literature, only one of which was in the Haynes sample of sixteen. These six studies, reviewed more extensively elsewhere in Roccella (786), had good methodological ratings and great success both in compliance and in cost-benefit payoff. I would like to defuse whatever debate* may have been occasioned by the divergent views of

---

*Readers interested in this debate are advised to review the articles cited above and consider their particular relev?nce to issues of patient compliance. [Ed.]

TABLE 10.1. Parallel principles in behavior modification and patient education

Behavioral therapeutics*	Learning principles in patient education†
1. "Identifying accurately the target behavior . . . that is ongoing and readily observable" (p. 106).	1. "Understanding of objectives: learning is more rapid and more efficient if the learner understands clearly what he is expected to learn" (p. 85).
2. "The use of all members of the health delivery team . . . who may see the patient during intervening periods" (p. 107).	2. "Feedback: learning is facilitated by rapid and complete individual feedback on the extent to which required learning is being accomplished" (p. 84).
3. "Providing social control in the form of the patient contract . . . totally individualized . . . through which the patient can exercise increased countercontrol . . . the conditions of the relationship are negotiated" (p. 107).	3. "Individualization: that is, learning is an individual process accomplished . . . at individual rates by individual means" (p. 84). "Relevance: learning is more efficient and effective when the student perceives that what she is expected to learn has relevance to her" (p. 84). "Motivation: learning is enchanced when the student is motivated . . . significant differences in the effect of internal as opposed to external motivating forces" (p. 85).

SOURCES: *From Barofsky 1976 (597);
         †from Neufeld 1976 (765).

Haynes and Rosenberg. I have sided with the latter author in my own previous reviews in concluding that health education indeed does have considerable potential in terms of cost-effectiveness and cost-benefits (681, 952, 955, 959); but, like Neufeld and Rosenberg, I have been terribly concerned with the narrow concepts sometimes applied in the name of health education (954, 958), the quality of practice in the implementation of it (960), the tendency to export educational methods from one problem or situation to another without an adequate assessment of educational needs peculiar to that problem or situation (680, 963), and with the primitive state of the measurement tools and the research literature (679, 956, 959, 961, 964, 966). These I take to be problems in the understanding, application, and testing of educational principles rather than flaws in the principles themselves. One final word on understanding: much of the difference in the interpretations reached by the study reviews alluded to above may stem from semantics alone. The implication that "education" is merely information exchange (with or without a "motivational appeal") (695) is simply incomplete. As shown in Table 10.1, an analysis of the learning principles involved in "behavioral therapeutics" (597) reveals that they closely parallel those involved in patient "education." In fact, *both* information exchange and behavioral therapeutics employ educational techniques, and distinctions between them blur because of this.

Having thus divulged my bias and referenced my previous assessment of the state of the art, this review will test some of these assessments against the recently emerging literature.

DEFINITIONS AND PARAMETERS

If it is not uniquely characterized by information transmission, what then is the distinguishing feature of education as a strategy to influence health behavior? To be consistent with the five principles of learning adapted by Neufeld (765), a definition of health education must include a provision for informed consent from those patients or citizens whose health-related behavior is in question. It is precisely the process of fostering healthy behavior through participation and informed consent, I believe, that defines the boundaries of health education in relation to the overlapping technologies of communication, motivation, and behavior modification, and in conjunction with medical procedures at the clinical level or with political and legal processes at the community level. Hence, *health education* is defined here as any combination of learning opportunities designed to facilitate voluntary adaptations of behavior conducive to health.

The operational terms for practitioners at the clinical or community level are *combination* and *designed*. How can learning opportunities be designed and combined to facilitate health maintenance most efficiently without coercing behavior? At the policy level, the issues are less with methods and design than with selecting those areas of health behavior in which health education can be most effective, and those illnesses or risk factors on which behavioral adaptations can have the greatest impact in cost-benefit terms for individuals and for society. I must leave the societal aspects to the epidemiologists and economists and will concentrate on answering the question for individuals with health problems.

The criterion of "combination" requires that the strategy include more than one element in order to assure that the several determinants of a given health behavior are addressed. It assumes multicausality (955). For any health behavior there are at least three types of determinants which an educational strategy can and should influence. These include a motivational or predisposing factor, an enabling factor, and a reinforcing factor. Only rarely does one find a situation in which one of these factors alone requires support; thus, it is unrealistic to expect that health education can achieve a lasting behavioral change with only one method. For this reason I find it necessary to define health education in terms of the combination of methods.

TABLE 10.2.   Use of contraceptives in Venezuela

Predisposing factor (Attitude)	Reinforcing factor (Social Support)	Enabling factor	
		Accessible	Inaccessible
Favorable towards family planning	High	90.9%	73.1%
	Low	77.6%	47.9%
Unfavorable towards family planning	High	84.3%	67.8%
	Low	48.1%	28.2%

SOURCE: Based on Kar 1977 (979). F =46.22, N = 1124, P < .001.

A recent study emphasizing the importance of the combined influence of predisposing, enabling, and reinforcing factors is provided by Kar (979, 980). In a large sample survey of the determinants of contraceptive behavior by 2,864 Venezuelan women, data were collected on over 700 variables. The three categories of variables that explained the largest proportions of variance in use of contraceptives were social support (reinforcement of spouses, friends, and relatives), awareness and perceived accessibility of services (enabling factor), and specific family planning attitudes and intentions (predisposing factor). The importance of the combinational or interactive effects of the three factors are clear in Table 10.2.

The second defining characteristic of health education is that it be "designed." This criterion requires that the methods employed have been developed or selected and combined on the basis of clearly delineated objectives derived from a diagnosis of the behavior in question.

The criterion of facilitating "voluntary" changes requires that the behavior occur under conditions of informed consent in which the patient's own health goals are being served.

Finally, "adaptations of behavior" refers to compliance with therapeutic and preventive regimens in this context. The term *adaptations* is preferred over *changes* because some health behaviors, especially in children, are developed *de novo* rather than by replacement.

Some of the confusion about what is and what is not health education no doubt stems from the fact that the boundaries of programs, activities, and methods that may be characterized as educational are vague. Most health education activities are embedded in other programs and many are not identified as health education. Indeed, those responsible for programs or studies sometimes disavow any association with health education in an attempt to distinguish their efforts as more innovative, modern, technological, behavioristic, client-centered, or scientific than they perceive health education to be. Alternative labeling occurs even when the methods employed clearly derive their philosophical, technical, and theoretical or scientific approaches from education, educational psychology, educational technology, or health education itself.

The alternative labels used for health education programs and activities reveal the scope and diversity of educational applications in health.

Motivation Programs

The term *motivation programs* has been used, especially in family planning, to refer to the activities generally included in health education programs (940, 942), and also to "incentive schemes" designed to appeal more directly to economic motives for family limitation (1008). From a formal psychological standpoint, the term *motivation* is incorrectly applied when it refers to programatic activities, because motivation is a construct intended to refer to the internal dynamics of behavior, not the external stimuli. The more correct designation for these methods is *motive-arousing appeals.*

Behavior Modification

The term *behavior modification* has been extended from its original applications in behavioral psychology (982, 1001) to include educational and political strategies for which the priority objectives are changes in behavior (597, 695, 1025). Purist behavioral psychologists would not categorize as behavior modification an educational method that is designed to achieve behavioral changes by means of changing knowledge or attitudes. But behavior modification (operant conditioning) techniques do qualify as educational methods so long as the subjects voluntarily submit to the conditioning procedures to achieve changes they desire in their own behavior. Beyond informed consent, they further qualify as educational strategies to the extent that they require training, self-instruction, and premeditated structuring of the subjects' environment, of their thoughts before and after behavioral events, and of rewards (941, 1000, 1004).

Health Counseling

Health counseling and its variants (genetic counseling, diet counseling, patient counseling) constitute another subset of health education insofar as they represent an approach to voluntary change in health behavior. Most counseling methods of education have their theoretical and philosophical roots in ego psychology, which is at extreme variance with behaviorism. Counseling is outside the defined scope of health education when it is more psychotherapeutic than informational in its method and content because the emotional state of the patient renders him or her unable to process information normally or effectively.

Communications

As an interdisciplinary concern of social psychologists, marketing and public opinion researchers, media specialists, health educators, and others, communications are applied and their effects on behavior are studied in every sphere of human endeavor (1015). Their applications in relation to health behavior are usually within the scope of health education programing (957, 1007, 1014), except when they are used to advertise or promote products or causes inconsistent with the health needs of consumers (954, 1020).

Other forms and methods of health education which define its scope are community organization, in-service training, consultation, group work, computer-assisted instruction (CAI), other teaching machines, programmed instruction, audio-visual methods, bibliotherapy, patient teaching, health fairs, exhibits, libraries, conferences, and routine health provider-consumer interactions.

EVALUATION OF HEALTH EDUCATION PROGRAMS

While firmly grounded in learning theory, the principle that two or more educational maneuvers be combined to promote healthful behavior requires much more empirical validation than it has received.

Behavioral scientists have made and continue to make significant contributions to the scientific base of health education through basic research on the processes of learning and behavioral change. The "applied research" of most behavioral scientists, however, seeks to isolate single variables that "predict" behavior rather than multiple variables represented in health or medical programs (931). As laboratory studies in psychology and survey research in sociology accumulate an increasingly lengthy inventory of "predictors" and "correlates" of health behavior, the practitioner and planner is further bewildered in deciding upon which factors to intervene. In terms of evaluation, the recommendation that two or more educational techniques be combined is intended to encourage a shift in research resources from highly controlled laboratory studies of singular methods of health education to field studies or clinical trials of health education strategies that combine several methods and are directed at multiple factors.

Randomized factorial experiments provide the best design for studying the merit of this recommendation. Where such randomization is not possible, quasi-experimental evaluations of demonstrations should be supported where most recipients receive a comprehensive educational program and comparison groups receive everything *but* selected experimental methods (678). Where prospective experimental control is not possible, cross-lagged correlation analysis is recommended (86, 962).

There are several dimensions and criteria on which the goals and outcomes of health education can be measured. In practical terms, it it helpful to consider maneuvers and measures according to the temporal span of outcomes sought, namely, immediate, intermediate, and ultimate outcomes.

Immediate Outcomes

The immediate outcomes of health education programs should be changes (improvements) in the key predisposing, enabling, and reinforcing factors which are known or expected to be causally related to the health behavior in question (925, 955). The general components of health education strategies that are found to be most effective with each of these factors are identified as follows.

Predisposing Factors.

Communication methods directed at the patient or the general public are most effective in achieving changes in predisposing factors such as knowledge, attitudes, beliefs, and values (603, 1007, 1014, 1015).

Enabling Factors.

Community organization and organizational development methods directed at other agencies and institutions are generally most effective in achieving changes in the enabling factors that facilitate or inhibit health practices. These factors include availability and accessibility of services, referral mechanisms, third party payment mechanisms, and clinic hours (925, 939, 1007).

Reinforcing Factors.

Training and consultation methods directed at the health providers and others who interact with the consumers (parents, employers, teachers) are most effective in achieving changes in the *reinforcing factors*. These factors include the attitudes and actions of clinic personnel toward walk-in patients, as well as the rewards and punishments that parents and teachers provide children in response to health actions, or that employers provide employees in response to safety practices (264, 604, 926, 937, 938, 987, 1028, 1031).

Intermediate Goals

Intermediate goals of health education programs are the behavioral outcomes expected to occur if the immediate goals are achieved (826). If, for example, a program successfully increases public awareness of a health problem (predisposing factor), improves the accessibility of services or resources to take action (enabling factors), and increases support for the behavior from parents or employers (reinforcing factors), it will be more likely to achieve changes in behavior than if only one or two of these immediate goals are achieved.

Different emphases of programs are known to have varying effectiveness in achieving the following five dimensions of behavior change.

Frequency.

If a health action must recur periodically and the goal of the program is to establish a pattern of regularity, then health education methods which provide cues at appropriate intervals tend to be more effective than one-shot or sporadic methods. Well-child visits, dental checkups, annual Pap smears, and prenatal visits have all been shown to improve in frequency with a telephone or mailing system that reminds consumers, parents, or patients of their next appointment (34, 168, 172, 173, 184, 453, 461). Similarly, the systematic incorporation of cues in the home or work site can improve the frequency of compliance behavior (843, 852).

Persistence.

If the required health behavior is one that must be continued over a long period, as with medical regimens for hypertension or diabetes, then health education methods which provide social supports in the clinic and home environments are most effective. Several studies on compliance with medical regimens confirm the importance of the doctor-patient relationship and the patient's perception of support from family members, especially the spouse (86, 604, 848, 946, 948, 1027). Persistence with diet and smoking cessation regimens depends on similar social influences and on the effectiveness of normative health education strategies (353, 954, 957, 963, 1003).

Promptness.

The behavioral goal in many health education programs is primarily to reduce delay in seeking medical treatment for selected symptoms or to reduce delay in adopting a preventive practice such as immunization, prenatal care, or contraception. Success in achieving the former goal appears to be heavily influenced by family support and by the relationship with a health care provider. It is therefore most effectively achieved through health education directed at reinforcing factors in the home and clinic environments, as was the case in the preceding dimension of behavior (927, 965). There are site- and symptom-specific variations in this rule, however (680, 928). Reduced delay in adopting preventive health actions, on the other hand, appears to be responsive to less intensive health education programs. Mass media campaigns, for example, have demonstrated their effectiveness in recruiting new clinic users in subsequent months, and the characteristics of the patients recruited indicate that the media are triggering earlier action in those who were already motivated and who would have come to the clinics at later dates (928, 1026). Thus, the mass media are useful in health education when the specific goals are to reduce delay in preventive health actions, but less effective when the goal is to reduce delay with illness or sick-role behavior.

Quality.

When the behavioral goal of a health education program is to improve the appropriateness of health actions, that is, when the consumer must choose between alternative products, sources of care, or types of symptom response, the evidence suggests that prior experience with the product or source of care is most influential in determining the quality of the choice. Health education directed at reinforcing factors in the health care system is most likely to influence appropriate utilization of health services (820, 928). Starting with failure to acknowledge and meet patient expectations on the first visit (186, 1036), through failure to take family and work situations into account in prescribing therapeutic regimens (604, 852), several points in the health care system can be identified where health education can strengthen the probability of appropriate health actions on subsequent occasions. Community organization methods are an essential component of health education when the quality of consumer choices is a function of the availability or accessibility of quality health products or services (939).

Range.

When the behavioral goals of health education are highly complex because an individual is expected to adopt a range of different health practices, more intensive health education methods are required. Individualized counseling, home visits and reinforcement of graduated steps in the behavioral repertoire may be required. Rehabilitation counseling, diet therapy, and education of parents of disabled children are most effective when they include these several elements. Health practices which are routine for middle class housewives may be highly complex for rural poor homemakers, and more intensive and long-term educational interventions are generally required for the latter (1027).

Ultimate Goals

The ultimate goals of health education programs, as with other "compliance-improving strategies," consist of reducing mortality and morbidity. These are usually measured as outcomes in community programs, on an aggregate rather than individual scale using vital statistics of incidence, prevalence, and distribution. When epidemiological measures are not accessible, or when the program is on a smaller scale, medical records, clinic or household interviews, and measures of symptoms or risk factors such as weight, blood pressure, blood or urine tests may serve to assess progress toward long-range goals beyond behavioral changes.

Evaluations of health education in terms of these longer-range goals have been rare because of the following difficulties:

1. Most health education programs have been too limited in time or resources to seek measures of these longer-range outcomes (969).
2. Community health education programs, by the nature of their employment of mass media and community organization methods, often preclude the availability of control groups unexposed to the program (961).
3. Some of the most extensive health education campaigns have promoted in good faith selected health practices later found by epidemiologists to be unhealthful, as in the nutrition education programs of the 1940s and 1950s urging people to eat eggs, red meats, and shellfish (957).
4. Health education programs are usually embedded in a larger program effort so that it is often impossible to unravel the effects attributable to other program components (679).

To overcome these problems, investigators are sometimes tempted to go to methodological extremes that make their results entirely ungeneralizable. It is a mistake, for example, to attempt to isolate the health education component of a total health program and to test that component by itself either in the community or in a psychology laboratory. The consistent failure of such "programs" to achieve the changes sought attests to the necessity of supporting health education with administrative and institutional arrangements conducive to the behavioral changes sought, and the importance of coordinating health education activities with other program components.

A further consideration arising from the difficulties outlined above is that judgment of the effectiveness of health education should not have to depend entirely on criteria for which measurement may not be available for many years and which may be overwhelmingly influenced by other circumstances over which health education could have no control. To take this one step further, I do not believe that health education should be held responsible for failure to achieve changes in vital rates if behaviors are successfully changed in accordance with medically recommended practices. Indeed, health education may cause some medically recommended practices to be called into question (986). The "bottom line" here is that health education can only be called to account for failure to achieve the behavioral changes recommended by health care workers and not for inadequacies of the recommendations themselves.

Time Frame for Goals

The foregoing classification of health education goals into immediate (improvements in predisposing, enabling, and reinforcing factors), intermediate (behavioral changes), and ultimate (reductions in morbidity and mortality) outcomes is concerned with causal priorities. The first must be achieved before the second can be achieved because the first causes the second, and so on from second to third. There is another time dimension on which health education goals may be framed and the effectiveness of programs judged; namely, how soon the goal is to be achieved. Some health education goals, even reduction in morbidity, can be achieved quickly, whereas others, including some changes in predisposing factors, require months, years, or decades to realize (679).

Health education programs vary in their capacity to achieve different rates of change, but these variations cannot be analyzed without considering two other dimensions of goal statements: extensivity (how many people are expected to change), and target populations (which groups or individuals in the population are expected to change). Thus, goal statements in health education, when formally stated as program objectives, contain four elements: who is to undergo change, how much change is desired, what kind of change is required, and when is the change required. For example, a health education program goal might be stated as follows: by 1980, the national percentage of former smokers among men in the twenty-one to twenty-four age range will increase from 20% to 40%. The time over which the change is expected to occur is largely a function of the level at which the program begins (the baseline level) and the amount of change expected. The first consideration can be analyzed independently as a function of timing; the second is a more complex issue to be analyzed in connection with population, cost, and other considerations.

The relative rates of change to be expected from community health education programs can be stated simply. Early in the introduction of a new idea or new program the rate of change (goal achievement) will be slow; as the program progresses the rate of change in the population will speed up until it has included the majority of potential consumers or subjects; then the rate of change will slow as the program attempts to reach the more socially isolated, poorer, and more resistant subgroups. This pattern of rate change in program achievement has been observed consistently across a wide range of program goals where the unit of change was percentage of the population adopting a new practice or "innovation" (936, 947, 957, 997, 1014).

The baseline level of adoption for the health practice in a community (town, industry, clinic) at the time a program is introduced determines the rate of goal achievement to be expected. If the health education program is introduced before anyone in the community has had an opportunity to adopt the practice recommended (zero baseline), it will tend to start slowly. Most programs, however, start in populations where at least some of the people have already adopted the recommended practice and many others are predisposed to adopt it but need some information, social support, or a cue to act. In these circumstances, there tends to be a temporary leap in the rate of adoption or change. This is sometimes referred to as "skimming the cream off the top" of the community, where the cream consists of those who are awaiting the program.

Programs that attempt to change attitudes and behavior in "hard to reach" groups (situations where the baseline level of acceptance for the larger community is high but recalcitrants remain) will have slow rates of change. Efforts will have to be more intensive and the educational cost per new acceptor will be high, but the benefits per new acceptor will also be high because these tend to be high-risk groups.

Because of these considerations, assessments of the relative impact of a given type of health education strategy should use measures which give greater weight to changes when baseline levels are higher than to equal changes from lower baseline levels.

One index of relative impact that may be applied to data from different health education programs in order to make the comparisons conform to the criterion in this recommendation is the Effectiveness Index (EI):

$$EI = \frac{P_2 - P_1}{100 - P_1}$$

Here, P_1 is the proportion of the population that has previously adopted the recommended health practice at the baseline, P_2 is the corresponding proportion at a later date (after at least part of the program). The denominator of this equation represents potential change and the numerator actual change (955). This measure will tend to favor programs reaching the poor.

The variable levels of achievement and rates of change for health education programs may be classified according to the following additional sources of variation: the nature of the behavioral changes sought and of the symptoms or diagnoses to which they relate, and the circumstances surrounding the behavior or the health problem; the characteristics of the population exposed to the program and the source (provider) of the educational communication; and the level of spending on the educational components to the program.

DECIDING WHAT BEHAVIORS TO MODIFY

Three facts interfere with gearing health education to deal with specific health problems. First, the prevention or reduction of many health problems (for example, heart disease) involves more than one health behavior. Second, many health practices (such as diet) relate to several health problems, conditions, diagnoses, and symptoms. Finally, many health practices are motivated by beliefs, values, fears, and aspirations unrelated to the specific health problems affected by the behavior.

Given these considerations, it has sometimes been more productive to assess health practices and develop preventive communication in terms of specific populations and their perceptions of the health practices rather than the health problems themselves. The analysis will focus here on behavioral problems.

It is sometimes difficult to find demonstration and evaluation funding for school health education, health exhibits, mass media programs, health education resource centers, and generalized patient education and community organization programs because these do not relate exclusively to the concerns of one of the institutes, bureaus, or divisions of governments.

In such situations, health care providers should allow for health education innovations which do not fit conveniently under categorical medical problems. This may be accomplished by pooling and channeling some of the categorical disease-specific effort into health education programs directed at changing practices, beliefs, and attitudes associated with several health problems.

Among the perceived attributes of practices that may influence the rate and extent of adoption of a new health behavior or regimen are its relative advantage over the practice it supercedes; its compatability with the existing values, past experiences, and needs of the receivers; its complexity; its trial potential in terms of being divisible into less complex parts; and its observability to other people who may reinforce or disapprove of the behavior.

National surveys on smoking between 1964 and 1970 indicate that the diffusion of smoking cessation has been responsive to these variables, as shown by attitudes and practices in three surveys (1010). Schwartz and Dubitzsky (1018) compared the expressed willingness of smokers to try ten different smoking cessation methods. They found that smokers were not willing to use methods most frequently offered by physicians, psychologists, and public health workers. The preferred methods were the more individualized (low observability) methods.

In contrast, it is bewildering to note the apparent popularity of group methods for weight control (1024) and for exercise programs (386). Thus, there is evidently an interaction between the characteristics of the innovation and the social circumstances surrounding its introduction or promotion.

The acceptibility of different health practices is reflected partially in the relative levels of recall knowledge in the public of specific heart-risk factors. The Harris (968) survey of American adults revealed major differences in the salience of specific risk reduction possibilities available to them. A recent community survey in Calgary, Alberta serves as a rough comparison. Mackie (999) found that 53% of her Canadian sample could recall overweight and 42% mentioned smoking as a risk factor, but only 12% mentioned cholesterol. Insufficient exercise was mentioned by 25% of the Canadian respondents. The Harris survey asked Americans what they thought were the best ways to prevent heart trouble and got almost the reverse order of risk-factor salience: 44% mentioned proper diet, 34% exercise, 17% smoking, and 16% mentioned weight. The US-Canadian differences most likely reflect differences in the dissemination of information within the two countries.

PRACTICAL RECOMMENDATIONS TO
IMPROVE COMPREHENSION, RECALL, AND COMPLIANCE

Those who wish to apply the general educational principles outlined above can maximize the effectiveness of their communications by designing them according to some practical, empirically validated guidelines.

The Principle of Brevity

We know from patient education studies that the number of statements forgotten increases with the number presented at a rate predicted by the linear regression equation

$$Y = 0.56X - 0.94$$

where Y is the number of statements likely to be forgotten and X is the number of statements made to a patient (989). The formula means that roughly one-half of the statements made to a patient will be forgotten within five minutes (990). It has been tested primarily in clinical settings where it predicts with 77% accuracy the number of verbal instructions forgotten plus or minus one. In one clinic, for example, doctors presented an average of 7.15 statements and patients were able to recall an average of only 3.60 within five minutes of the consultation (991).

The point in presenting these statistics is not to disparage information giving, but rather to emphasize the importance of selectivity in presenting information that the patient may be expected to recall. This will require separating that part of the communication that discloses detailed information for informed consent purposes from the part that presents advice to the patient on using the medicine.

The Principle of Organization

The foregoing recommendation leads to a concern with the structure of the information. Joubert and Lasagna (975) asked 133 people how detailed they thought patient package inserts should be. Most agreed that detailed information should be included even if it made the insert very long, but 15.3% wanted a short summary only, and 59.9% wanted both a detailed *and* a summary statement. The percentage who wanted only a summary varied significantly with age, with 6.1% of those under age 31 desiring only a summary, but 31.6% of those over 50 wanting only a summary (976).

Preferences aside, the advisability of summarized and clearly categorized information is supported by basic and applied educational research where the forgetting of fictitious medical information by student volunteers closely parallels forgetting of actual medical information by patients (992). By a simple re-organization of 15 medical statements into "labeled" categories, Philip Ley and his associates (991) were able to increase recall by 50%.

The Primacy Principle

A special case of the principle of organization is the retention and recall advantage gained by the medical information first presented to patients over information presented later in the same communication. Ley (993), experimenting with serial order of medical information presented variously by oral,

TABLE 10.3. Weight loss in groups receiving ordinary or experimental (super-memory) leaflet

| | Mean weight loss in pounds at | | | |
	2 weeks	4 weeks	8 weeks	16 weeks
Ordinary leaflet	2.7	4.7	7.7	8.2
Experimental leaflet	4.4	8.6	12.3	15.4
Ordinary versus experimental leaflet:	$P < 0.10$			

visual, and oral plus written methods, found significantly greater mean recall scores for information presented in the first third of the communication, regardless of communication mode.

The Readability Principle

Pyrczak and Roth (1013) recently applied a standardized readability formula to a sample of warnings and cautions on the labels of over-the-counter drugs and found only one below the eleventh grade level of reading ease. Only one among eleven caution and warning statements tested could be read with ease at the fourth grade level. In America it has been found that approximately 12 million people over the age of thirteen cannot read as well as the average fourth grader (945). The implication for preparing written materials is obvious.

The Principle of Repetition

Supplementing oral instructions with written communication is an application of the educational principle that information which is repeated will be retained and recalled more readily than information that is not repeated. Written instructions can be referred to repeatedly by the patient (460). But beyond these de facto applications of the principle of repetition, written communications might be strengthened in their impact on compliance behavior by selectively and strategically repeating messages and advice that have known relationships to medication error.

The Principle of Specificity

In general, it is more persuasive to say "lose ten pounds" than to say "lose weight." An inherent disadvantage of written instructions is that they must be sufficiently general to apply to most people, but wherever there is an option to present a more specific or less specific instruction or item of information, the more specific should be considered the more powerful communication in terms of retention and effect on behavior (994).

The foregoing principles are demonstrated in combination in an experiment reported by Ley (733) in which two versions of the same leaflet were designed to help women keep to a low carbohydrate diet for weight loss. One had a moderate readability level (control), whereas the other was very easy and contained explicit categorization of information and repetition. Weight reductions after sixteen weeks for the two groups are shown in Table 10.3. Thus, application of a few principles to enhance communication can substantially improve treatment outcomes even for the very difficult problem of weight reduction.

EXTENDING PATIENT EDUCATION TO THE COMMUNITY

All the foregoing principles of information transmission are subject to the inherent limitations of the medium or channel of communication. Their effect on health can be enhanced substantially by coordinating patient education in clinical and pharmaceutical settings with health education in the media, schools, home visits, and occupational health programs. The combination of written and verbal instruction has been demonstrated to be superior to either alone (101), but a more extensive concept of combination is intended here.

The major conclusion from this analysis is that the potential effects of improved communications on patients are great, but not without a broader concept of the health education task to which they are addressed. That task is to bring relevant, comprehensible, useful information to bear at the time and place where it is most likely to motivate, enable, or reinforce health behavior. The times and places for such educational effects are as often outside the medical encounter as within.

11

Behavioral
Strategies for
Improving Compliance

Jacqueline M. Dunbar,
Gary D. Marshall, and Mel F. Hovell

INTRODUCTION

Broadly speaking, the strategies for improving compliance discussed in this book fall within the categories educational, behavioral, and organizational. For the purpose of the discussion which follows we would like to make somewhat arbitrary distinctions among these techniques, recognizing that in practice they are often difficult to distinguish precisely and that others may not concur with our definitions. *Educational interventions* are defined here as those that rely most heavily on transmission of information and instructions as a means of changing behavior, for example, pill container labeling, written instructions, and health education classes. *Organizational interventions* focus primarily on clinic and regimen convenience and on the utilization of personnel, including minimizing waiting time and employing nurses for follow-up care. *Behavioral strategies* are those procedures that attempt to influence specific noncompliant behaviors directly through the use of techniques such as reminders, self-monitoring, and reinforcement, but with information and instruction playing a secondary role. Elements of each would and should be utilized in most intervention programs, as illustrated in Figure 11.1. Educational strategies were discussed in the preceding chapter by Lawrence Green (who uses a more comprehensive definition of education than we have used here), and organizational strategies are described in Chapter 17 by Edward Gibson. This chapter will focus on behavioral strategies.

It is helpful in approaching the topic of compliance-improving strategies to consider the goal of the intervention. Is it prevention, remediation of low compliance, or maintenance of high compliance? For the goal of prevention, the target of intervention is an entire patient population. The purpose is to shift the current or expected compliance distribution toward high compliance. This is

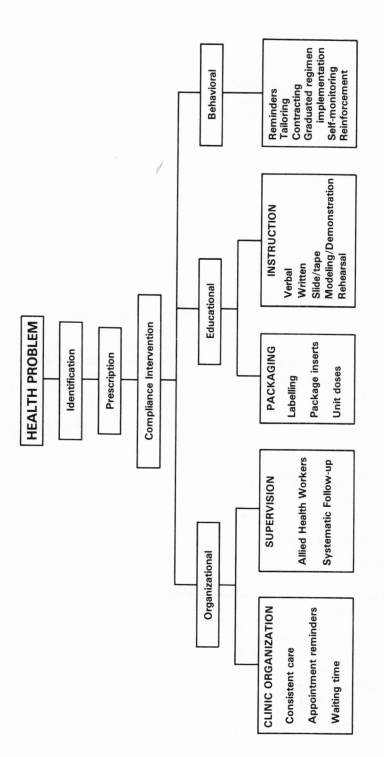

FIGURE 11.1. A process model of compliance intervention.

typically attempted with patient education or clinic management strategies. The success of such approaches is measured best by comparing the resulting compliance distribution with that of a similar untreated population or with the expected distribution for that regimen.*

The second goal is remediation. Here the target of the intervention is that group of individuals with identified compliance problems. The goal is individual improvement, typically through behavioral strategies. Success at this level of intervention can be evaluated by either single case or controlled group designs.* Currently, there is a paucity of such investigations in the compliance literature.

The third goal, maintenance, represents a dilemma to all in the field. Although one can anticipate that approximately one-third of all patients will achieve and maintain good compliance without systematic intervention, maintenance is clearly a problem for the person whose low compliance has been increased through the application of some compliance improving strategy (228, 1047). Declines in adherence over time are also seen with patients on long-term preventive regimens (200, 442, 505). The goal, of course, is to sustain good and improved compliance. Success would be evaluated by comparing the compliance trends over time with those of a similar but untreated group. Although there have been studies with follow-up data that suggest effective maintenance strategies (1045, 1047), no investigation has been undertaken to evaluate compliance-maintaining techniques per se.

Behavioral strategies may be used to improve compliance at each level. However, organizational and educational procedures have predominated in the prevention phase with behavioral strategies more commonly used for remediation.

Keeping in mind these definitions and goals of intervention, let us consider specific behavioral strategies in depth. The strategies which have been investigated in controlled studies include: reminders, tailoring, contracting, graduated regimen implementation, self-monitoring, and reinforcement.

PREVENTIVE AND REMEDIAL INTERVENTIONS

Reminders

Reminders have a well substantiated role in behavior therapy. They are useful when the problem is a failure of the behavior to occur, for they prompt or cue the occurrence of the desired behavior. It should be noted that the value of such stimulus events in improving compliance depends upon the presupposition that forgetting is a major component of the problem.

Reminders have been used to prevent appointment breaking (375, 1043, 1066, 1068) and, to a lesser degree, to improve medication compliance (312). All of these controlled studies have reported better compliance in a group where

---

*See Chapter 21 for detailed comments on research designs.

reminders were used than in a comparable control group. The gains seen with appointment keeping are fairly consistent across studies—an increase of 13% to 20% with reminders.

There did not appear to be any substantial differences between the effect of mailed and telephone prompting in the studies compared in Table 11.1, although this was not systematically examined. Brigg and Mudd (1043) did find telephone prompting by the professional staff a useful method of resolving prospective clients' doubts and anxieties about counseling as well as encouraging early cancellations by those who had "second thoughts" about keeping the original appointment. Thus, not only did appointment keeping itself improve, but earlier canceled appointments allowed time to schedule other clients. Turner and Vernon (1068) also reported this advantage in telephone prompting by a clinic receptionist.

It should be noted that each of four studies included canceled and kept appointments in the keep rate. Only "no shows," or in the case of the Brigg and Mudd (1043) study, last-minute cancellations were counted as unkept appointments. The studies do not indicate whether clients who cancel appointments subsequently make them up. That study remains to be done. It is also not known whether the improved keep rate is due to more appointments actually being kept or to an increase in cancellations with a corresponding decrease in no shows or to a combination of factors.

At any rate, appointment reminders appear to benefit a clinic economically, if for no other reason than that canceled appointments can be rescheduled for different patients. Turner and Vernon (1068) reported that the monthly cost of the telephone reminder procedure was recovered in their clinic when just six additional appointments were kept. If their findings were transferable to other settings, the return on the reminder system investment would be considerable.

The use of a reminder system to improve medication compliance has been reported in a number of investigations (16, 341, 365, 1061). However, just one controled study has been reported. Lima et al. (312) utilized two devices in a three-group controled comparison study with outpatients in antimicrobial therapy. In one group the reminder consisted of a prescription label with a clock face, with hours of administration circled; in the second group a sticker with directions on administration was provided for posting in a convenient place. Physicians were blinded to the patient's group assignment. The clinic pharmacist enrolled patients and instructed them on the use of the reminders or, in the case of the control group, repeated usual medication administration instructions. Assessment of compliance was by pill or liquid count during a home visit on the ninth or tenth day of antimicrobial treatment.

The authors reported a significant improvement in compliance among the reminder group, as compared with the control group (clock: $\chi^2 = 5.4$, P $<.025$; sticker: $\chi^2 = 11.3$, P $< .005$). The difference between the two reminders, however, was not statistically significant. Interestingly, the effect of the reminders was greater in the pediatric population (where 24% of the control group and

TABLE 11.1. Effect of reminders on appointment keeping

Authors	Type of setting	Type of appointment	Type of reminder	Keep rate	
				Before	After
Brigg and Mudd (1043)	Marriage counseling	Intake	Telephone	65%	78%
Nazarian et al. (375)	Multispecialty health center	Follow-up	Mail	48%	64%
Shmarak (1066)	Dental clinic	Follow-up	Telephone or Mail	72%	92%
Turner and Vernon (1068)*	Mental health clinic	Intake	Telephone	70%	87%
				75%	85%

*This study used a reversal design in which reminders were introduced (87%) in the clinic after an assessment of the keep rate (70%), then withheld (75%), then reintroduced (85%). The other three studies used control group comparison designs.

57% to 59% of the reminder groups were above 70% compliance) than in the adult population (where 40% of the controls and 67% of the reminder treated patients were above this criterion). It should be noted that in the control group considerably fewer children (24%) were compliant than adults (40%), thus allowing for greater improvement within the pediatric population. Differences in the type of infections experienced by the children and adults did not create this discrepancy, for the authors reported no relationship between disease and compliance.

This study indicates that compliance with short-term antibiotic regimens can be improved with reminders. Still, a substantial portion of the group did not reach the 70% compliance criterion. This suggests that the reminder strategy is useful, but only for a portion of patients, perhaps a third of the pediatric and a quarter of the adult group. This may represent that portion of the problem of compliance with short-term regimens that is primarily accounted for by "forgetting." The study did not identify specific reasons for poor compliance nor did it determine which types of problems responded to the reminder. It also did not address the utility of reminders for long-term regimens. One might speculate that a reminder would lose its effectiveness with time, as its saliency in the environment diminishes. The Lima et al. (312) study, however, does open an avenue of investigation into compliance interventions as well as present a tested strategy for improving compliance with short-term medication in an important segment of the population.

Tailoring

Tailoring refers to a process of fitting the prescribed regimen and intervention strategies to specific patient characteristics. For example, a patient having difficulty adhering to a weight loss program and expressing concern about a lack of social support might be referred to a support group such as Weight Watchers or TOPS rather than placed on a self-managed regimen. In this case, several interventions might be appropriate for managing obesity, but the provision of social support would make the group program best for this patient. A second example of this concept appears in Chapter 14 on programs for alcoholism.

Another way of tailoring is to adapt a standard treatment to an individual's unique characteristics and circumstances. For example, Best (49; see Chapter 13 as well) reports that in smoking withdrawal procedures, the efficacy of attitude change procedures depends on their timing. That is, attitude change manipulations will tend to be more effective with the less motivated smoker *after* abstinence is achieved, while the highly motivated patient is more likely to profit from *early* attitude change efforts. Thus, the sequencing of treatment steps can be tailored to the patient. Similarly, the patient's conduct of a regimen can be adapted to his personal habits and routines. In the forgetful patient, twice-daily medications might be prescribed at tooth brushing time—if the patient brushes his teeth twice a day, of course. Similarly, the hypertensive patient who tends to skip breakfast might have his medication prescribed before dinner.

Best, as mentioned above, examined the effect of tailoring smoking with-drawal procedures using a research design that included matching and mismatch-ing the treatment and timing of attitude change efforts with the subjects' locus of control and motivation to quit smoking. All subjects used a rapid smoking—concentrated smoke procedure. Best reported that his data supported a tailoring hypothesis. However, abstinence in the control group was not significantly dif-ferent from that in the experimental groups.

Hallburg (1049) utilized a tailoring approach as a preventive strategy to re-duce medication errors in elderly ambulatory patients. Although she refers to her intervention as a "decision-making approach," she essentially tailored the patients' prescribed medication regimen to their routines, living patterns, abilities, and other unique circumstances. She cites the example of developing a pill-an-hour regimen that was in accord with the prescriptions for one patient who was on numerous medications but felt he could not take more than one at a time. Hallburg reports that the results favored the tailoring approach. Serious errors were made by 23.5% of the control patients but just 11.5% of the experi-mental group. However, as with the Best study, the differences between the control and experimental groups were not significant.

Tailoring has also been included as a component of a remedial behavioral package designed to improve compliance in noncompliant uncontrolled hyper-tensive men (228). In this instance tailoring referred to the process of matching medication administration times and places to the patient's daily habits or rituals. The authors do report a significant improvement in compliance and dias-tolic blood pressure. However, it should be noted that tailoring was just one of six components* in the intervention, and the research design did not allow for an analysis of the effectiveness of individual components.

Basically, tailoring treats patients as unique individuals, not as members of a uniform group. Thus, it is not assumed that a standard regimen or a uniform method of carrying out a regimen applies equally well to all patients; but rather that treatment and regimen scheduling must be individualized. However, while tailoring has much intuitive appeal, the limited research on it suggests that it does not have a strong effect, at least as it has been applied in studies to date. It may be that many patients tailor regimens for themselves so that the benefit of doing so for them may make little quantitative difference in group studies. As a result, the application of tailoring must itself be tailored to those who need it. It is not clear at this time if there are certain types of patients who respond well to tailoring, nor do we know the most effective guidelines to follow in fitting

---

*The components included: (1) tailoring, (2) home blood pressure measurement, (3) home blood pressure charting, (4) home medication charting, (5) increased supervision, and (6) monetary reinforcement.

regimens to patients' circumstances. These areas require careful study if we are to determine when and how tailoring can be effective as a compliance–improving strategy.

Contracting

Contracting refers to a process of specifying a set of rules regarding some behavior of interest and formalizing a commitment to adhere to them. Typically, these take the form of "if-then" rules: *if* a behavior occurs, *then* X consequence is to follow; *if* the behavior does not occur, *then* Y consequence and not X is to follow. For example, Mr. B. (who enjoys a glass of wine after dinner) might contract to use margarine on his bread at dinner, as called for on his low saturated fat diet, in exchange for a glass of wine after his meal. In these contingency rules, a positive consequence occurs after the desired behavior and does not occur if the desired behavior does not occur.

Mahoney and Thoresen (1058) list five guidelines for developing a contract:
1. The contract should be fair.
2. The terms of the contract should be very clear.
3. The contract should be generally positive.
4. Procedures should be systematic and consistent.
5. At least one other person should participate.

While noting that a contract may be a self-contract in which the person administers his own rewards and punishments, Mahoney and Thoresen suggest that the individual might be more successful if he receives the positive consequence initially from another person.

The positive and negative consequences would, of course, have to be tailored to the individual. However, they should be readily available and follow, not precede, the behavior itself. Tokens, which could be exchanged for a reward at another time, or the reward itself should be given immediately after the patient has complied with the contracted behavior.

Contingency contracts offer a number of advantages. First, the process of developing the contract involves the patient in the planning of his regimen. This provides an opportunity to individualize treatment as well as to correct inappropriate expectations or misconceptions. Second, the contract provides a written outline of the behavioral expectations. Thus, forgetting details of the regimen can be circumvented. Third, a formal, public commitment is elicited. Kanfer et al. (1054) suggest that making promises and intentions explicit and public may foster the development of self-control over that behavior. And, fourth, the contract provides incentive value through the establishment of rewards for attainment of a self-established goal.

In addition to their contribution to the management of a variety of behavior problems, contracts have been used with modest success in the treatment of obesity (225, 1046, 1060). In these studies weight losses of 1.1 to 4.3 pounds per week were obtained under the contracting procedure. The greatest weekly loss (4.3 pounds per week) was reported in a single case study of a grossly obese ten year old with the use of successive contracts (1046), that is, subgoals for weight loss were set and as each goal was met the contract was renegotiated. In the two studies that reported follow-up data, the losses were not maintained following termination of the contract (225, 1060). Indeed, subjects in these studies subsequently gained an average of 0.9 to 1.9 pounds per week.

Success with contracts as a preventive strategy to improve blood pressure control has been reported in one controlled study (477). Patients chose the specific blood pressure intervention to emphasize, e.g., medication compliance, weight loss, stress management. The clinic nurse provided inexpensive tangible reinforcers for meeting the specific contract goals. The authors noted that these contracts resulted in lower blood pressure as well as greater weight loss, and that more appointments were kept. It should be noted that few patients contracted to improve their medication compliance. Although it is possible that compliance improved even when not specifically contracted for (as suggested by the lower blood pressures), the authors do not indicate whether this occurred.

Remediation of medication compliance was specifically addressed by Bigelow et al. (1042) in a study of disulfiram ingestion in alcoholic outpatients. In this study the patient's behavior was compared before and after the contract procedure. The contracts differed from those reported by Steckels and Swain (477). First, alternative treatments were not available to the patients. All patients were to report to the clinic daily for fourteen days and then on alternate days for a minimum of three months to receive 0.5 grams of disulfiram. Second, rather than supplying a positive reinforcer, patients placed a financial security deposit with the investigators. Failure to report to the clinic and ingest the medication resulted in forfeiture of a portion of the deposit, which was then sent to a charity. The remainder was returned to the patient at the end of the study. Thus, the patient did not have a choice of treatment modalities, and negative rather than positive reinforcement was used.

The authors reported a greater duration of alcohol abstinence using the contract procedure. Abstinence was measured by a breath-alcohol reading, alcohol-disulfiram reaction, self-report, or report of a significant other. Subjects had a median abstinence of four and one-half months during the contracting period, compared with the median of one month in over three years preceding the study. Some portion (up to $150) of the deposit was forfeited by 35% of the subjects, and 7.8% of scheduled visits were missed. That the patients themselves found contracts beneficial was apparent in that 70% of them entered into a second contract after the study period.

These studies suggest that contracts offer promise as a modality for altering health behaviors, although research is still needed in the specific area of medication compliance. Maintenance following the use of contracts remains a problem.

Graduated Regimen Implementation

Graduated regimen implementation refers to the process of introducing components of the regimen sequentially as the patient successfully masters prior steps in the sequence. The steps are graded in order of difficulty to the patient. For example, a patient with an ultimate goal of a 1000-calorie weight loss diet might begin with a 250-calorie breakfast, eating as usual the rest of the day. When he has successfully adhered to that component of the diet regimen, he adds a 250-calorie lunch, and so on. With medication, this might mean beginning with one pill a day and gradually increasing the number of pills and/or times per day medication is taken, up to the full dose. This approach assumes, of course, that a delay in reaching full medication dosage is not medically harmful.

Along with graduated regimen introduction, other principles of "shaping" (from behavioral therapy) are employed. Reinforcement is used to alter behavior gradually by systematically increasing the criteria for adequate performance and reinforcement. Matching the performance criteria to what can reasonably be expected of the patient is critical. Kanfer and Phillips (1055) claim that not doing so is a prominent cause of failure.

This sort of procedure is in wide use with a variety of behavior problems. The notion is not new to medical practice either. Gradually increasing medication doses has purportedly reduced the incidence of the side effects of prednisone in the treatment of myasthenia gravis (1065) and of progestrogen in combined oral contraception (1044). Its use as a compliance-improving strategy has been examined in just one study where it formed a single component of an intervention package (1047).

In this controlled study, cholestyramine or placebo ingestion was gradually increased to improve the compliance of poorly adhering participants in the National Heart, Lung, and Blood Institute's Lipid Research Clinics Program, the Coronary Primary Prevention Trial. The procedure worked in the following manner. Subjects recorded their daily medication taking for a three-week period. Included in the record were the number of packets taken, the time at which they were taken, and various pieces of information on the circumstances surrounding medication taking or the failure to do so. These records were reviewed with a medication counselor who then requested the participant to take a number of packets during the next week equal to or slightly less than his baseline average at the most frequent baseline time to insure the probability of successful adherence. Thus, criteria were set according to the individual's capabilities. If the participant achieved 75% compliance with that quantity, the next week his dosage was increased by one packet. When the patient reached four packets on one occasion, a second time per day was introduced at the second most commonly occurring time during baseline and so on until the full dose required by the study protocol was achieved.

During a six-week intervention period, significantly more participants in the group described above attained or exceeded a 75% compliance rate in the full study dose than in control and attention control groups which did not receive the intervention (P < .01); the former also achieved greater reductions in cholesterol levels (P < .05). However, as the group was followed beyond the intervention period, a slow but persistent rise in cholesterol levels was seen.

Like tailoring, gradual regimen inplementation does have intuitive appeal when the prescription requires a complex set of behaviors. It is clearly an avenue worth further exploration both as a remedial strategy and as a method of introducing patients to a complicated regimen.

Self-monitoring

Self-monitoring is a process of observing and recording one's own behavior. It has been widely used in various behavioral strategies and has formed a component of most self-control programs (1067). Its utility has been primarily as a data collection device.

Evidence has grown, however, that self-monitoring or record keeping may be a useful intervention strategy (1052, 1059, 1063). One hypothesis is that self-monitoring alters behavior (1053). That is, the individual observes one of his behaviors, evaluates it, and then regulates it. If this is so, then it should be an effective procedure with the individual who misperceives his own actions. There is, indeed, some evidence for this. In a study of medication compliance in which self-monitoring and increased attention comprised the intervention for one of the groups, improvement was noted in a subset of patients who both overestimated their compliance rates and showed greater variability in the amount of medication taken daily (1047). Further, since misperceptions of compliance were associated with greater variability in compliance, it was quite possible that the clients' erratic performance led them to misperceive the quantity of medication they were actually taking. Self-monitoring might have provided the corrective feedback needed for improvement.

Self-monitoring has been evaluated as an intervention technique in weight loss programs, but the results have been inconsistent. Romanczyk (1064) reported that monitoring of food intake was effective although monitoring of body weight was not. Others reported that recording what was about to be eaten rather than what had been eaten was effective when other forms of monitoring were not (1041). Thus, the effectiveness of self-monitoring might be a function of the behavior monitored: monitoring the behavior (eating) that leads to some goal (weight loss) was more effective than monitoring progress toward the goal (weight).

This theory receives support in the few compliance studies which used self-monitoring as the primary intervention. Carnahan and Nugent (88) examined the effect of home monitoring of blood pressure on hypertension control. The authors speculated that increased awareness of this asymptomatic condition through self-monitoring might increase drug compliance. They found, however, that diastolic blood pressures of experimental subjects were not significantly reduced compared to those of controls. Thus, as in weight loss, monitoring of the physiological outcome measure may not be the most effective process.

Moulding (365) suggested that daily medication displayed on a calendar might provide feedback similar to self-monitoring. He found that the use of such a calendar improved regular medication taking, but his study lacked concurrent control subjects. Similar results were found by Marshall et al. (1061) in a study using weekly medication dispensers. Neither of these studies, however, actually involved patients recording their behaviors.

As noted earlier, self-monitoring of medication was used by Dunbar (1047) with one group in a controlled study of low compliers. Following treatment, compliance did not differ significantly between experimental and control subjects. However, over six months of follow-up, experimental subjects made continuous and progressive gains in compliance with concomitant reductions in cholesterol which were not seen in the other groups. This suggests that although self-monitoring did not achieve dramatic immediate effects, its influence may become more apparent over time and produce an effect of longer duration. Maletzky (1059) also reported maintenance of weight loss following self-monitoring when a gradually tapering schedule of booster sessions was used during the follow-up period. This is contrary to Mahoney (1056) who suggested that the effects of self-monitoring tend to be short-lived. Mahoney, Moura, and Wade (1057) also found that the effects of self-monitoring alone were weak. Barlow (1040) has suggested that the influence of self-monitoring can be strengthened when: (1) the patient is motivated to change; (2) the behavior being observed is easy to discriminate; (3) recording materials are easy to use; (4) the patient is instructed in how to self-monitor; (5) recording occurs in close time proximity to the behavior; (6) feedback is provided; and (7) the patient knows the report will be checked for accuracy.

Reinforcement

An essential component in each of the preceding strategies to improve compliance is *reinforcement*, which refers to any consequence that increases the probability of the behavior being repeated. Reinforcement may include such techniques as praise for a job well done or a self-administered treat (positive reinforcement) for successful performance, paying some monetary penalty or foregoing that evening cocktail (aversive reinforcement or punishment) for failure to carry out the behavior. What reinforces a specific person's behavior is clearly an individual matter.

Behavior does tend to be regulated by its consequences, with the individual usually discarding activities that are punished or unrewarded and retaining those that are rewarded. It becomes easy to see, then, why patients on preventive regimens might be the poorest compliers. Their daily health activities go unrewarded, with the only motivating factor being some increased probability of avoiding an aversive consequence in the distant future (e.g., stroke for the hypertensive patient or myocardial infarction for the hypercholesterolemic patient). This is not to say that reinforcement must always be immediate, for Bandura (1039) suggests that most behaviors are largely under "anticipatory control," that is, the anticipation of reward. However, more immediate reinforcements are important in building a new behavior into a person's life, e.g., taking a new long-term medication, reducing caloric intake, modifying the fat content in the diet. It should be noted that reinforcement *alone* would be an inefficient means of teaching a patient how to perform a new health behavior, but once the behavior has been taught through educational strategies, reinforcement is important to its continued performance. Early in the implementation of a regimen, the reinforcements ought to be immediate. Later on they might be delayed, with the anticipation of the delayed consequences sustaining the regimen. It is likely, however, that periodic tangible reinforcement is important to maintenance.

The value of reinforcement in behavioral intervention programs has been widely demonstrated (1041, 1050, 1057, 1060). Both Bellack (1041) and Mahoney et al. (1057) reported greater weight losses in self-reward groups than in groups which did not utilize positive reinforcement. Aversive reinforcements have been found useful as well in contingency contracting programs for weight loss (1060) and for medication compliance among alcoholics (1042). Mahoney et al. (1057) suggest, however, that positive reinforcement is superior to aversive consequences, at least when self-administered. One must, of course, question the willingness of individuals to self-administer punishment.

In addition to the self-administration of reinforcement, there is value to externally administered consequences, at least early in an intervention program. For the clinician, his time and attention to the patient may be the most powerful available reinforcer; there is evidence that the quantity of time a patient spends with the clinician is positively related to compliance (295, 1051).

External administration of reinforcements need not be limited to the clinician. In fact, they might be administered more powerfully by those persons in the patient's immediate environment, who are not only most significant to the patient but also most readily available at the time the health behavior occurs. Both family members and peers have been found to be important reinforcers in compliance programs (4, 384, 604, 1037, 1038, 1048). For example, in the work site studies by Alderman (4, 1037, 1038) it appears that the encouragement provided by other union members, family, and friends may have accounted for a large portion of the program's success in producing blood pressure control. Similarly, in a review of studies involving family members in medical compliance, Becker and Green (604) reported that support and encouragement (forms of positive reinforcement) were important to the patient's compliance with the regimen.

Thus, not only is reinforcement an important component in many preventive or remedial compliance-improving strategies, but it can come from a variety of sources. Initially, it might be offered by family, friends, and/or peers (suggesting the importance of educating these persons in the appropriate conduct of the regimen) and then by the patient himself (e.g., self-administration of a reward). The clinician should not forget his value as a contributor to and coordinator of compliance reinforcement for the patient.

MAINTENANCE INTERVENTIONS

One of the major problems in compliance is maintenance over the long term. A number of studies have demonstrated a persistent decline as time passes (200, 442, 505). Unfortunately, the compliance-improving strategies that have been tested generally have not shown evidence of continuing effects when the intervention is withdrawn (225, 228, 1047, 1060).

This, of course, is not an atypical finding with a variety of interventions and problems. In the investigation of behavioral interventions we may have created our own difficulties with the widespread use of reversal designs to demonstrate therapeutic efficacy. That is, studies in which behavior returned to baseline conditions when treatment was stopped after a treatment effect had been demonstrated were convenient for assessing alternative treatments, but the accompanying lack of maintenance was generally ignored. This may have had the undesirable result of selecting out techniques that were immediately powerful but that were without lasting effects.

As more attention has been paid to maintenance in recent years, considerable speculation has arisen regarding conditions that could foster a lasting effect of treatment. For example, Bandura (1039) states that behavior is least susceptible to varying situational inducements if the reinforcement is either intrinsic to the behavior itself or is self-generated. The question, then, is how can these best be incorporated into a behavioral strategy?

It has been postulated that in the early stages of behavior change self-reinforcement may be learned through reinforcement by others and by observing others reinforcing themselves (1039, 1062). Some activities also have naturally occurring intrinsic value, for example, the relief of muscle tension with relaxation exercises or the relief of hunger through eating. However, even many activities that individuals find rewarding in themselves may have no reinforcement value when coupled with uncomfortable regimens. For example, the runner who enjoys running for the sense of peacefulness and general well-being it brings has to persist through muscle pain, fatigue, and scheduling adjustments before running becomes a pleasure in itself. Thus, extrinsic reinforcers may be necessary during the initial stages. The implication is that the nature and source of the reinforcement and how it is applied may be important factors in inducing maintenance of treatment. Furthermore, the effects may differ depending on the stage of implemetation of the regimen. For instance, after initial external reinforcement, it may become important to switch the emphasis toward the development of self-reinforcement. Extrinsic reinforcement may then be reduced gradually to periodic "booster sessions" (1059). As noted above, concurrent with the initial external reinforcement the opportunity might be afforded for the patient to observe as others evaluate and reinforce their own related performance. Of course, research is still necessary to establish the efficacy of this approach.

Based on the research literature, two other strategies show some promise. One is the use of self-monitoring, although the results have been varied. As noted earlier, Mahoney (1056) contends that the effects of self-monitoring are not enduring, at least with weight loss. Dunbar (1047), however, reported greater long-term effects among a self-monitoring control group, in the three-group medication compliance study citied earlier, than was seen with the experimental group, despite better short-term results among experimental group subjects. There is some evidence, then, that given the patient with those characteristics noted earlier (misperception of own compliance and variability in performance), short-term self-monitoring might induce long-term change.

The other strategy that shows promise in producing maintenance is to involve the spouse in the treatment regimen. Brownell (1045), in an obesity study, examined the effect of cooperative participating spouses, cooperative nonparticipating spouses, and noncooperative spouses on weight loss using the same behavioral treatment package in all three groups. The unusual touch to Brownell's study was that the participating spouses not only attended the group sessions and learned about the weight loss regimen, but were also responsible for carrying it out themselves. The groups did not differ in weight loss immediately following treatment, but there were marked differences after a six month follow-up period with the participating spouse group clearly outperforming the others. An average of 29.6 pounds had been lost by this group, compared with 19.4 in the cooperative nonparticipating spouse group, and 15.1 in the noncooperative spouse group. The latter two groups did not differ significantly. Thus, the clinician might attempt to involve the spouse or other family members as participants in health behavior regimens such as dietary or exercise regimens, plaque control programs, or the use of seat belts. This, of course, would be less feasible in the case of medication taking. Here self-management strategies (e.g., self-monitoring, contracting, self-reinforcement) might be more useful, with the family assuming reinforcing roles.

While the problems of maintenance are far from being solved, at least three strategies appear capable of producing enduring change. Continuing research efforts are clearly needed in this aspect of compliance management.

TABLE 11.2. Selected controlled compliance-improving studies: behavioral interventions

Technique	Purpose	
	Prevention	Remediation
Reminders	Brigg and Mudd (1043) Lima et al. (312) Nazarian et al. (375) Shmarak (1066) Turner and Vernon (1068)	
Tailoring	Hallburg (1049)	Best (49) Haynes et al. (228)
Contracting	Dinoff et al. (1046) Harris and Bruner (225) Mann (1060) Steckel and Swain (477)	Bigelow et al.(1042)
Graduated regimen implementation		Dunbar (1047)
Self-monitoring	Bellak et al. (1041) Carnahan and Nugent (88) Mahoney et al. (1057) Maletzky (1059) Marshall (1061) Romanczyk (1064)	Dunbar (1047) Haynes et al (228)
Reinforcement	Bellak et al. (1041) Bigelow et al. (1042) Hladek and White (1050) Mahoney et al. (1057) Mann (1060)	
Family/peer support	Alderman (1037) Alderman et al. (1038) Brownell et al. (1045) Fass et al. (1048) Oakes et al. (348)	

CONCLUSIONS

The improvement of patient compliance is a major need in health care. The application of behavioral strategies to these problems has demonstrated utility. Among these strategies are reminders, tailoring, contracting, graduated regimen implementation, self-monitoring, and reinforcement, with self-reinforcement, self-monitoring, and spouse participation appearing especially useful in promoting enduing changes (see Table 11.2).

Although the independent effect of these strategies on compliance has not been dramatic, each has contributed to the improvement of compliance. There is a pressing need for further research into specific types of compliance problems, for matching patient characteristics to each strategy, and for generating guidelines for their administration. Until such time, the clinician is advised to utilize package interventions that are composed of multiple strategies, for these appear capable of achieving clinically meaningful improvements in compliance.

IV
ALTERING
HARMFUL LIFESTYLES

12

A Media Role for
Public Health Compliance?

A. Benjamin Kelley

"All of us who care so much and work so hard to make the people healthier and longer lived would be ever so much more effective—if only those people would cooperate!" That is a not unfair statement of a chief frustration among physicians, public health workers, safety activists, and medical researchers. It is a fact of life that human beings, with their countless differences in habits, biases, preferences, fears, and backgrounds, often seem to be the principal stumbling blocks to the effective implementation of health programs *intended to aid those very human beings.* "If it weren't for the people, think how much we could help them."

The most effective programs for producing desirable public health changes are those that, all other things being equal, do not depend on modifying the behavior of the beneficiaries or those around them. These "passive" approaches that work automatically without relying on individual cooperation (as opposed to "active" approaches that require changed behavior by individuals) have been shown repeatedly throughout public health history to have much higher payoffs, and over longer duration, than do the active alternatives (686, 1074, 1080).

For instance, the successful elimination of milk as a transmitter of bovine tuberculosis came not through "educational" efforts to persuade housewives to heat milk before serving it—such efforts had little if any effect—but through the pasteurization of all milk at source of production, thus automatically eliminating the public health hazard.

Nevertheless, in an imperfect world, much that will benefit people's health and longevity must be brought to them in active form, and so must depend for effectiveness on the cooperative participation of the people themselves.

A prerequisite to much behavioral change in humans is communicating to them information, concepts, instructions, analogs, and data. It thus follows that the media may have an important influence on what people think and do. Does it further follow that this influence can be harnessed in the interest of improving public health?

THE PRESENT STATE OF KNOWLEDGE

Research results, informed judgment, and the attitudes of both media and public health workers strongly suggest that although the media may have considerable influence over the public health attitudes, decisions, and actions of their audience, that influence is difficult to harness dependably to effect public health improvements.

It has traditionally been a premise, untested but widely held, that by transmitting exhortations for behavioral change, the media could serve as a catalyst between public health agencies (both governmental and private) and people at large in bringing about public health improvements. (For radio and television, this has been formalized in the United States by the provision of predetermined time slots for the airing of "public service messages.")

Before deciding whether to use the media for conveying information and exhortation intended to improve public health behaviors, however, medical and public health workers should ask the sorts of questions they would ask about the fielding of a new drug, a new surgical technique, or any other proposed countermeasure to a threat to life or health. The questions include these:

1. What is the intended result of the planned message campaign?

2. Is there a reasonable expectation that the campaign will lead to that result?

3. Can the effectiveness of the campaign be premeasured, at least roughly?

4. Can the effectiveness of the campaign be measured both during the campaign and after it?

5. Are there better ways to accomplish the same results?

These questions are rarely asked and practically never answered by users of "free" broadcast time and print space (431). Some recent studies, however, have attempted to determine whether the media in fact can promote attitudinal and behavioral changes leading to desirable predetermined improvements in public health.

MASS MEDIA CAMPAIGNS TO
PROMOTE SAFETY BELT USE IN AUTOMOBILES

The use of safety belts in automobiles greatly reduces the probability of death and injury in crashes (1082). However, the availability of safety belts does not guarantee their use. In October 1970 a study was conducted that included actual observation of drivers in their automobiles. In a metropolitan area only 6.5% of drivers of 1968 and later models were using lap and upper torso belts and an additional 16.3% were using lap belts only (432). Belts, even when present, were used less often in earlier models. In spite of a number of campaigns urging safety belt use, the proportion of vehicle occupants using them is so low that much of the reduction in death and injury that should be achieved by their use is not being realized.

Campaigns promoting the use of safety belts had been based on inadequate knowledge of the factors contributing to lack of use. Slogans such as "buckle up for safety," "lock it to me," "what's your excuse," and the like were the hallmarks of these campaigns. When the campaigns were evaluated at all in terms of effectiveness, the evaluations were faulty in design and execution (1077, 1078). Even with free public service time and space contributed by television, radio, and newspapers, the cost of these campaigns was usually high and the results inconclusive.

Although methodologically inadequate, previous studies of the effects of mass media efforts on safety belt use were not encouraging. A 1968 campaign by the National Safety Council used the equivalent of $51,509,034 in public service time and space in various media. Self-claimed use of safety belts, obtained by interviewing a national sample of 2,500 adults before and after the campaign, revealed no change in claimed usage (1071). However, random public service time is often the least desirable time in radio and television. Also, claimed use of safety belts has been shown to be an invalid measure of actual use (836).

In a 1971 study, Fleischer selected a number of radio and television safety belt messages from among those produced in recent years by the National Safety Council, the American Safety Belt Council, and the US Department of Transportation (1073). When these messages were exposed to expert and lay panels, there was wide disagreement over which messages the panel members thought would be effective. The experts emphasized entertainment value and avoidance of the "scare approach" while the lay panel rated highly those messages with "scare content".

Subsequently, safety belt use was studied in three communities by Fleischer during a radio and television campaign using materials selected according to the panel ratings. A mix of those messages rated highly by experts and laymen was employed. Similar in demographic characteristics, the three communities were given intensive exposure, moderate exposure, and no exposure, respectively, in a five-week campaign on local radio and television. Observed safety belt use increased slightly in the intensive and no-exposure communities but not in the one receiving moderate exposure. Postcampaign use was about the same as precampaign use in all three communities.

These seemingly paradoxical results may be a result of insufficient control on the part of observers rather than differences in safety belt usage. The observers in Fleischer's study were allowed to choose or change observation sites at their convenience, for example, to avoid having the sun in their eyes. We have found that safety belt use rates can vary among sites in the same community by an order of magnitude larger than that found between communities in the Fleischer study.

In the work in this area with which I have been involved, we attempted, I believe successfully, to overcome many of the methodologic problems of previous studies. The studies we carried out under the auspices of the Insurance Institute for Highway Safety sought to determine the effectiveness of a television commercial campaign to increase safety belt use (431). Our aim was to design and execute as definitive a test of mass media as present knowledge and technology would allow.

In preparation for this study, investigation was undertaken to determine some of the factors influencing safety belt use. It is worthwhile considering the methods and findings of this developmental study before describing the main study further.

The preliminary survey consisted of interviews with safety belt users as detected by trained roadside observers and a random sample of nonusers observed at the same sites and times. We found that the higher the respondent's education, the greater the likelihood that he was observed wearing a safety belt. Those who rated safety belts as relatively more comfortable and convenient, those who said that they did not smoke while driving, and those who had a friend or relative injured but not killed in an automobile crash were also more likely to use belts. Furthermore, these factors were additive, that is, the presence of each factor increased the probability of use independent of other factors (432).

We utilized the findings from this study to develop the content of television commercials to promote safety belt use. For example, the finding that a friend's injury but not death increased the probability of use suggested to us that the fear of being disfigured or disabled is more motivating in the use of safety belts than fear of death in a crash. Thus, we decided to emphasize the efficacy of safety belts in decreasing disfigurement and disability.

We were more wary of the comfort and convenience factor. Realizing that because of poor design, the safety belts in many automobiles are uncomfortable and inconvenient, we did not want to reinforce the tendency not to use belts because of this factor. Since smoking while driving and educational background probably reflect a number of differences in personal characteristics including risk-taking behavior and self-esteem, which we do not believe are readily manipulable by television messages, these factors were not considered in the creation of the messages.

In addition to the information gained from the preliminary study, we also decided to utilize techniques that are said in the advertising industry to be successful in product marketing, for example, physician endorsement and a family responsibility theme.

Television messages were then written and produced in collaboration with an advertising agency that had a record of success in advertising commercial products as well as experience with public service material. The preliminary study and some ideas for messages were shared with the writers from the agency.

These writers then outlined many messages, some of which were selected and modified in subsequent discussion. Six basic messages were eventually developed and filmed.

By industry standards, the messages were of high quality. Of the two messages entered in advertising industry competition, one was judged the best among 30 entries in the public service category of the TV-Radio Advertisers Club of Philadelphia and the other was among the ten finalists of 400 entries in the public service category of the Advertising Club of New York. The latter was also chosen as a finalist among the public service entries in the American TV and Radio Commercials Festival and National Print Advertising Competition. An informal opinion was obtained from the Director of the National Association of Broadcasters Code Authority that the messages were in compliance with the code.

The messages were not shown indiscriminately. Each was placed on or adjacent to a program likely to have an audience to whom the message would most likely appeal. For example, "the witch" was shown on network children's programs, "the father and son" on National Football League games, and "the scarred faces" on popular soap operas. No attempt was made to control what was shown in addition to our messages. For example, a number of automobile manufacturers had "tag lines" urging safety belt use at the end of their commercials throughout the study period. Of course, these were shown to both experimental and control groups and are thus constant for both audiences.

To evaluate the impact of these messages, they were shown on one cable of a unique dual cable television system designed for marketing studies (1070). Located in a county of 230,000 people (1970 census), the two cables feed television signals to 13,800 households. There are 6,400 of these households on Cable A, on which our messages were shown, and 7,400 on Cable B, which is, in this case, the control cable. Each cable contains the full range of channels available from local stations as well as special movie and weather channels.

The two cables are distributed in a checkerboard fashion among blocks of homes in the community that have chosen to pay for the improved signal that the cable provides. Although the assignment of households to one or another cable is not strictly random, the various marketing studies done in the community have found no significant differences between the two service populations in terms of demographic characteristics, ownership of automobiles and other consumer goods, and pretest purchasing behavior for a large number of products (1069).

To assess safety belt utilization, we used maps of the cable distribution among the streets and traffic flow maps obtained from the local traffic engineer and chose observation sites at points that maximized the likelihood of observing automobiles from the neighborhoods where the cables were installed. Observers were assigned to a particlar site for a given number of hours on a given day. No deviation from the observation sites was allowed.

TABLE 12.1. Number of safety belt messages shown by month and time of day

| | 1971 | | | | | | | 1972 | | |
	June	July	Aug.	Sept.	Oct.	Nov.	Dec.	Jan.	Feb.	Total
Sign-on to noon	30	31	40	53	32	32	12	14	33	277
	21%	28%	29%	48%	30%	33%	17%	19%	34%	
12:01 to 6:00 p.m.	105	68	78	43	50	25	26	41	43	479
	73%	62%	57%	39%	48%	26%	38%	55%	45%	
6:01 p.m. to sign-off	8	11	19	15	23	40	31	20	20	187
	6%	10%	14%	13%	22%	41%	45%	27%	21%	
Total	143	110	137	111	105	97	69	75	96	943

NOTE: Percentages are based on the total number of messages in a given month.

Observing the driver only, observers stood at designated sites on the opposite side from the driver of an approaching automobile. Using a small hand-held tape recorder, the driver's sex, racial appearance, and approximate age were recorded. The driver's use or nonuse of lap or lap-and-shoulder belts was observed as the automobile passed the observer. The automobile license number was then obtained as the automobile moved away.

The license plate numbers were matched with the owner's names and addresses using the files of the state department of motor vehicles. The names and addresses were then matched to the file specifying which cable was assigned to given households. In those cases where the household was not on a cable, the household was specified as to whether or not it was in the same county as the cable groups. Thus, there are four groups for comparison: Cable A households where the messages were shown; Cable B households, which constitute a control group; noncable households in the same county as the cable households; and out-of-county households.

The messages were shown for nine months on Cable A exclusively. Table 12.1 presents the distribution of the messages by time of day over the nine-month period from 7 June 1971 through 5 March 1972. For the first few months the messages were shown mainly in daytime hours. In the late fall and winter more "prime" evening time became available through the courtesy of insurance companies and other advertisers who were running test advertising dealing with other subjects on Cable B and were willing to have public service advertising on Cable A. These arrangements were made with the parent companies so that local affiliates of the companies were unaware of the experiment. The local television station managers were aware of the campaign, as they are of all tests on the experimental cable system.

There were fewer exposures in the later months because more people can be reached by exposures in prime time. We estimate, on the basis of audience ratings for the programs on which the messages were shown, that the average television viewer saw one or another of the messages two or three times per

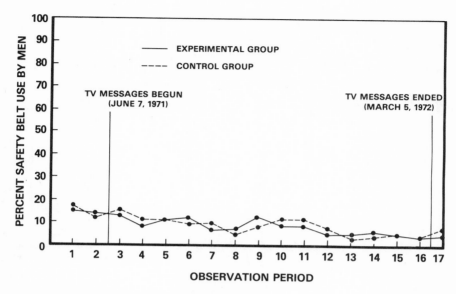

FIGURE 12.1. Percent safety belt use by men.

week. In total, the campaign was equivalent to the type of major advertising effort that companies use to promote a new product. If this campaign had been sponsored on a national basis, it would have cost approximately $7,000,000.

The results of the study were clearcut. The campaign had no effect whatsoever on safety belt use. Figure 12.1 shows the percentage of observed male drivers using lap or lap-and-shoulder belts for each of the time periods necessary to observe drivers at all of the designated sites. Only 1964 and later cars are included. The number of observations on which the percentage is based is shown beside each percentage.

There were no significant differences between drivers from households on the experimental cable and drivers from households on the control cable in any of the observation periods. Also, there were no differences in use between those on the cables and other drivers observed at the same sites whether from in or out of the county. The same conclusions must be reached when the data for females are viewed in Figure 12.2.

There was a downward drift in safety belt use from the spring through the winter months, more remarkable among male than among female drivers. However, this decline occurred in the control and noncable groups as much as in the experimental group. Therefore, it cannot be argued that the messages had a deleterious effect on safety belt use. Some unknown factor or factors contributed to decreased use of safety belts in the winter months in all of the groups studied. The overall use rates were significantly lower for black persons (3%)

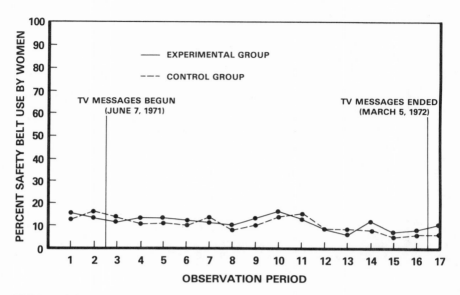

FIGURE 12.2. Percent safety belt use by women.

than for whites (10%), as was found in earlier studies (1072). Age differences were small and not statistically significant.

The failure of these campaigns to increase safety belt use adds evidence to the argument that mass media approaches are inefficient and ineffective means of reducing highway losses (1081). Passive approaches (1075), such as air bags that inflate on impact and do not depend on voluntary action, show greater promise for reducing deaths and injuries in crashes, just as such passive approaches have historically proven more successful in closely analogous public health situations. Some passive devices, for example, energy-absorbing steering columns and wind-shields that perform like fire nets, have been required by US federal standards since 1968 and have been shown to produce large reductions in fatalities and injuries (1076).

The apparent failure of a number of mass media safety belt campaigns to increase use beyond precampaign levels may not mean that it is impossible to create a campaign that will increase safety belt use. However, the negative evidence is sufficiently strong that the burden of proof of substantial gains in belt usage resulting from such campaigns is on those who advocate use of mass media for this purpose.

Mass Media Campaigns to Reduce Cardiovascular Risk

A recently completed project, the Stanford Heart Disease Prevention Pro-gram, has sought to use combinations of face-to-face influence, mass media information, and each in isolation to influence behavioral patterns bearing on tendencies toward cardiovascular disease. Although the project has just been completed and has not been evaluated finally at this time, the researchers conducting it believe that the use of mass media to change such behaviors has been effective in their project. They have concluded:

> Mass media are potentially much more cost-effective than face-to-face education methods. Our results show that mass media can increase knowledge and change various health habits, but we believe that the power of this instrument could be considerably enhanced if we could find ways to use mass media to stimulate and coordinate programs of interpersonal instruction in natural communities (such as towns and factories) and to deliver forms of specialized training and counselling about weight-loss and smoking avoidance (156).

Unfortunately, follow-up in this study was complete for only about two-thirds of the original participants and it remains to be demonstrated that mass media are indeed cost-effective in changing health habits. Readers interested in determining the value of mass media in promoting healthful behaviors should certanly seek the final evaluation of the Stanford project.

CONCLUSION AND RESEARCH PRIORITIES

While the appeal of mass media campaigns is widespread among those who wish to promote healthful behaviors in the general community, there is no solid evidence on which to base endorsements of this method. On the contrary, there is good evidence that the media have little or no impact on such elementary health practices as safety belt use. The preliminary results of the Stanford Heart Disease Prevetion Program are more encouraging, but this study is already flawed by incomplete follow-up of participants.

I would strongly urge those who promote the use of mass media for public health purposes to evaluate their programs according to the questions posed earlier in this article. Potential buyers or users of mass media should demand nothing short of rigorous evaluation before proceeding along this route.

Pending the final results of the Stanford Project, I would think that research into this area has relatively low priority in view of our experience. The passive approaches alluded to in this article are quite obviously superior, in terms of morbidity and mortality, to methods such as persuasion through mass media, which require active ongoing changes in the behavior of individuals.

13

Compliance
in the Control
of Cigarette Smoking

J. Allan Best and Maurice Bloch

INTRODUCTION

The concept of compliance is utilized in a variety of empirical literatures (1112). Each has its own methodology, research questions, and unique contribution to make to our understanding of compliance. We therefore need to clarify the way the concept of compliance applies to smoking modification.

Studies in smoking modification differ from most other compliance investigations in that the focus has been on outcomes rather than on regimen adherence. Many researchers have myopically evaluated the results of different intervention strategies with no consideration of the extent to which smokers actually followed treatment recommendations in reaching these outcomes.

There are several factors contributing to the smoking literature's focus on outcomes or effectiveness. First, most compliance studies deal with well-established medical procedures. In contrast, we do not have smoking techniques that produce such reliable therapeutic effects. Second, medical regimens and smoking modification techniques differ in nature, and most regimens in the compliance literature involve the taking of medications. The concern is with a pharmacological prescription designed to produce biophysical effects. With smoking, on the other hand, we have behavioral prescriptions (e.g., instructing the client to smoke only in certain circumstances) that we hope will produce behavioral effects (reducing smoking). These behavioral effects may lead in turn to biophysical effects but our concern is with initiating behavior-behavior relationships. Such behavior-behavior relationships may be inherently less reliable than pharmacological-biophysical relationships. Furthermore, regimen adherence and

Preparation of this chapter was facilitated by grant 1212-9-42-1 from the Non-Medical Use of Drugs Directorate, Health and Welfare Canada. The address of the first author is now Department of Health Studies, University of Waterloo, Waterloo, Ontario, Canada, N2L 3G1.

the effects of such adherence are far from independent. If the client begins to follow a regimen, he or she may receive immediate feedback on the effect of compliance. This experience of the regimen's outcome in part determines the degree of continuing compliance. This consideration seems especially cogent with respect to lifestyle change regimens. In sum, the study of compliance in smoking and other lifestyle modification programs is particularly challenging since factors affecting regimen adherence and outcome must be considered jointly.

Our health delivery system is rapidly moving toward a more integrated consideration of the full range of factors affecting morbidity and mortality. We are increasingly concerned with prevention and health lifestyle (1160). A consideration of the problems and promises in the smoking modification literature may thus contribute to our understanding of compliance in this broader context.

PRESENT STATE OF KNOWLEDGE

Research in the smoking modification area has grown explosively in the past ten to fifteen years as a function of our increasing knowledge of the serious health consequences associated with chronic cigarette consumption. There are several comprehensive reviews documenting the lack of success in early attempts to modify smoking behavior (1091, 1156, 1172, 1178, 1220). Similarly, there are excellent reviews detailing more recent progress (736, 1093, 1176).

The aims of the present review are (1) to summarize the empirical data on a variety of therapeutic approaches to smoking modification, including studies published since prior reviews; (2) to focus on issues particularly related to the study of compliance; and (3) to identify general trends in the results that give rise to guidelines for clinical practice.

The smoking literature is a good starting point in a consideration of compliance and lifestyle modification for two reasons. On the one hand, it is a convenient lifestyle to study. On the other hand, it is a complex lifestyle, one that is difficult to change, and thus one from which we can learn a great deal as we increase our understanding and improve the effectiveness of change procedures.

The Study of Smoking

Smoking is convenient to study: it is observable, occurs in discrete units, and has an absolute zero. Thus it can be quantified and measured reliably. We have an absolute standard—abstinence—against which to evaluate our success. Furthermore, smoking is a problem that occurs at a high rate in the general population, represents a very serious health risk, and is an aspect of lifestyle that many people would like to change. Nine out of ten smokers claim they either have tried to quit or would try if effective means were available (1240).

Determinants of Smoking

However, smoking is complex. We only partially understand the factors that control its occurrence. The pharmacological effects of nicotine certainly play a role (1120), and they may interact with individual physiological differences in promoting smoking behavior (1124). Furthermore, a person's mood or affective state may determine smoking (1237, 1238). There are also social influences on smoking (1134, 1147, 1180, 1181, 1186, 1215). As a result of the individual's learning history, smoking may be associated with a need to relax, to relieve boredom, or to have a reward. To a large extent, smoking occurs for no "good" reason at all; rather, it occurs because it is a habit associated through experience with a wide variety of smoking situations, such as the end of a meal or a cup of coffee (705, 1145). Because it is an "overlearned" habit, smoking often occurs so automatically that the individual is unaware of what factors control his smoking behavior (1145).

Thus, smoking is controlled by a diverse set of factors including pharmacological, environmental, affective, and cognitive cues and consequences. Smoking seems tied to a wide variety of specific situations (1095). The pattern of reasons for smoking varies considerably across individuals and is typically complex for any one smoker. This multifaceted view of factors controlling smoking behavior has major implications for studies of smoking modification and compliance. As with any behavioral excess, the design of an effective therapeutic regimen is likely to necessitate consideration of those factors currently controlling the behavior. The degree of regimen compliance and ultimate success of the program thus will depend on the institution of competing forms of control that result in alternative (nonsmoking) behaviors.

Client Characteristics

The smoker brings with him to treatment not only an idiosyncratic and complicated set of reasons for smoking but also a variety of personality, attitudinal, and motivational characteristics that affect his response to treatment. Such individual differences generally have not been good predictors of compliance (605, 1112), although conceptually these factors may affect both regimen adherence and the effectiveness of the compliance-improving strategy. In the smoking literature, demographic variables such as age and sex have been related to the outcome of smoking modification programs (119, 280, 415, 447, 1118, 1122, 1138). The typical positive finding is that older, male smokers tend to be more successful in quitting and/or remaining abstinent. However, as will be found true for all client characteristics reviewed, a large number of studies have failed to demonstrate the age and sex relationship. Furthermore, in those cases where a significant effect was demonstrated, the magnitude of the effect was usually small and of little clinical value.

Many smoking modification studies have administered at least some, if not a host, of personality measures. Unhappily, the results of these attempts are decidedly negative with respect to the consistent contribution of a specific trait to success in quitting (47, 48, 49, 1096, 1097, 1171, 1184, 1219, 1227).

Success in giving up smoking has been shown to vary directly with motivation to change and expectations of success (47, 48, 1097, 1122, 1178, 1218), and inversely with pretreatment smoking rate (48, 1118, 1122). Again, however, a far larger number of studies have failed to find these relationships.

In sum, it must be concluded that demographic, personality, and motivational factors have not been shown to predict success in smoking modification programs. This conclusion holds true despite the common finding, noted below, that the particular form of treatment also contributes little to success. (Surely some treatment or client variables must give rise to the fact that some smokers quit while others do not!) The possibility remains that individual differences do contribute to outcome, but that these are sufficiently idiosyncratic and complex as to have thus far eluded attempts at empirical specification.

A few studies have examined the interaction between client and treatment variables. Client characteristics may combine with aspects of the treatment program such that successful outcome can be facilitated by tailoring treatment to the individual. For example, we have demonstrated statistically significant benefits from matching clients to modification regimens on the basis of both motivational and personality measures (49, 1096, 1097). Similarly, Hildebrandt and Feldman (1146) suggest that smokers initially low on "commitment" benefit more from a commitment training procedure. Conway (1107) suggested that individuals who generally tend to feel in control of the consequences of their actions may make better use of a self-control training manual. Pechacek (1199) found that anxious smokers tended to benefit more from stress management training procedures, although the work of Levenberg and Wagner (1164) did not reveal this interaction. Unfortunately, although the proportion of positive associations seems high when we study client-treatment interaction, the magnitude of the relationships remains small. This is consistent with the broader literature on individual differences, which finds only weak relationships between general trait measures and responses to specific circumstances (1100, 1190). We are more likely to find interactions between variations in the individual's smoking pattern and analysis of his response to treatment (48, 651, 1091, 1117, 1135, 1185, 1202), and some preliminary work in this area is described below.

SMOKING MODIFICATION STRATEGIES

In a determined effort to help smokers quit, clinicians of differing persuasions have used a wide variety of strategies. These may be grouped roughly into five classes: (1) group strategies, (2) educational and attitude change strategies,

(3) pharmacological strategies, (4) hypnotic strategies, and (5) behavior modification strategies.

Group Strategies

Group meetings are a popular context for smoking modification efforts. They vary widely as to specific content but may be characterized broadly as a means for smokers to come together for help from clinic organizers and from each other. Free discussion is common and it is assumed that the discussion per se (as well as the dynamics typically operative in small groups, i.e., encouragement, moral support, and social pressure) may facilitate quitting. These factors are frequently augmented by health information and specific tips from the organizers.

In general, the results of such clinics are quite consistent, suggesting long-term smoking cessation rates of between 15% and 20% (303, 1138, 1151, 1205, 1221, 1239, 1246). On occasion, long-term results have been nearer 30%. This higher rate may be associated with a major medical involvement in the clinic and/or inclusion of various specific change procedures (267, 280, 1118).

Many of the group approaches have not been properly evaluated with appropriate controls. Thus, when waiting lists or minimal treatment controls have been incorporated into the evaluations, the results suggest that group approaches add little to the smoker's unaided efforts to quit. However, this does not mean that groups are of no value. The social context and interaction may well provide a vehicle for effective impact. It does mean that group meetings must include effective content, perhaps drawn from some of the alternatives described below, if they are to promote cessation.

Education and Attitude Change Strategies

Health behavior change can be viewed as a two-step process. First, the individual must become motivated to change. This can occur as the individual acquires information about the health risk associated with a behavior and accepts the degree of personal risk. Second, the individual must take action to change. The preliminary action of requesting help with smoking cessation does not assure that the individual is well motivated for change, and many clinic attenders express ambivalence toward quitting. Procedures that are educative and/or produce attitude change are important in this context.

Most research in this area has explored the effects of persuasive communications designed to produce fear about the health hazards of smoking (334, 1150, 1165, 1173, 1202, 1211, 1228). Typically, smokers have taken part in the role playing of a patient/physician interaction during which the smoker is given the distressing news that he has lung cancer and that surgery is indicated.

The modal finding is that the procedure produces considerable fearfulness and attitude change but has little enduring effect on smoking. Many physicians can testify to this all-too-frequent outcome with their own patients.

The recent use of sensory deprivation as an alternative to role playing provides the exception to the negative results for attitude change techniques. Suedfeld and his colleagues (1229, 1231, 1232, 1233) reported good results when a variety of antismoking and prosmoking messages were presented during twenty-four hours of sensory deprivation (which the smoker spends lying quietly on a bed in a light- and sound-proofed chamber). Initial abstinence is as high as 100%, although the long-term results may not be much greater than are typically achieved with other methods.

The limitation to all education and attitude change approaches is that, while they underscore *what* the smoker should do (i.e., quit), they do not specify *how* this is to take place. If combined with effective "how to" procedures, education and attitude change techniques may play an important role. As an example, preliminary data from a series of case reports (1230) and from a controlled study presently being conducted, suggest 80% abstinence at six months follow-up when sensory deprivation is combined with behavior change procedures. Certainly, a pervasive major shortcoming of other approaches to smoking modification has been a failure to consider attitudinal and motivational factors.

Pharmacological Strategies

What are some of the direct ways of changing smoking behavior? Consideration of the role played by nicotine in controlling smoking has led to two approaches. The first prescribes a nicotinomimetic compound, lobeline sulphate, commercially available in a buffered form as Bantron or Nikoban, during the initial withdrawal period. This can indeed reduce tobacco consumption, thus attesting to the role nicotine plays in smoking (1206). However, the effects are both weak and temporary, often no greater than those of placebos (1113, 1121, 1127, 1148, 1189).

The second, more recent, approach involves a newly developed chewing gum containing nicotine. An initial double-blind study reported a statistically significantly greater reduction of cigarette smoking with nicotine gum than with placebo gum (1102). A well-controlled study by Russell, Wilson, Feyerabend, and Cole (447) demonstrated a statistically significant nicotine gum effect when clients were instructed to smoke normally but no advantage of the nicotine gum over the placebo while subjects were trying to reduce their smoking. They concluded that the specific effect of the nicotine was small, explaining only 7% of the variance in smoking reduction.

In summary, the unaided use of pharmacological regimens is ineffective. It seems clear the problems of smoking modification extend well beyond those arising from pharmacological dependence.

Hypnotic Strategies

Outcomes from the use of hypnosis vary dramatically. There are reports of long-term cessation rates ranging from 60% to nearly 100% (1108, 1157, 1196, 1242, 1244). Others studies have had almost no success (400, 1200, 1226). Most of the successful studies have combined hypnosis with a wide variety of other (poorly specified) procedures. Hypnosis is used for multiple purposes, and its use can parallel the fear-induction role described earlier. If it is used only for the latter purpose, it appears ineffective. However, it may also be used to aid the teaching of alternative behaviors in smoking situations; for example, teaching other ways of dealing with tension, anger, or a desire to have something to do with one's hands (1244). In the adjunct role, hypnosis may well make a contribution to reduced smoking. There is need for better controlled studies to evaluate both the specific role of hypnosis and the circumstances under which it can be beneficial.

Behavior Modification Strategies

Behavior modification represents not one treatment procedure but a host of techniques bound loosely together by allegiance to social learning principles and to a common set of assumptions. In this context, smoking is viewed as an overlearned habit and smoking cessation as a learning process. Although behavior modifiers have traditionally preferred to focus on environmental determinants of behavior, the recent growth of cognitive behavior modification (1182, 1188) has had a major influence in the smoking cessation area. In addition, the pharmacological, affective, and cognitive variables described above as in part controlling smoking behavior are included in this approach (1095).

Thus, smoking is conceptualized as a chain of behaviors and events, as illustrated in Figure 13.1. Some of the behavioral techniques aim primarily at the antecedents of smoking behavior—the smoking situation, the urge to smoke, and the decision to smoke process. Others are concerned more with the consequences of smoking and endeavor to change the contingencies associated with the behavior.

Antecedent Techniques of Behavior Modification

1. *Aversion Techniques.* The use of aversive conditioning techniques is commonly documented in the smoking literature. The basic rationale rests on the principle that situations elicit smoking because they have become associated with smoking through experience and because smoking has often proved rewarding in these circumstances. In a similar way, the experience of repeated aversive consequences for smoking should create an urge *not* to smoke in these situations. It is hoped that ultimately the urge not to smoke will prove of

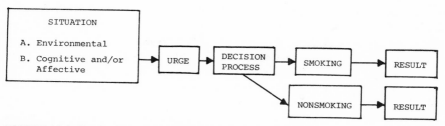

FIGURE 13.1. Sequential events and behavior in the smoking chain.

sufficient strength to counter the urge to smoke and thus prevent smoking behavior.

Electric shock is a common form of aversion. Smokers have been shocked while smoking in the laboratory (448, 1083, 1096, 1107, 1166, 1214). They have been shocked in the natural environment (1197, 1203, 1247). Furthermore, instead of shocking smoking behavior, other researchers have shocked the urge to smoke (1086, 1087, 1088, 1227). In general, the use of electric shock for smoking itself has not proved effective, although there is some suggestion that shocking the urge to smoke has promise; Berecz (1089, 1090) has argued this position, but better controlled research is required for confirmation. Shock also may be effective when combined with self-management techniques (1105); there are commercial smoking cessation programs based on the program these authors originally developed. These commerical operations claim considerable success, but the high level of motivation engendered by large fees may comprise a substantial portion of their contribution. Furthermore, these operations have not been systematically evaluated.

Two forms of aversive oversmoking have been used instead of electric shock. The rationale for them is similar, but it also includes the suggestion that an aversive agent more closely related to the problem behavior will enhance the strategy's effectiveness. The first aversive strategy is called *rapid smoking*. As developed by Lichtenstein and his colleagues at the University of Oregon, it requires the smoker to sit down, at first once a day and then gradually less frequently, and chain smoke as many cigarettes as possible, taking puffs every six seconds (1171, 1219). Clients are instructed to remain abstinent between sessions. Reports on rapid smoking indicated up to 100% abstinence at termination and 60% at six-month follow-up. The technique has now been shown dependent upon a good relationship between smoker and therapist (1141). Indeed, the Oregon group's data suggest that it may be most effective when administered in the laboratory rather than at home. Furthermore, rapid smoking appears more effective when treatment is continued until the client is abstinent and reporting little difficulty in managing urges (1159, 1245).

The effectiveness of rapid smoking has stood up well on several replications, although long-term levels of abstinence have been somewhat lower, ranging between 30% and 50% (49, 298, 1161, 1191, 1195, 1207, 1222). When results were less impressive, deviation from the recommended procedure may have been the cause (119, 299, 1116, 1126, 1128, 1129, 1162, 1164, 1235), since it does appear effective as developed by the Oregon group. However, concerns have been raised as to the medical safety of the technique (690, 1114, 1140), since smoking affects the cardiovascular system in two ways: (1) via the pharmacological action of nicotine, and (2) more indirectly as the result of increased carboxyhemoglobin production. There is an immediate increase in heart rate and arterial blood pressure during smoking, and cigarette smoke also contains a relatively high level of carbon monoxide which produces increased carboxyhemoglobin levels and reduces the blood's oxygen carrying capacity. Rapid smoking might exaggerate these effects and thus in theory might produce cardiovascular harm in certain smokers. However, available data suggest that the procedure does *not* produce effects of clinical significance when administered to healthy smokers (1111, 1115, 1170). Nevertheless, prior medical evaluation is called for and prudence dictates that the technique should not at present be used on smokers with cardiovascular disease.

The second form of aversive oversmoking is called *satiation*. This technique requires smokers to double or triple their usual smoking rates for several days. Resnick (1208, 1209) originally reported success rates from satiation comparable to the best of those published for rapid smoking. However, efforts to repeat this high success rate have generally been disappointing (1097, 1106, 1177, 1183, 1184, 1234). Two recent studies do suggest that satiation may be as effective as rapid smoking when combined with self-management training procedures (48, 1117). Furthermore, there have been methodologic differences between satiation and rapid smoking studies that may have contributed to the apparent superiority of rapid smoking. In the satiation studies, treatment time has been shorter, there has been less emphasis on the good therapist-client relationship shown to be critical for rapid smoking (1141), and there has been less attention to the cognitive components of the oversmoking experience. This last different is of particular interest. Lichtenstein and Danaher (736) have argued that oversmoking is effective because it provides the smoker with unpleasant experiences that can be reinstated subsequently or rehearsed cognitively in coping with urges. Thus, the strategy can be continued after formal treatment ends. This is important in view of the theoretical limitation inherent in aversion procedures when they are applied to behavioral excesses. If the individual does not have alternative responses available, the suppressant effect may be only temporary (1085, 1152). Thus, the maintenance of smoking change may be dependent upon factors quite distinct from those that influence the initial behavior change (49, 705, 1110).

This distinction also provides a rationale for the final aversive technique to be reviewed. *Covert sensitization* uses cognitive imagery to provide the aversive associations with smoking. The technique has the advantages of being cheap, easy to apply, and medically safe. As described by Cautela (1104), the smoker is directed repeatedly to imagine himself in a typical smoking situation and to conjure up vivid and powerful negative consequences (e.g., becoming nauseous and throwing up on the cigarette pack in his hand). This cognitive imagery may be alternated with a scenario in which the client decides not to smoke and experiences positive consequences. Research designed to evaluate the technique and its variations has produced poor results (1163, 1177, 1198, 1216, 1225, 1243, 1250). However, Severson and Hynd (1222) recently demonstrated that covert sensitization may be a useful adjunctive technique to rapid smoking, especially with respect to the *maintenance* of change. This is consistent with a cognitive explanation of the rapid smoking effect and underscores the potential importance of cognitive variables in long-term compliance with nonsmoking regimens.

In summary, the effectiveness of aversion techniques varies considerably. Rapid smoking in a socially supportive context produces the most consistent positive findings and seems to produce good short-term abstinence and moderately favorable long-term effects. We can speculate that aversion techniques may be most effective when the smoker can cognitively rehearse the unpleasant effect in coping with smoking urges. Aversion techniques thus may be viewed most appropriately as contributing to the initial change in smoking behavior. Maintenance of this change appears to be due to different processes, however. Cognitive rehearsal of aversion effects may be one way to promote maintenance. Furthermore, variations of the aversion experience that encourage such rehearsal may enhance treatment outcome. Alternatively, aversion techniques may be more effective if they are combined with some of the self-management procedures described below.

2. *Stimulus Control.* Aversion techniques are not the only strategies aimed at producing change at the "situation-urge" stage of the smoking behavior chain. A variety of other strategies are designed to alter the stimulus control of smoking. Two steps are involved: (1) smoking is first restricted to a few, often novel, cues so as to extinguish associations with previous smoking situations, and (2) there is a gradual reduction of smoking in the presence of even these few cues. Azrin and Powell (1084) used a cigarette box that locked automatically and permitted smoking only at designated time intervals. Others have used pocket timers, planned intersmoking intervals, or specific smoking times to accomplish much the same end (44, 1097, 1106, 1128, 1167, 1223, 1241). In another version of this approach clients were instructed first to refrain from smoking in easy situations or for short time periods and then progressively to eliminate their smoking in more difficult situations (1184, 1216, 1249). In yet another approach, the effects of posters on smoking has been studied (588) as has the restriction of smoking to a designated "smoking" chair (1194, 1210).

Unfortunately, the results of these studies are generally negative. The failure of stimulus control procedures may be in part a function of their requirement of a gradual reduction in smoking. For example, Flaxman (1126) has demonstrated the inferiority of gradual compared with abrupt quitting. Furthermore, many investigators have noted that, as the smoking rate decreases, the reinforcement value of each remaining cigarette increases accordingly. Thus, there seems to be a floor of about ten cigarettes per day below which smokers find it difficult to continue a gradual reduction.

3. *Self-monitoring.* Self-regulation requires a feedback loop such that the individual becomes aware of his or her actions and of their consequences and is therefore in a position to behave differently on subsequent similar occasions (1153). Self-monitoring techniques require clients to monitor their smoking behavior formally by writing down some aspects of it. That the recording of cigarette smoking reduces its occurrence is well documented (1155). For example, Rozensky (1213) demonstrated greater reduction in smoking when a subject recorded the behavior before, rather than after, its occurrence. This result is consistent with a self-regulation notion since, with presmoking recording, the act of monitoring itself may occasion different behavior. Kantorowitz and Walters (1154) compared the effects of monitoring smoking during treatment with those of monitoring successfully resisted urges to smoke. They replicated McFall and Hammen's (1178) earlier demonstration of similar results with the two forms of self-monitoring (although both groups were superior to a waiting list control).

The benefits of self-monitoring tend to be transitory and do not extend much beyond treatment termination. The technique is therefore perhaps best thought of as an adjunct that may be a prerequisite for the effective use of other self-control techniques. The coverant control model developed by Danaher provides a fuller discussion of this issue (1109, 1110).

4. *Anxiety Management.* The final strategy for modifying the relationship between antecedent events and the decision to smoke focuses on smoking that is associated with anxiety and tension. Systematic desensitization, in which anxiety-producing situations that lead to smoking are paired with relaxation, has been found ineffective in eliminating cigarette smoking (1133, 1158, 1164, 1204, 1243). This negative result might have been expected. Although tension is perhaps the most common perceived reason for smoking, the anxiety management strategy does nothing to affect those cigarettes not associated with tension or anxiety.

Consequence Techniques of Behavior Modification.

We turn now to procedures primarily designed to produce changes at, or subsequent to, the point in the smoking chain at which the decision to smoke is made. It should be emphasized that this distinction between antecedent and consequence techniques is drawn for a discursive and not explanatory purpose. Certainly, the techniques already discussed may have their effect, at least in part, at a later point in the smoking chain, yet all effective procedures presumably will result ultimately in the extinction of the urge in former smoking situations. The distinction in part highlights the quality of activity on the part of the smoker. Most of the strategies discussed to this point might be expected to permit a relatively passive response to the smoking situation. Once an aversive response has been conditioned, anxiety extinguished, or stimulus control developed, nonsmoking will presumably result more or less automatically. In contrast, the following procedures call for an active effort in smoking situations. They require the use of self-management procedures that raise a different set of issues with respect to compliance. For example, laboratory-based aversion techniques theoretically require relatively little compliance beyond appointment keeping. In contrast, compliance (often of a considerable magnitude and under adverse circumstances) is a prerequisite for the self-management program.

1. *Response Substitution.* Response substitution techniques are based on an understanding of factors controlling an individual's smoking; they are of two types. First, the nonsmoking response may be functional in that it is equivalent to smoking; for example, an alternative way of relaxing or coping with boredom might be substituted. On the other hand, the nonsmoking response may be nonfunctional. In this case, it will be effective to the extent that its occurrence decreases the probability of smoking behavior (1125, 1174, 1175). For example, if an individual experiences a strong urge to smoke while at a party, he or she might cope with that urge by going for a walk until the urge diminishes.

There are compelling theoretical arguments for the power of response substitution procedures (48, 705, 1092), and a variety of successful smoking cessation programs have included such techniques without isolating their specific contribution (47, 48, 1103, 1105, 1191, 1202). Preliminary data from a study in our own clinic show significantly improved outcomes when response substitution procedures are added to the oversmoking techniques previously described (1098).

2. *Contingency Management.* The simple procedure of instituting monetary penalties or rewards for smoking or not smoking has proved surprisingly effective when considered against the background of repeated failures to modify smoking documented to this point. Elliott and Tighe (1123) reported that 84% of former smokers were abstinent at the end of treatment and 38% abstinent at a later follow-up when a deposit was collected, to be forfeited if the client smoked. Similar response-cost conditions have been shown superior to those of "no cost" controls, but the differences between these groups have disappeared with long-term follow-up (299, 1249). Overall, monetary and social rewards for not smoking seem relatively effective over the short run (1212, 1217). However, their long-term effects are less certain and their most appropriate applications may be as useful additions to other strategies.

3. *Social Support.* An alternative positive consequence of not smoking can come from social interactions. The contribution of such social support has rarely been evaluated despite the common emphasis on social support in conjunction with other techniques (1099, 1163, 1236). Janis and Hoffman (1149) compared the relative effectiveness of daily versus weekly contact between pairs of smokers. The high contact group maintained a 75% mean reduction in smoking twelve months later, a reduction that compares favorably with the best in the literature. Similarly, Lewittes and Israel (1168) described a case study with two undergraduate roommates both of whom quit successfully and remained abstinent as a result of the rapid smoking technique, then were made responsible for each other's nonsmoking. On the other hand, results among married couples have been less impressive (1139, 1193).

In sum, the systematic planning of social support and reinforcement is a promising approach to maintenance. Such social techniques may be particularly relevant, since recent data suggest the relapse often occurs in social situations (1169). Nonetheless, more research is required to specify the important parameters in these complex social relationships.

4. *Maintenance Procedures.* The relative independence of factors affecting initial and long-term achievement of abstinence have been noted. It also seems clear that long-term maintenance is the larger problem, since many clinics document good short-term results but extensive relapse. Furthermore, Hunt and his colleagues (704, 1144) noted a similar independence for other addictions. In their review of clients initally abstinent, approximately 75% relapsed within six months.

Researchers have increasingly focused attention on the problem of maintenance and have begun to assess possible strategies for improving it. Continuing clinic contact has been included in some relatively effective programs (1099, 1101, 1105, 1202). However, supportive telephone calls during and after treatment, as well as more frequent post-treatment follow-up, have led to significantly poorer long-term results in other investigations (47, 1219).

Although smokers have been asked to return for "booster" treatment, to call a "hot line," or to use maintenance procedures themselves if they start to experience problems, they tend not to make use of such support (49, 808). In addition, direct tests of the utility of booster sessions show no incremental effect (1207). Gordon and Katz (1137) recently assessed the relative effects of three maintenance procedures when added to rapid smoking: contingency management, group social support, and continued rapid smoking. Both contingency management and group social support were significantly superior to rapid smoking on follow-up.

Many of the self-management strategies discussed earlier are conceptually well suited to promoting maintenance. For example, Bloch and Best (1098) found that a complex response substitution package produced better maintenance than rapid smoking alone. Nevertheless, the effects of maintenance

procedures are still poorly understood and considerably more research is required.

Treatment Packages of Behavior Modification Strategies.

The increased recognition that smoking cessation is a multifaceted process
requiring diverse strategies has prompted use of treatment packages rather than
single techniques. Results have often been encouraging (47, 48, 280, 1099,
1103, 1105, 1117, 1191, 1202), although less successful programs have also
been documented (1126, 1142, 1179, 1224). There is considerable variation in
the contents of such packages. These differences arise in part from theoretical
predilections but may also reflect our very preliminary state of understanding
of the cessation process. For example, we know almost nothing about the
means by which millions of North Americans have quit on their own, and we
have just begun to identify those factors that affect relapse. Until more complete
and empirically based conceptual models are developed, treatment packages will
inevitably remain something of a hit-and-miss affair. Despite their shortcomings,
however, there are reasons to encourage their use.

Davidson (1115) has reviewed the compliance literature and stressed the
significance of the internal attribution of change upon long-term compliance.
This view supports programs in which packages are served up "cafeteria style";
that is, clients focus their efforts on those procedures that seem best suited to
their individual styles and needs. There are data to suggest that therapeutic outcome is better when smokers receive their preferred treatment (1119). Thus,
treatment packages are likely to be effective because (1) they include diverse
strategies, thereby increasing the probability that signficant problems will be
addressed and (2) the element of choice will promote self-attribution of change
and thereby better maintenance.

Looking back over the smoking cessation studies reviewed here, it is noted
that the focus has been on therapeutic outcome, not regimen compliance. By
inference, one might suppose that potentially more effective programs will
induce greater compliance, but this needs to be established empirically. There
are only two bits of data bearing directly on the issue of regimen compliance.
First, the probability of success in quitting smoking is greater if clients do comply with treatment demands (1094, 1097). Second, clients are more likely to
comply if the therapeutic regimen is presented in writing rather than just verbally (1094).

PRACTICAL APPLICATIONS

What are we to make of this welter of variable findings? Is there any guidance
for the practicing health professional? Several practical applications do emerge.

First, treatment is more likely to be effective if it is multifaceted. Several considerations dictate this need. The reasons for smoking behavior are complex and variable across individuals. Furthermore, strategies effective in producing initial change may be quite distinct from those facilitating maintenance of change. Moreover, problems in smoking cessation tend to vary from one individual to another. Finally, self-attribution of change can be promoted by providing the smoker with a range of treatment alternatives.

Second, it must be recognized by both client and health professional that the real problem in smoking modification is one of maintenance. There is an understandable tendency to focus on the considerable effort and withdrawal pains associated with achieving initial abstinence. However, it has been clear for some time that almost any well-designed program can achieve high levels of initial change (1091). Although the difficulty in quitting initially may be real, it diverts attention from long-range problems. It is not yet clear what strategies are most effective in promoting maintenance. Options include (1) provision of a supportive physical and social environment, (2) emphasis on cognitive strategies for dealing with problem urges, (3) self-attribution of change, and (4) the development of effective alternative behaviors that collectively comprise a new, nonsmoking lifestyle.

Third, it is likely that treatment will be more effective if it is individualized. Tailoring strategies to the individual will require that considerably more attention be given to the assessment and conceptualization of factors that control smoking behavior and the change process.

A Sample Program

The treatment package we have recently developed illustrates these principles. The program is designed for potential utilization in public health and preventive medical settings (47, 48). Thus, on the one hand the program strives to be sufficiently comprehensive to ensure high levels of treatment effectiveness. On the other hand, it requires relatively little professional time, no special equipment, and only brief specialized training. The program consists of five weekly sessions, each lasting between thirty and ninety minutes. Clients are seen either individually or in small groups of up to eight; there is some evidence that although group administration of the strategies saves time, it is less effective (47).

The three phases of treatment are described in Table 13.1. The first phase concerns planning for change; it begins with a conceptual introduction to both smoking and change and then introduces the strategy of self-monitoring. Self-monitoring requires that the smoker record the time, place, activity, and perceived reason for each cigarette, thus increasing the kind of awareness of the smoking act that is a prerequisite for later self-control efforts. This technique also provides data for determining the factors that control the individual's smoking and thereby facilitates the selection of appropriate strategies.

TABLE 13.1. Objectives and strategies in an approach to the planning, initiation, and maintenance of smoking cessation

Planning change	Initiating change	Maintaining change
Objective:	*Objective:*	*Objective:*
Functional analysis of smoking behavior	Conditioned aversion	Analysis of problem situations
Increased cognitive mediation	Rapid behavior change	Alternative response programming or training
Preliminary testing of alternatives to smoking		Planning of coping strategies
		Practice and reinforcement of non-smoking behavior
Strategies:	*Strategies:*	*Strategies:*
Self-monitoring	Satiation	Relaxation training
Individualized experimentation with alternatives to smoking	Rapid smoking	Contingency management
		Social support
		Coverant control
		Stimulus control
		Behavioral rehearsal

Armed with these records, the second session is devoted to planning, with the health professional serving as a consultant who describes a general approach to treatment and provides some expert advice but leaves primary responsibility for decision making and change in the smoker's hands. Reasons for smoking and possible alternative behaviors are discussed as an introduction to a problem-solving model for smoking cessation in which the urge to smoke becomes the occasion for such problem solving. Four steps are involved: the smoker should try to (1) pinpoint those factors contributing to the urge to smoke, (2) consider the possible alternative actions that might serve similar functions, (3) try out possible alternatives to assess their adequacy, and (4) practice viable alternatives until they become a well-established, nonsmoking lifestyle.

A detailed example will clarify this process. Suppose the client is a forty-five-year-old manager of a small advertising firm. His self-monitoring records show that 40% of his smoking occurs in tension situations. Some of these occur at the office, when the pressure starts to build; others occur in the presence of other people, when there is an element of social evaluation. A possible alternative in the office situation would be to pause for a few moments and use deep breathing techniques in a concerted effort to relax. A more likely option for the social occasion might be self-instructional training (1187), to change what individuals say to themselves about evaluative aspects of the situation.

Boredom was a second common reason for smoking in our example. It typically occurs after a period of doing straight paperwork. The alternative action here might be frequent, but brief, active breaks, which serve the same stimulatory function as the cigarettes.

Finally, many cigarettes were smoked in habit situations—with a morning cup of coffee, on the telephone, in the car, or after meals. A change in these routines—switching from coffee to tea or having the morning coffee in the dining room instead of the kitchen—may prove an adequate coping strategy.

Towards the end of the second session the smoker is usually fairly certain of his reasons for smoking and is beginning to see some possible alternatives. The final four days of the planning stage are devoted to clarifying these reasons and trying out the alternatives.

The second phase is devoted to initiating change. As noted earlier, aversive oversmoking procedures are the most effective and reliable strategies thus far developed for achieving cessation. We use both rapid smoking and satiation, as described above, having previously screened for cardiovascular problems and obtained written consent from the smoker's physician. Clients are instructed to increase their smoking rate as much as possible for three days just prior to quitting; the guideline given is to double their normal smoking rate, but it is stressed that subjective discomfort is the primary criterion. At the end of each day of satiation, clients complete a form in which they rate the severity of each of twenty-four possible reactions to oversmoking (e.g., dry mouth, dizziness, sore throat). They then decide upon the number of cigarettes for the next day's oversmoking and allocate them on an hourly quota basis.

Clients are instructed to stop smoking abruptly on the morning following the conclusion of the satiation period; for many, it's a relief to no longer *have to* smoke! They attend the third treatment session that day and towards the end of that session the second oversmoking procedure, rapid smoking, is demonstrated. It requires that the client (1) continue smoking cigarettes, taking puffs every five to six seconds, until he or she can tolerate no more and (2) focus attention between trials on reactions to oversmoking, on the assumption that increased cognitive involvement will enhance the procedure's effectiveness (48). Clients subsequently perform rapid smoking at home, at first daily and then gradually less frequently, for a total of seven trials during the first two weeks off other cigarettes. This procedure closely parallels that described by Lichtenstein (1171, 1219) except that it is take-home in nature and the total number of sessions is fixed.

The oversmoking procedures seem to do their job. They typically create a strong aversion to cigarettes and clients usually report a considerable reduction in their urge to smoke. Conceptually, however, we distinguish between those procedures designed to initiate and maintain change. Thus, an effective initiation procedure should both suppress smoking behavior and reduce the intensity and frequency of the urge, creating optimal circumstances for the development of the maintenance procedures introduced in the final phase.

The third phase of the treatment is aimed at maintaining change. Nonsmoking is then viewed as a set of actively performed alternative behaviors to smoking.

A wide variety of strategies are used on an ad lib basis. These include: relaxation training (1136), contingency management, and social support. Clients are also encouraged to rehearse coping strategies (e.g., ways of turning down cigarettes) cognitively or behaviorally before they are needed in a problem situation.

There is an increasing focus on cognitive techniques. For example, an urge-management procedure requires that strong urges be (1) considered first through statements or images that emphasize negative consequences of smoking, (2) followed by a covert decision to not smoke, and finally, (3) associated with positive images or statements related to nonsmoking. Clients are asked to generate their own lists of positive and negative associations and to vary them in applying the technique.

The treatment program is designed to be flexible enough to respond to individual needs, yet highly structured. Thus, although the specific strategies vary for different clients, there are always detailed tasks to be completed between sessions (e.g., self-monitoring, rapid smoking, practicing relaxation, discussing problem situations with a spouse). All of these tasks are written down and most require a specific product to be presented at the next session (e.g., ratings of rapid smoking reactions, a list of positive and negative associations to smoking). Such a structure increases compliance (1094), and it also aids in identifying problems with noncompliance. Clinically, therefore, we treat noncompliance as a motivational problem. The first time a client fails to follow through on a task, we point out the failure and its implications for ultimate treatment success. In our experience, repeated noncompliance is consistently associated with failure to achieve and maintain cessation. Accordingly, the second time a client fails to follow through, we depart from the normal session format to discuss the problem in detail. Sometimes the problem can be resolved; for example, a previous unspoken concern about possible weight gain after quitting may be allayed. Sometimes, however, the noncompliance is associated with ambivalence about quitting and the client often decides to discontinue treatment until he or she is better motivated for change.

The program consistently stresses the importance of self-management. At the end of treatment, clients will still experience urges to smoke. However, at this point they have mastered the strategies needed to manage their nonsmoking and the clinic's part in the process is complete. It is then assumed that clients will continue to practice the new repertoire of nonsmoking skills until they are well established and the urge to smoke is eventually extinguished.

PRIORITIES FOR FUTURE RESEARCH

Research on compliance with healthy lifestyles is really just beginning. There is much to be done. Three broad priorities can be identified. We need research aimed at (1) improving the effectiveness of lifestyle change programs, (2) improving compliance with the behavioral prescriptions included in such programs, and (3) improving our communities' lifestyle services.

Improving Effectiveness

Clients are more likely to comply with the requirements of a treatment program if they believe it to be effective. Although there have been recent advances in smoking modification, even the best programs still can expect roughly half the participants to relapse ultimately. What lines of investigation may be expected to improve this picture?

A fundamental distinction researchers need to make here is that between the initiation and maintenance of change. It seems likely that relatively independent processes contribute to each and that smoking modification thus requires two distinct, although interrelated, technologies. We can define a procedure's initiation effects operationally as those occurring *during* the change program, and its maintenance effects as those occurring *after* the program ends. Criteria for effectiveness may be similar for initation and maintenance. For example, an effective initiation procedure is one that decreases the smoking rate (ideally to zero) and decreases the frequency and intensity of urges to smoke. Similarly, maintenance procedures are effective to the extent that they maintain a reduced smoking rate, urge intensity, or urge rate. In other circumstances, the criteria for effective initiation and maintenance procedures may differ. For example, maintenance may be facilitated if there is a restriction in the range of circumstances under which smoking urges occur, or if a procedure tends to result in continuing the active practice of nonsmoking skills. In contrast, one initiation procedure might be preferred over another if it produces rapid rather than gradual reduction in smoking behavior. Therefore, our research designs should include a range of measures that will allow us to assess the separate and joint effects of initiation and maintenance procedures. This is an ambitious undertaking, going far beyond previous calls for more standardized, although still basic, program evaluation (1192). However, the fact is that we know very little about the process of smoking change and we may not find out much more unless we use measures that can reflect that process.

In a similar vein, we need to study the process of relapse. We know almost nothing about relapse despite the clear fact that it is the biggest problem facing smoking modification programs. What kinds of factors control relapse? Is it related to noncompliance, to a failure to follow treatment recommendations after the program ends? Fortunately, a beginning has now been made (1169). Nonetheless, this kind of study needs to have a much higher priority than it has been afforded to date.

Smoking modification researchers must also come to grips with the fact that they are studying a very complex and difficult problem. It is inappropriate to prescribe treatment with no attempt at diagnosis, that is, with no consideration of factors currently maintaining the individual's smoking. Programs are more likely to be effective if they are tailored to these individual differences. Positive steps in this direction include the recent trend toward use of treatment packages and the strategy, proposed by Lichtenstein and Danaher (736), of focusing initially on intensive pilot work with individuals or very small groups.

Improving Compliance

We can start by beginning to measure compliance. The same kinds of measurement problems will arise here as with other compliance studies. However, our recent demonstration of differential compliance as a function of treatment condition, and of a relationship between compliance and outcome, argues that meaningful measurement is possible (48, 1097), even though the measures of compliance used in these studies were primitive. For example, we argued that the client was complying with the regimen if he or she submitted the requested records of tasks completed between sessions. The therapist then used a five-point scale to rate compliance from the client's description of efforts to complete these prescribed tasks. The complexity of these tasks gave rise to significant variation in performance, thereby yielding a sensitive measure of compliance.

The complex nature of smoking modification regimens also has some advantages when it comes to studying factors affecting compliance. We can begin to ask why clients comply with some aspects of the program and not with others. Similarly, we can examine the relationship between specific acts of compliance and treatment effectiveness.

An additional research priority stems from the insularity of smoking modification research. There has been almost no consideration of the existing compliance literature or the relationship between smoking change and other aspects of health lifestyle. As increased attention in smoking modification research is paid to compliance variables, a corresponding consideration of the broader health lifestyle context seems indicated. For example, promotion of positive health values may be an important prerequisite to compliance with smoking modification programs. It may be that an individual is more likely to change his smoking behavior after he has experienced the benefits and sense of control gained from changes in other lifestyle areas.

Improving Community Services

While the effectiveness of our smoking modification technology has begun to improve, community programs remain largely unchanged. In part, this shortcoming arises from factors outside our present concern, e.g. inadequate governmental funding of preventive programs. However, researchers also must assume some of the responsibility. Best et al. (47) have described problems arising from researchers' inadequate attention to the requirements of program development research, in contrast to those for controlled outcome studies.

There is also a need for the systematic study of the population's perceptions of smoking modification programs and of factors affecting their utilization of these services. The consumer has been left out of program development efforts and the consequences of his exclusion may be serious. For example, although nine of ten smokers apparently have some interest in modifying their smoking habits (1240), results from a recent pilot survey of ours suggest that only one in five smokers who are currently trying to change their habits would consider going to a clinic. Why are we not reaching those who ought to be using the service? Frederiksen and Peterson (1130, 1131, 1132) have argued that it is in part because we are not offering the services they want. Most smokers do not really want to quit smoking; they want to rid themselves of the associated health risks. Many would choose to do so by reducing their smoking rate, but researchers have frequently pointed to the apparent inability of smokers to maintain a reduced rate as an alternative to abstinence. However, it is to be expected that controlled smoking might require different strategies and the development of different skills. There has not yet been a systematic attempt to develop effective controlled or reduced smoking programs, even though they might meet with much wider acceptance than the current abstinence programs.

We are making advances in the areas of smoking modification. Greater consideration of compliance issues promises to add to our knowledge about which services to offer and how they should be offered. Our belief is that these services will be improved further through more sophisticated research and more attention to the broader health promotion context of smoking modification.

14

Compliance
in the
Control of Alcohol Abuse

Edward M. Sellers,
Howard D. Cappell, and Joan A. Marshman

INTRODUCTION

The problem of promoting compliance in accepting and adhering to treatment is not identical where medical and behavioral interventions are concerned.
In medical practice, one may wish to promote compliance in order that a treatment regimen of known efficacy will be followed by the patient; a physician
can safely promise relief from certain infections, for example, if the patient will
only take his penicillin. Behavioral and medical practitioners treating alcoholism
are faced with a special problem: not only must they persuade a patient to
accept treatment, but they must often do this without knowing in advance that
the treatment they decide to offer will be efficacious in a particular case (1253,
1254).

This chapter reviews some current developments in treatment research,
promoting retention in treatment, developing efficacious treatments, and measuring outcomes for alcoholism (Figure 14.1). Complete reviews concerning
treatment have been published recently and material contained in them is not
reiterated in detail (613, 648, 1253, 1254, 1279, 1281, 1284). The acceptance
of treatment, adherence, efficacy, and the assessment of outcome are inevitably
intertwined. Therefore, the topic is complex. In addition, societal attitudes and
perceptions are important, ever-present variables confounding the promotion
of compliance in this area.

Acknowledgment: We thank Dr. Frederick B. Glaser for his careful reviews and helpful
comments and particularly for the ideas relating to the Core Shell Treatment system.

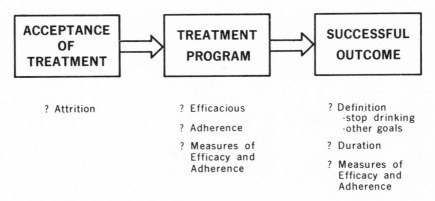

FIGURE 14.1. Steps in alcohol treatment.

FACTORS INFLUENCING THE CONSUMPTION OF ALCOHOL

Social factors, including prevailing attitudes and beliefs, influence not only the level of alcohol consumption and the subsequent prevalence of alcohol-related problems but also the acceptance of and adherence to alcohol treatment programs (1257, 1263, 1282).

Patterns and Extent of Consumption

"Alcoholism" is not the exclusive property of an aberrant group in society but represents one pole of a continuum between abstinence and heavy consumption. Consumption frequency has a log-normal distribution. A fairly predictable relationship exists for many countries, indicating that the proportion of heavy drinkers (>80 g absolute ethanol per day) increases as the average per capita consumption in the society increases. In the industrialized world, at least, the overall trend in alcohol consumption shows a remarkable increase since World War II, particularly during the 1960s. In the United States, average yearly per capita intake among those over fifteen years of age increased by 30% (from 7.5 to 9.8 liters of absolute alcohol) between 1950 and 1973 and by 8.4% between 1968 and 1974. In Canada, 1973 consumption was 10.3 liters and the increases in the same intervals were 58% and 22%, respectively (1251, 1270).

Consequences

Heavy users of alcohol have a substantially elevated risk of premature death. The etiologic importance of alcohol is clear with respect to deaths from cirrhosis of the liver, accidents, and certain cancers. Furthermore, at least for cirrhosis, the relationship between heavy consumption and excess mortality is manifest in the general population in a covariance of liver cirrhosis and per capita alcohol consumption (1257).

Determinants of Consumption Level

In general, the overall availability of alcohol seems to have an independent effect on the general level of alcohol consumption in a society. There are examples in which restrictions on availability have led to a decrease in consumption and instances where relaxation of restriction has led to an increase (1257, 1263, 1282). These instances involve changes in age limits, outlet frequency, beverage strength, marketing regulation, and prices. In most instances alcoholic beverages behave like other commodities; a rise in alcohol prices leads to a decrease in alcohol consumption. The average price of alcoholic beverages relative to the consumer price index has fallen 25% since 1949 and has represented a smaller and smaller fraction of disposable income (1270). Obviously, this is one among a number of reasons why it is easy for individuals to continue to consume harmful amounts of ethanol.

REHABILITATION OF PERSONS WITH ALCOHOL-RELATED PROBLEMS

The Therapeutic Problem

The management of alcoholism involves a wide range of measures aimed at reducing the patient's level of alcohol consumption and/or promoting a higher level of adaptation in various areas of functioning. These measures are ordinarily introduced after the patient has recovered from intoxication or withdrawal reactions. They are therefore aimed primarily at correction of a behavioral rather than a pharmacological or physiological problem. Accordingly, the measures employed consist largely of social or psychological therapy; pharmacological agents are of secondary importance. Since the causes of alcohol-related problems are multiple and complex, the therapeutic strategies are accordingly multiple and, in the ideal situation, should be adapted to the specific constellation of causal factors in the individual case.

Therapeutic Strategies

In general terms, there are two groups of strategies: those aimed at alleviating preexisting emotional problems, of which excessive alcohol consumption is seen as a symptom or a consequence; and those aimed directly at altering drinking behavior, so that drinking is replaced by some less harmful response, whatever the underlying causes may have been.

Among the more commonly cited emotional or personality problems alleged to lead to excessive alcohol consumption are anxiety, depression, low frustration tolerance, latent homosexuality, dependence, and immaturity in assessing long-term consequences. For most of these, the treatment, if any, must rest on various forms of psychosocial intervention.

Similarly, behavior modification techniques which seek to prevent excessive drinking rest primarily on psychosocial rather than pharmacological bases. The object is to reduce excessive drinking and to reward some alternative behavior. Drugs may be the means of suppressing consumption, as in the conditioned aversion methods based on disulfiram, apomorphine, or succinylcholine. The role of drug treatments will be discussed in detail later.

There is little evidence to distinguish among various emotionally and behaviorally oriented strategies in terms of outcome success. This may well be due to the fact that none of them have proven successful, but it could also be due to inappropriate application of the techniques. It is important to consider such problems before dismissing available strategies out of hand.

Acceptance of Treatment and Subsequent Attrition

Recent reviews of the literature on dropout rates in alcoholism treatment (1253, 1254, 1272, 1273) confirm that the prospect of "success" in treating alcoholism is crippled by the failure of a huge proportion of patients to present for treatment or to remain in it for very long. For example, Larkin (1273) estimated attrition rates in alcoholism treatment programs to be as high as 75% before many visits with therapists were completed. The rates of attrition are relatively independent of age, sex, duration of drinking, type of treatment program, social class, and inpatient or outpatient status.

Attrition rates for patients attending the Clinical Institute's Addiction Research Foundation in Toronto, Canada during 1975 (Figure 14.2) were developed by applying the life table method of Cutler and Ederer (1260, 1287). For the period 1 October 1974 to 31 March 1976, patient information was transcribed onto data cards for entry into the BMD Life Table Program (BMCX76). A patient was considered to be still attending if he was seen within the period of follow-up. If he was seen at least once between the 30 December 1975 closing date, and 31 March 1976, he was considered still active at the closing date. A patient was considered lost to treatment through attrition if he was not seen on at least one occasion between the date of his last appointment prior to the closing date and the end of 31 March 1976. For 9% of the patients the interval between these two contacts was more than three months. Therefore "lost to attrition" is a less stable entity than is "dead," the more common focus of life table studies. The error introduced by using a shorter and less final measure is small, and it tends in the direction of lower attrition rates.

The data for all cases registered from 1 January 1975 to 30 December 1975 are presented in Figure 14.2 The fate of each individual cohort can be followed on the triangle diagram for each period of follow-up. The overall gross attrition rate for the sample is 83% for the first three months of patient contact, and 95%

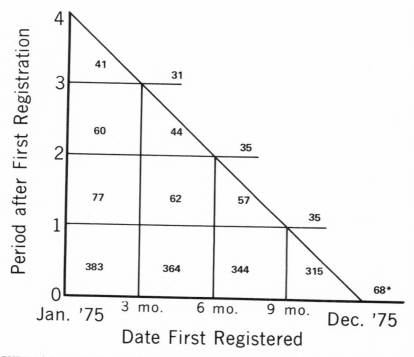

FIGURE 14.2. Life table attrition for attendees at the Clinical Institute's Addiction Research Foundation from 1 January to 30 December 1975.

for the year. As shown in Table 14.1, the results were quite uniform across all parameters of data collected (age, sex, and type of drug used). While attrition was most marked during the initial period of contact, significant attrition also occurred subsequently. Of the patients who remained beyond the first three months, only 28% were in attendance nine months later.

*Still active at closing date. The period of the study, on the abscissa, is divided into quartiles. Patients entering the study are grouped within each quartile to form cohorts. The number of persons remaining in the cohort can be followed until the closing date (represented by the hypotenuse of the triangle) by moving vertically, parallel to the ordinate. The first quartile cohort is followed for four three-month periods, or the whole period of the study, whereas the last quartile cohort is followed for only the last three-month period until the closing date.

Attrition for each cohort can be calculated for periods of follow-up by subtracting from the number of patients remaining at the beginning of the chosen period the number of such patients still remaining at the subsequent period of follow-up. For example, for the first quartile cohort, the attrition in the third period of follow-up is found by subtracting from the number attending at the beginning of the third period (60) the number of patients still in attendance at the beginning of the four period (41), namely 60-41 = 19. The numbers at the right of the hypotenuse count the patients still attending at the closing date. In the last quartile of the year of study 315 new patients registered, and 68 were still attending at the closing date.

TABLE 14.1. Cumulative rates of attrition

PERIOD (MONTHS)	ALL	MALES	FEMALES	ALCOHOL	DRUGS	YOUNGER (-35)	OLDER (36+)
0-3	83%	84%	80%	83%	84%	82%	85%
3-6	89%	89%	85%	88%	89%	87%	90%
6-9	92%	93%	89%	92%	92%	91%	94%
9-12	95%	95%	94%	95%	97%	94%	96%
S.E. (12 mo.)	1%	1%	2%	1%	2%	1%	1%
N	1406	1135	271	1072	320	732	674

The results are in accord with the reports of almost all other treatment programs. Glaser (1264) estimated for the inpatient therapeutic community in his study that only 5% of clients admitted would eventually become successful graduates and cited similar data from comparable programs. Results from the Phoenix House Program have also suggested an important relationship between outcome and time in treatment (1261, 1262). Reports of the fate of alcoholic dropouts are lacking despite similar rates of attrition. Some cautions are in order concerning these data. First, only instances (visits) are counted, not patients. Therefore, patients may reenter later for successful rehabilitation. Second, the high early attrition rate almost certainly means that for many patients no "treatment" could have been started. Therefore, high attrition is not necessarily synonymous with treatment failure.

While present data do not permit us to say why attrition is so high, it is evident that present programs are not successful in convincing this reluctant population to remain in treatment. Speculation as to the causes of high attrition leads to two considerations. First, it is likely that these patients have something in common that contributes to their lack of inclination to return for more definitive intervention. Second, treatment programs may be seen by some clients as the instruments of powerful social forces attempting to control deviance and promote social compliance. To the extent that alcoholism represents a protest against social compliance, attrition may be a measure of social recalcitrance. However, there is hope that the rapid provision of primary care and closer matching of program capabilities with a patient's needs may prove helpful in reducing early attrition, regardless of the underlying reason, and thus permit the program to operate effectively.

The Current System of Alcoholism Treatment

A major initial goal of any treatment system should be simply to retain patients long enough for assessment and treatment to be initiated. However, acceptance of treatment by a patient can be undermined seriously by a wide variety of factors, some of them individual, others concerned with program content or format, and still others related to the setting where treatment is to be given. There is no general treatment known that can be effective for all patients with alcohol-related problems (1266, 1267). With only a few exceptions, there is not much evidence that treatment programs for the rehabilitation of alcoholics are effective in more than 20% to 30% of the overall chronic alcoholic population (1253, 1254, 1281, 1284). Ironically, such a rate might prevail spontaneously, in the absence of any program at all. Admittedly, there is wide variation in the reported effectiveness of various treatment programs. However, those programs reporting the highest effectiveness typically have been evaluated improperly or not at all. Among those programs having the lowest improvement rates are those that have been studied in the most detail and those with the best research designs. There are even several studies demonstrating programs that have caused harm to patients.

A notable exception with respect to treatment success is the alcohol rehabilitation programs in industry. These programs are effective in some settings for over 70% of employed individuals (1253, 1254, 1281, 1284). The reasons for this remarkable efficacy compared to other treatment settings and tactics may lie partly in the highly coercive element that exists. Usually the basis for treatment is an implicit or explicit agreement between employer and employee that continued employment is dependent upon abstinence or moderation in drinking. In addition, a person still fully integrated into a working role and only beginning to experience alcohol-related problems is obviously more likely to be rehabilitated.

Why is the treatment of chronic alcoholism relatively ineffective? A review of existing treatment programs suggests the following sorts of assumptions and recurrent problems in the treatment of chronic alcoholism (1266, 1267).

1. A common assumption of treatment programs is that the client population is homogeneous. However, this population is as heterogeneous as any other group of people in society. These individuals drink different amounts of alcohol and have done so over widely differing periods of time. Therefore, they are likely to vary widely with respect to the effect of alcohol on their physical health, mental health, marital and family life, employment status, social and recreational life, and financial stability. These are among the most common factors affected by chronic alcoholism or problem drinking. Because of these differences, it is unreasonable to expect uniform responses to a single treatment modality. Typically, however, there is no attempt to select individuals for a particular treatment. For example, if a program is religiously oriented and an individual's major problem is financial, a favorable outcome could not be expected. Mismatches between patient's problems and treatment modalities can result in considerable distortions in evaluating the effectiveness of different treatment options.

2. To compound the mismatching problem mentioned above, treatment programs usually offer one or a very limited number of treatment choices. As a consequence, it is difficult to tailor treatment to a group of clients who vary widely among themselves with respect to need. Moreover, even when alternative interventions are available, many programs assume that a single modality of treatment will suffice for an individual patient when it may well be that different modalities are more effective during various times in the course of rehabilitation. It is also often assumed that the goals of education programs, disulfiram treatment programs, counseling programs, inpatient programs, and outpatient programs should all be comparable. These assumptions seem highly improbable.

3. Most treatment programs ignore the possibility that continuity of care is

important. Short-term treatment is far less likely to succeed than a program employing long-term reinforcement of whatever behavioral changes have been achieved.

4. While lip service is usually paid to the notion that program evaluation should be an intrinsic part of alcoholism intervention projects, in fact the research (evaluation) component is commonly viewed as being imposed from without and in conflict with the delivery of treatment. To be effective, research must be an integral part of all alcoholism treatment activities. At the same time, however, individuals giving treatment are not in a good position to evaluate their own work and should be left to do what they do best—treat. Thus, we must seek to meld evaluation with treatment without distorting the basic process of either. Unfortunately, this goal is not easily accomplished.

5. Most treatment programs consider that an assessment of outcome success at a single point in time is an adequate predictor of future performance. Given what is known about continued attrition it is important that treatment research be longitudinal and continuous, and that it incorporate a means of modifying program function on the basis of information that has been gained.

These are but a few of the possible reasons why an unsystematic approach to treatment (depicted in Figure 14.3) is unlikely to be effective for many patients and why compliance is so poor.

A Model Treatment System

It is easy to identify potential and actual problems in the delivery of various methods of treatment in alcoholism. It is much more difficult to provide solutions. What follows is a brief outline of the current state of our own program which we feel addresses many and solves some of the issues raised.

Since patient acceptance of treatment and treatment efficacy may be seriously undermined by existing approaches to treatment (Figure 14.3), a model treatment *system* (Core Shell Treatment) has been developed by the Addiction Research Foundation (Figure 14.4). The components of the system are: only one point of entry for all patients to any treatment program(s); ongoing care of each patient by his or her own primary care worker; full social, psychological, and physical assessment (core) over two to three days as a prerequiste to offering definitive treatment; assignment of patients to the treatment(s) (shell programs) they need and wish; and long-term follow-up. Operational research to improve the efficacy of patient matches to treatment and research on optimal treatment methods are conducted by individuals not involved in the treating process. This approach appears to overcome many of the disadvantages of current alcohol treatment programs. Whether or not it will lower rates of attrition from treatment is not known at present, but it is reasonable to think that it may. Specific studies are planned for the future.

ALCOHOL TREATMENT ?

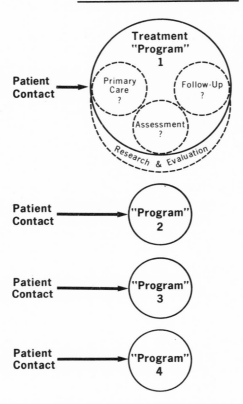

FIGURE 14.3. Typical isolated alcoholism treatment programs.

Manipulation of Alcoholic Behavior by Contingency Management

In the preceding section, a systematic approach to organizing entry into available treatment modalities was described. Organization can help reduce attrition and patient-treatment mismatch and thus can permit individual treatments to operate at maximum effectiveness. However, organization cannot transform failure into success if the basic treatments are worthless. We have already raised the possibility that this may be the case. In this section we discuss a behavioral approach that we believe can actually overcome some of the deficiences of current treatment. There is evidence to support the use of this approach, but it is far from rigorous, and we are again in the position of advising the reader to apply caution in interpreting the material that follows.

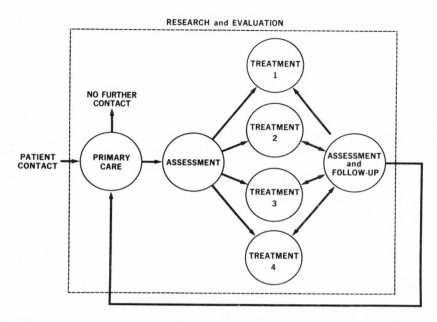

FIGURE 14.4. Core shell health care delivery and treatment system.

The Rationale of a Behavioral Approach.

The essential tenet of an operant analysis of behavior is that behavior is affected by its consequences. Reinforcing consequences are those that maintain behavior, and punishing consequences are those that suppress it. In this scheme, plans for the manipulation of behavior flow from a functional analysis of the relationship between a target behavior of interest (drinking, for example) and some consequence that might be expected to influence the probability of occurrence of a target behavior. This approach is firmly rooted in behavior theory; at a practical level, the implementation of a behavioral treatment regimen is rigorously empirical. If we wish to talk about modifying a behavior, we must be able to define and measure it. If we wish to manipulate behavior, we must be able to specify consequences and apply them systematically in an explicit relationship to a behavior targeted for change. What follow are some illustrations of how these principles have been applied in the treatment of alcoholism, and how they might be relevant to the problem of compliance in general.

If we view the treating agency as a source of potential reinforcers for the patient, and remaining in treatment as a behavioral response, dropout becomes eminently explicable. It is well known that behavior is not readily maintained without reinforcing consequences; this process is described technically as extinction. We should not be surprised if treatments that do not take into account the behavioral circumstances and capacities of the patient fail to maintain the desired responses (i.e., presentation for treatment) if they can in turn offer little by way of reinforcement.

This analysis simply provides a more elegant way of asserting that patients will not continue to be present for treatment if they do not get some payoff from it. To reiterate, little research has been done to explore this notion where attrition is concerned, but there is some suggestive evidence. Patients who expressed a preference for treatment specifically focused on alcohol and drinking were more likely to terminate treatment prematurely to the extent that therapists failed to discuss these issues during initial interviews (1272). Patients prescribed minor tranquilizers were more likely to remain in treatment during its early stages than those who were not (1254). Since it is known that minor tranquilizers can act as powerful reinforcers (1256), it may be that the relatively higher retention rates occurred because the pharmacological "reinforcement" maintained the behavior (i.e., presentation for treatment) upon which its continued availability depended. In fact, this is one justification for offering methadone in maintenance programs: it provides pharmacological reinforcement for remaining in treatment long enough for psychosocial rehabilitation efforts to become effective (1268). However, making continued access to pharmacological reinforcement contingent upon remaining in treatment raises ethical questions. These considerations render a direct experimental test of this behavioral maneuver contentious, although such a procedure has been tested (see below).

These illustrations are amenable to alternative interpretation, and in themselves provide support only for the plausibility of behavioral analysis. More compelling than attrition studies are those of the efficacy of treatments derived from a behavioral analysis.

Contingency Management.

There is a growing literature on the use of contingency management in the control of behaviors related to alcoholism (1280). A mandatory requirement of contingency management is that a contingent relationship between change and the application of some consequence be specified and enforced. This strategy has been employed with considerable efficacy in both laboratory and field settings. In one study, chronic alcoholic subjects lived on a hospital ward where they could obtain alcohol (1259). On some days, the alcohol was freely available without any contingency in effect, but on others the subjects were offered a cash payment for abstinence. Although there were individual differences in the price of abstinence, drinking could be suppressed by payment even when alcohol was available. It was important to apply the rewarding contingency close in time to the abstinent behavior, because a delay of payment disrupted the effectiveness of positive reinforcement on managing drinking. Others have shown that aversive consequences can suppress drinking as well. Moderate drinking was maintained in alcoholics when access to hospital ward privileges was made contingent on moderation or, alternatively, when consignment to a relatively unpleasant life on the ward was a consequence of exceeding a drinking limitation (1255). It has also been found that drinking can be suppressed if a brief period of social isolation is made contingent upon taking a drink (1269).

Research like this has practical implications for treatment. It demonstrates that a major feature of alcoholism, namely self-administration of the agent, can be brought under control when a specific environmental consequence is applied in a carefully prescribed way to a clearly defined and measurable behavior. This specificity distinguishes the operant behavioral approach from most alternatives.

An obvious question is whether comparable procedures can be applied in the natural environment. The small amount of evidence on this issue is positive. One such study, in the field setting, concerned patients in a methadone maintenance program who drank alcohol excessively (1274). The investigators compared a group of patients who were given their daily dose of methadone contingent upon ingesting disulfiram with a control group that was given and urged to take disulfiram but not required to do so in order to receive methadone. During this time the experimental (contingent methadone) group drank much less than the control group, thus attesting to the effectiveness of the management procedure.

A comparable procedure has been applied very effectively in the industrial setting to promote the ingestion of disulfiram by patients whose primary problem was excessive drinking (1280). Some such approaches entail extreme degrees of coercion which a patient must accept. For instance, four individuals who were employees of a hospital faced loss of employment because of excessive drinking. A treatment regimen was developed in which these patients were required to report to the alcoholism clinic of the hospital daily and ingest disulfiram if they were to work on that day. Failure to meet this contingency resulted in the loss of the opportunity to work and a corresponding loss of salary. The regimen was very effective, and it was reported that none of the patients ever failed to comply with the contingency. Absenteeism among these patients dropped dramatically. Results of equally impressive success were obtained with another group of patients who were required to attend a clinic and ingest disulfiram or lose a cash deposit left in trust with a therapist.

Another interesting application of contingency management in a natural setting was reported by Miller (1276). In this case study, a husband and wife contracted to control the husband's drinking. When drinking occurred outside situations that were agreed upon as acceptable the husband was required to pay the wife a fine of $20.00 to be spent frivolously. The wife also left the husband's presence immediately upon discovery of inappropriate drinking. Drinking was suppressed by this agreement and remained so during a six-month follow-up.

Contingency management procedures appear to be among the most effective in managing undesirable behaviors associated with alcoholism, whether in a laboratory or a natural treatment setting. They have the great advantage that a preformance "contract" is specified in terms such that there can be little doubt about what is expected and what the consequences of failure to fulfill the contract will be. It follows that an objective source of data for monitoring the effectiveness of the procedure is automatically built into the design of such treatments. A comment on the general issue of compliance is in order here. Published reports on this method typically have not reported explicit attempts to retain clients in treatment as such, but rather to obtain particular results among those who are willing to submit to contingency management. Yet it is not difficult to see how such methods might be used to promote retention in treatment, whatever the nature of the treatment. Beyond the willingness of the patient to accept contingency management, the therapist must clearly have available the material basis for contingency management, such as a spouse or an employer willing to cooperate with the treatment procedure, and a reward that is more appealing to the patient than the factors that promoted the problem in need of treatment in the first place.

The focus of contingency management can be varied. In the case of alcoholism, it can select as the target behavior drinking itself. In this case, the index of compliance and treatment outcome are the same. Additionally, the procedure can focus on compliance in taking a particular treatment (disulfiram) that in turn may produce the desired outcome. The latter instance is most analogous to the more traditional medical situation, in which the problem is to promote acceptance of a treatment with known efficacy.

Adjunct Pharmacotherapy

Often pharmacotherapy is used alone or in conjunction with behavioral or other psychosocial maneuvers. In general, expectations of drug therapy are unrealistic. In some situations drugs are an inappropriate substitute for proper assessment and treatment. However, drugs can be employed for at least two important purposes in the management of alcoholism. The first, involving drugs such as disulfiram, is to interact pharmacologically with ethanol in such a way as to discourage its use. The second, involving various psychopharmacological agents, is to alleviate emotional disturbances that may contribute to the need for alcohol consumption. Both of these uses relate to compliance: the first, by contingency and coercion, and the second, by promoting a patient's ability to participate in treatment (1284).

Aversive Pharmacotherapy.

In simple classical aversive conditioning, the sight, smell, taste, or thought of alcohol (conditioned stimulus) is linked to an inherently aversive sensation such as nausea and vomiting, or apnea (unconditioned stimulus). For conditioning to occur, the conditioned stimulus must usually precede the unconditioned stimulus by a short and rather narrowly limited interval. Drugs are sometimes used as an adjunct in order to generate the unconditioned stimulus. It is important to note that all studies of these agents include preselected, willing, and motivated patients and therapists. Thus positive results can hardly be generalized to the alcoholic (or therapist) community at large.

Apomorphine and emetine induce nausea and vomiting. Once they have been given, alcohol is offered to the patients just before the effects of the drugs are expected to appear. However, it is difficult to gauge the time precisely, and properly designed studies with these agents are virtually impossible. It is not surprising, therefore, that the reported results with these agents are no better than those of other hospital treatment methods in similar patients. Moreover, apomorphine and emetine are not without some risk.

Succinylcholine is a depolarizing neuromuscular blocking agent that can be injected intravenously in a dose that paralyzes all skeletal muscle, including the diaphragm and intercostal muscles, within one to two minutes. By monitoring the prodromal fasciculation of the muscles, it is possible to time the presentation of alcohol to occur within a few seconds of the onset of paralysis and apnea. This dramatic aversive event is potentially dangerous, highly unpleasant, and has had little acceptance by therapists or patients. It is capable of generating a long-lasting conditioned anxiety response, but the results in relation to prevention of drinking have not yet proven sufficiently encouraging to warrant general use (1253, 1279, 1284).

Though disulfiram is used to discourage drinking by causing an aversive reaction when alcohol is consumed, the time relationships are not those of classical conditioning. Disulfiram is an inhibitor of aldehyde-NAD oxidoreductase, an enzyme located in liver mitochondria which is responsible for the biotransformation of acetaldehyde to acetate. Inhibition of the enzyme results in accumulation of acetaldehyde when ethanol is metabolized. Within five to fifteen minutes after ingesting 0.5 ounce or more of alcohol, the patient feels warm and begins to develop a blush or flush over the upper chest, neck, and malar region. Pulse pressure widens and heart rate increases. The reaction can become more severe and result in nausea and vomiting, hypotension, severe anxiety, and dyspnea. The reaction may last for several hours and has occasionally been fatal. It is the promise and threat of this reaction that establishes the tenuous basis upon which the alcoholic is encouraged to take the drug. On the other hand, the drug must be taken daily by a willing patient. Discontinuing disulfiram for several days will permit full drinking.

Even though there are about a dozen studies comparing disulfiram to a control treatment (1254), use of an appropriate placebo drug control is rare (1253, 1254, 1265, 1279). In all studies, disulfiram appears to be effective in reducing the incidence of relapse. The patient who does better on disulfiram is typically older, better motivated, has a longer drinking history associated with blackouts, and is compulsive and dependent. In each study there are differences between drug-treated and control groups that indicate possible important differences in motivation between the two groups. Therefore, the higher success rate cannot be attributed to disulfiram alone. The study by Gerrein et al. (1265) suggests that disulfiram (250 mg per day) when taken under direct supervision may result in better clinic attendance and identification with the clinic by patients. A program that included supervised disulfiram ingestion, combined with four counseling or group therapy sessions a week, was more effective than programs involving unsupervised ingestion of disulfiram. Unfortunately, this study confounds the effects of supervised administration of disulfiram with those of much more intensive counseling.

The efficacy of disulfiram therapy appears to be determined by patient motivation and by the amount of coercion to continue taking the drug brought to bear on the patient by legal obligation, by a family member, or by an employer. There is no conclusive proof of drug efficacy as distinct from the coercive or motivational elements. In this respect, the subcutaneous implantation of disulfiram seems a reasonable way of ensuring patient compliance. Various accounts of disulfiram implants exist. No double-blind study with random patient assignment to drug and placebo implant conditions has been reported. A high incidence of infection in the implants and extrusion of tablets (14.9%) has been reported (1275). Improved compounding of disulfiram may circumvent these problems. Since it is questionable in some patients whether daily oral dosages of 250 mg to 500 mg of disulfiram produce an adverse reaction after alcohol, it is puzzling why implants of 500 mg to 1,000 mg should be expected to persist and be effective for up to a month. Analysis of drug and metabolites in blood is an essential requirement for any acceptable disulfiram efficacy study. Such assays are now available (1258) and will permit proper studies of disulfiram to be undertaken.

The evidence for disulfiram efficacy is sketchy, the disposition of the drug and its mechanisms of action are unknown, and its potential toxicity and side effects are considerable. Much more study of this agent is therefore required.

Metronidazole, a drug for the treatment of amebiasis, anaerobic infection, and trichomonas vaginalis, is reported to produce a disulfiram-like reaction when alcohol is ingested. Such reactions occur inconsistently, are often mild when they do occur, and are not a particularly effective deterrent to alcohol ingestion. Indeed, animal experiments have failed to confirm a significant effect on acetaldehyde metabolism. Furthermore, short-term studies (one to three months) and longer follow-up studies (six months to one year) have failed to show that this drug is effective (1253, 1279). In addition, the drug is carcinogenic in rodents, mutagenic in bacteria, and should be regarded as potentially dangerous in humans, particularly during chronic ingestion. Further investigation of this agent or its use in the treatment of chronic alcoholic patients should be discouraged (1284).

Citrated calcium carbimide can produce a physiologic interaction with ethanol similar to that of disulfiram, but the reaction is milder, of more rapid onset, and of only half the duration. There are no controlled studies of its efficacy compared to a proper placebo condition or to disulfiram (1284).

Nonaversive Pharmacotherapy.

A wide variety of psychoactive drugs have been employed in attempts to overcome emotional disturbances presumed to cause or contribute to the need for alcohol. These include benzodiazepines, tricyclic antidepressants, and lithium.

Long-term studies with benzodiazepines have failed to provide clear evidence that drug therapy prevents relapse in chronic alcholics who are in remission, or that it assists their longer term behavioral adaption (1253, 1279, 1284). On the other hand, if one is content with shorter term therapeutic goals, there is some evidence that, over six to eight weeks, chlordiazepoxide, prazepam, oxazepam, and diazepam are superior to placebo with respect to patients' subjective improvement in anxiety symptoms and/or physicians' global rating. At best these changes are minimal; and contradictory results do exist. The rate of attrition among patients treated with chlordiazepoxide has been found to be lower than with thioridazine, methocarbamol, or placebo at six weeks. In another study an unselected group of inpatients was started on therapy with chlorprothixene (60 mg to 120 mg daily for two weeks), oxazepam (120 mg to 240 mg daily), or placebo immediately upon admission. Dosages were decreased during the third week and placebo only was given in the fourth week. Oxazepam was significantly more effective in reducing anxiety symptoms than was chlorprothixene, which was more effective than placebo. Chlorprothixene therapy was associated with a significantly greater number of adverse drug effects than the other treatments. Long-term studies (over one year) have failed to show any differences ascribable to the drugs. There appear to be no differences among the various benzodiazepines even during the short term.*

The tricyclic antidepressant drugs are effective in the treatment of endogenous depression if given in adequate dosage. Pharmaceutical claims and clinical preference notwithstanding, all have similar antidepressant activity and would be expected to provide essentially the same symptomatic improvement in chronic alcoholics suffering from depression. Only a few studies have attempted to indentify alcoholic patients with primary endogenous depression to prove this point.

Imipramine was shown to be more effective than placebo in a six-week trial in depressed female alcoholic outpatients and at three weeks in depressed

---

*A preliminary analysis of this issue appears in Bliding A: Efficacy of antianxiety drug therapy in alcohol post-intoxication symptoms. *Brit J Psychiatry* 122:465-468, 1973.

alcoholic inpatients (1253, 1284). In a study of mixed anxiety and depression, doxepin (25 mg t.i.d.) was more effective than diazepam (5 mg t.i.d.) after three weeks in male alcoholic inpatients. In a group of 100 unselected patients both diazepam (5 mg t.i.d.) and doxepin (50 mg t.i.d.) appeared more effective than placebo. However, the placebo group had fewer drug side effects. Other studies, typically with unselected patients or in outpatient settings with high dropout rates, have failed to find even short-term beneficial effects of tricyclic antidepressants.

Since the benzodiazepines are not effective in endogenous depression, and the tricyclics are not indicated for anxiety, comparisons among these agents make little sense.

Lithium may be more effective than placebo in decreasing drinking episodes and rehospitalizations in depressed alcoholics (1290). The studies reported to date have not examined the effects on attrition and there is reason to suspect that patients assigned to drug and placebo groups have not been equivalent. Nevertheless, additional studies of lithium seem warranted in order to define whether and to what degree it helps patients. Until such results are available, lithium has no established general role.

Miscellaneous Pharmacologic Agents.

In addition to its peripheral-blocking action, propranolol has effects in the central nervous system. Results are conflicting with propranolol in the treatment of chronic alcoholism. Some studies suggest a short-term global improvement in symptoms, but others indicate no influence on level of alcohol consumption (1284). Further studies with propranolol are justified since in usual dosages it is a relatively nontoxic drug and does not cause physical dependence.

Several studies suggest that some phenothiazines in low doses are effective in controlling anxiety symptoms. Phenothiazines have never been shown to be as effective and safe as other agents in the chronic alcoholic. In virtually no study have drug-induced abnormalities been analyzed as carefully as have beneficial effects (1253).

A host of other agents have been studied in reasonably well controlled investigations. There is no evidence to justify the long-term use of carbamazepine, methoxydone, cyproheptadine, tybamate, nialamide, phenaglycodol, or hydroxyzine (1284).

Conclusions on Adjunct Pharmacotherapy.

Drugs are unlikely ever to play a primary role in the rehabilitation of the chronic alcoholic. On the other hand, for inpatients with primary affective disorders the short-term usefulness of minor tranquilizers and antidepressants may maximize the patient's ability to participate in other programs. In outpatient studies they may retain patients in treatment for a longer time. A number of precautions seem judicious for future studies of drug efficacy. The therapeutic goal of drug treatment must be defined. Studies must be controlled appropriately and should be double-blind wherever possible. Heterogeneous patient groups should not be studied; rather, patients should be assigned to receive drugs appropriate to the treatment of their individual affective disorders. A measure of patient compliance with medication instruction must be included, and measurements of drug concentrations in blood or plasma should be included wherever possible. In outpatient studies, adverse effects of the drugs must be looked for in detail. High dropout situations should be avoided, since they bias the results negatively. Effects on attrition rates should be sought. Only with precautions such as these will we be able to define more exactly the adjunct role of drug therapies and ensure that potentially effective drug therapies are not judged inadequate and discarded because of faulty trial design.

MONITORING PARTICIPATION, COMPLIANCE, AND OUTCOME

Some of the confusion about which treatments work and which do not stems from inadequate measurement of the process variables of participation in and compliance with treatment programs and from incomplete documentation of treatment outcomes, both in the short and long run. We will remain in ignorance until such assessments are performed. The situation is all the more lamentable, since some of the important variables involved can be measured in a straightforward fashion in alcoholism. In this section we present our recommendations for appropriate evaluation of the success of alcoholism treatment programs.

Retention

Since retention in a treatment program is closely related to outcome, the use of attrition rates may provide a convenient first approximation of treatment program success. Comprehensive evaluation of programs is difficult and expensive, and at present we have not developed the necessary expertise. Obviously, a statistical measure of retention is preferred. Compared with more traditional outcome measures, the life table method illustrated earlier is a simple, inexpensive starting point from which to evaluate the efficacy of programs.

Behavioral Methods for Monitoring Compliance

Behavioral methods to measure compliance directly have not been developed. The reason for this failure, as stated earlier, is that compliance with treatment is sometimes difficult to disentangle from outcome. Such methods are still at a primitive stage of development and the major emphasis has been on the assessment of drinking behavior per se. One important development in this area has stemmed from the rejection of the traditional disease concept of alcoholism. Although extensive discussion of this controversy is not warranted here, Sobell and Sobell (1288) argued that the disease concept of alcoholism as "uncontrollable drinking" tended to limit thinking concerning outcome measures to two categories: abstinence and nonabstinence. These investigators reasoned that to the extent that abstinence is the only criterion of improvement, progress in treatment short of abstinence would not be acknowledged or even sought. To rectify this deficiency they developed follow-up measures that incorporated operationally defined outcomes ranging through the categories of abstinence, controlled drinking (less than 6 ounces of spirits in a day), and drinking of sufficient severity to result in arrest or hospitalization. Moreover, they attempted to obtain these measures for each day of follow-up so that they could construct an outcome index based on the number of days each patient was observed to fall into a particular category. The data were corroborated by sources other than the patients themselves (e.g., friends, family, official records) in an attempt to increase their validity. By recognizing "drinking disposition" as a continuous rather than a dichotomous variable, Sobell and Sobell were able to construct a much more sensitive measure of outcome than has been reported before. A similar approach has been used to assess the effects of a different program with good success (1252).

Another assessment method that has been applied with some success in evaluating treatment outcome involves the direct observation of drinking behavior in the laboratory. One study attempted to evaluate the effectiveness of electrical aversion therapy in suppressing drinking in an alcoholic subject (1277). Efficacy of treatment was observed directly by permitting the subject to drink alcoholic or nonalcoholic beverages in what was presented as a "taste test," but was really a method designed to assess surrepetitiously disposition to drink. The preference for alcohol was markedly reduced as a consequence of the aversive conditioning procedure. In another study (1278), a different measure of disposition to drink was used in an attempt to predict responsiveness to a behavioral treatment procedure. Drinking disposition was measured by allowing subjects to perform the simple response of operating a switch in order to earn points that could be converted to alcohol. Of the 20 subjects tested, it was found that the ten who responded least in order to obtain alcohol were subsequently judged to have improved the most following an eight-week behavioral treatment program.

More examples could be cited to show how laboratory assessments of drinking have been used to measure the efficacy of treatment interventions (see reference 1280). What is important to note is that by using drinking behavior as an indicator, it has been possible to select a variable that is clearly specified and readily measurable. Obviously, a basic assumption of the validity of this technique is that alcohol consumption per se provides a good index of the current degree of an individual's "alcohol problem."

Biochemical Measures

Reduction in alcohol consumption is the main goal of alcoholism rehabilitation. It is surprising to note then, that the various direct and indirect biochemical or pharmacologic measures of alcohol consumption seldom have been incorporated into treatment programs despite their widespread availability. The application of sensitive, reliable, and inexpensive measures of alcohol consumption should receive high research priority. Monitoring alcohol consumption could be applied effectively in conjunction with contingency management techniques. Measurements of blood alcohol concentration could be made in a fashion similar to that for urine testing in methadone clients. Unfortunately, ethanol is rapidly biotransformed, and even heavy drinking twelve hours previously will not be detected. Methods that provide a measure of alcohol consumption over longer periods are promising but insufficiently developed and tested. They include the collection of sweat over seven days and measurement of sweat ethanol concentration (1289), and measurement of the liver mitochondrial enzyme glutamic deyhydrogenase (GDH) (1285, 1286). Methods for assessment of the other liver enzymes and of the metabolic consequences of alcohol (1271) are not sufficiently sensitive or reliable either to detect or to follow intermittent or even chronic excessive alcohol consumption.

To the assessment of blood or breath alcohol levels should be added methods of following compliance with medications prescribed as adjuncts in treatment. This would aid greatly in assessing the efficacy of such agents and, for those of established efficacy, would permit early detection of compliance problems and rational remedial intervention.

CONCLUSIONS AND PRIORITIES FOR FUTURE RESEARCH

In contrast to the usual medical treatment situation, the treatment of alcoholism involves unusually complex problems of acceptance of treatment, initial attrition, adherence, efficacy, and assessment of outcome. This review suggests that, in future, patient compliance may be enhanced by the development of systematic, comprehensive approaches to treatment; by the increased development and use of behavioral techniques; and by the more precise use of drugs and of biochemical indicators of alcohol consumption. The need for careful evaluation of old and new therapeutic interventions has been emphasized repeatedly throughout this chapter.

V
COMPLIANCE
PROVIDERS AND PLACES

15

Nursing
and
Compliance
Carol C. Hogue

INTRODUCTION

This chapter offers a nursing perspective of compliance. It describes, through several examples, how nurses have been involved in promoting or studying compliance, then indicates what that knowledge, coupled with our understanding of nursing, contributes to recommendations for nursing practice and for future research.

There is, of course, no one nursing view of compliance; there is not even a unitary perspective of what nursing is. Nurses are an extremely heterogeneous group of providers, partly because of a wide range of educational preparation. The practice of nursing has changed markedly in recent years, and it is likely that this change will continue. It goes without saying, then, that what follows represents the perspective of one nurse, rather than that of all nurses or even of any particular subgroup.

It is important to appreciate the different facets of nursing care and the breadth and diversity of the nursing profession in order to gain insight into the actual and potential contributions of nursing to the understanding and management of compliance problems. Several authors have given useful characterizations of nursing roles. Hall (1309) describes nursing as an integration of many processes in which *both* the client and the nurse participate.

She outlines three levels of nursing skills:

1) basic process skills, which include perceiving, communicating, caring, knowing, problem solving, creating, and valuing;
2) the components of nursing practice, including assessment, intervention, and evaluation; and
3) change process skills—inquiring, helping, teaching, supervising, coordinating, collaborating, consulting, bargaining, confronting, and lobbying.

An open systems paradigm guides the perceding view of nursing. This approach holds that a person is the concatenation or linking of many different systems in which a disturbance in one system may produce disturbances in other systems. Such a paradigm has encouraged nurses and others to seek "comprehensive care" or what is now often called "holistic care."

Sociologists have described nursing as both *instrumental*, that is, including techniques and procedures directed toward treatment of disease, and also *expressive*, or attending to the provision of emotional support. Discussing the physician-nurse-patient triad, Skipper notes that the instrumental activities may lead to emotional tension in the patient, that this tension may be counterproductive, and the "nurse's role in this three-way relationship is expressive, one of system integration, rather than mainly instrumental." Skipper continues, emphasizing the expressive aspects of nursing:

> By her explanations, by willingness to listen and understand . . . by providing comforting *care*, the nurse functions not so much to cure the patient as to maintain the necessary motivational balance while the patient is undergoing the technical processes designed to return him to health. Therefore, the nurse must treat the patient as a *person* (1335).

Several theories or conceptions that help to describe nursing have been advanced by nurses themselves (1316, 1319, 1330). These fomulations do not exclude instrumental considerations, but they do emphasize expressive roles, and they tend to introduce another dimension, that of self-care, a patient's "personal, continuous contribution to his own health and well-being" (1328).

It should be clear from the introductory remarks above that while the focus of this chapter is compliance from a nursing perspective, nurses view compliance (as do other health providers) within the broader context of a relationship with a patient or client, as a means to an end, and not as an end in itself. Nurses are interested in helping people participate effectively in plans to promote health, treat disease, or effect rehabilitation.

THE PRESENT STATE OF KNOWLEDGE

In this section we will review attempts by nurses to illuminate the phenomenon of compliance. We will then examine the practical contributions of nursing to improving compliance.

The Problem of Compliance

Nurses have long been aware of discrepancies between what is prescribed for patients and what they actually experience. Schwartz (455), for example, studied problems in medication taking by elderly, ambulatory individuals with chronic disease several years before the problem of compliance was more generally appreciated by investigators in other disciplines. One of the earliest comprehensive reviews of compliance with medical regimens is the work of Marston (741), which appeared in the nursing literature in 1970. In a later general review paper, Hogue described the compliance problem and addressed conceptual and methodologic issues in compliance research (703).

Several empirical studies by nurses have attempted to shed light on the compliance problem. Triplett (1340) interviewed 40 poor, white, urban mothers of preschool children to see if good and poor users of health services perceived interactions with health workers differently. Poor users were more likely to perceive threat in past interactions with professional workers, but no relationship was uncovered between use and perceptions of present threat. In another study of low income mothers, Lindstrom (313) conducted focused interviews with 30 Mexican-American mothers who had been identified as attenders, nonattenders, or sporadic attenders at a child health clinic. Factors related to ethnicity and poverty were described, but the study design.did not allow any firm conclusions to be drawn.

Vincent (505) interviewed patients with glaucoma for whom eye drops had been prescribed. The aim of the study was "to examine and analyze variations in the behaviors of conforming and nonconforming medically diagnosed individuals, with reference to the sick role construct formulated by Parsons." The study was designed to describe rather than to test a hypothesis, but it led to several interesting propositions for situational nursing interventions and to the overall impression that "conflict inherent in the sick role may be confounded by conflicts between this role and the normal social role obligations of the individuals involved." We will refer to Vincent's study again when we offer suggestions for clinical practice and research.

Along somewhat different lines, Bille (54) studied body image, patient education, and compliance in 24 men who were treated for myocardial infarction. The results indicated no association between knowledge and compliance, although there was a positive association between body image and reported compliance with posthospitalization prescriptions.

A number of nursing studies of compliance have attempted to test propositions arising from the Health Belief Model (as described by Marshall H. Becker in Chapter 6). Stillman studied 122 women's health beliefs about breast cancer and their practice of breast self-examination (BSE). Eighty-seven percent scored high in perceived susceptibility to breast cancer and 97% scored high in perceived benefits of BSE in reducing the threat of breast cancer. However, only 40% practiced BSE monthly and over 20% of those who perceived the BSE to be beneficial were nonpracticers (1338).

Springer (1337) studied 38 male veterans with chronic obstructive pulmonary disease. All had been told to stop smoking; 20 continued to smoke. Using an interview schedule based on the Health Belief Model, Springer found no variable in the model associated with giving up smoking. In a similar study, Smith (1336) found no associations between health beliefs and compliance with anticonvulsants among 34 ambulatory male veterans. Unfortunately, the sample sizes in these two studies were rather small for firm conclusions to be drawn.

In a somewhat larger study by Hogue and Morgan, the postnatal health beliefs of mothers of all infants (N = 109) born during one month in a North Carolina county were assessed for comparison with the immunization status of the infants when they were between eight and eleven months old. All mothers who could be contacted and who were willing to participate were interviewed at home; complete data were obtained from 66, or 61% of the mothers. The compliance rate for three D.P.T. and polio immunizations was 64%. More than one-third of the respondents were thus identified as noncompliers, a level of noncompliance similar to that found in other studies. The only single or combined variables that were associated with compliance were those comprising the Attitude Toward Medical Authority Scale (247, 1327). Thus, in contrast to the results of some other investigators, this nursing study and the three citied before it have found little merit in the Health Belief Model.

The Role of Nursing Care in Improving Compliance

Nurses have figured prominently in successful strategies to promote compliance. Their contributions have been particularly important in this aspect of the management of chronic disease. One superlative example is the report of Wilber and Barrow (521) on the effect of reinforcement from public health nurses on compliance with antihypertensive regimens among 220 outpatients in rural Georgia. In the nursing care or experimental group the 15% with good blood pressure control at the beginning of the visitation program was increased to 80% after two years, compared to an increase in the control group from 15% to 34%. Two years after the visits stopped, the proportion with good control decreased in the experimental group from 80% to 29% (and from 34% to 21% in the control group). We cannot do more than guess why the nursing intervention was effective, but, as suggested by Brian Haynes in Chapter 8, extended supervision appears to be at least one of the active ingredients. This may account for the compliance drop-off when the special nursing service was discontinued.

Wilber and Barrow's study was one of the first to document the substantial patient benefits that can result from nurses acting in what has now become known as an "extended role." A postbaccalaureate program to prepare nurses to function in an expanded or extended role in child care was described by Ford and Silver more than a decade ago (1304, 1334). Since that time, more than 5,000 nurses have graduated from more than 250 formally organized nurse practitioner programs to practice in a wide variety of settings (1342). Many more registered nurses regard themselves as nurse practitioners even though they have not graduated from recognized programs. Levine (1321) estimated that more than 12,000 nurse practitioners, including those self-declared, were employed in the U.S. in 1977. A great deal of confusion and controversy has accompanied this development, both within nursing and in other groups. The discussions have included concerns about titles, functions, preparation, supervision, reimbursement, and even such basic issues as whether nurse practitioners practice nursing or medicine. In this presentation we simply ask if nurses identified as nurse practitioners have contributed to the improvement of compliance and, if so, in what way. We can identify several studies of nurse practitioners that have addressed patient compliance as an important if not central issue.

Lewis and his co-workers (1322, 1323, 1324) studied nurse clinics in major medical centers. In one study, patients (mainly women) were randomly allocated into two groups after initial testing and evaluation. One group received their care from a nurse, the other from a physician. Patients in the nurse-managed group had less disability, fewer symptoms, fewer broken appointments, fewer criticisms of care, and less use of other medical services than did those in the control (physician) group. The rate of broken appointments was 10.1% among the controls and 5.4% among those treated by the nurses (1323). The investigators reported that the nurses were "engaged primarily in supportive role functions, rather than the technical-diagnostic and therapeutic activities of internists." They suggested that the differences in patient outcomes noted above were related *not* to initial differences in the patients, nor to "the abilities of the practitioners [to] care for them, but to the different process of care emphasized by physicians and nurses" (1324).

Bessman (1292) built on the earlier work of Lewis and his colleagues in a study of the care of 550 diabetic patients. Half the patients (randomly allocated) received care from medical house officers supervised by physicians, and the others from nurse clinicians, also supervised by physicians. The quality of care in the two groups was found to be equivalent, as measured by biochemical parameters (blood sugar and BUN), morbidity (hospitalizations), and mortality after a follow-up period of approximately two years. The percentage of missed appointments in physician clinics was 26% and in the nurse clinics, 16%. It was found that the nurse took more time to educate the patient, paid more attention to social problems that could impinge on medical care, and was more likely to call in a visiting nurse. It should be noted that in the nurse clinics the patient saw the same nurse each time whenever possible, but that the medical house-staff rotation system made it unusual for the same physician to see the same patient twice in a row. Disadvantages noted for the nurse clinician program were recruitment, training, and adequate remuneration for the nurse participants.

Long-term management by nurses of health and illness problems among both children and adults has been described further by Charney and Kitzman

(1297), Alderman and Schoenbaum (4), Lewis et al. (1325), Burnip et al. (76), Flynn (1303), and by many others. We continue the review, however, by looking at nurses acting in roles more specifically related to compliance.

Compliance and Teaching by Nurses.

Teaching patients about the characteristics of their disease and the details of its treatment is a time-honored nursing approach to enhancing compliance. Unfortunately, a great deal of the nursing literature in this area has been prescriptive or descriptive, with little attention to evaluation, especially evaluation of outcome. There is evidence of progress in this area, however.

Hecht (229) studied the effect of nurse teaching on compliance in medication taking in 47 adults with tuberculosis who attended an outpatient clinic after hospital discharge. The teaching was individualized, but included three themes: the importance of the medication therapy, information about the drugs, and "how to achieve congruence between the drug regimen and each patient's lifestyle." One control group received no special teaching; three experimental groups received different levels of teaching. Compliance was assessed at two home visits made later by independent nurse observers. Patients who had the special teaching made fewer errors than did those who had none. Based on pill count, serious error was reduced from 53% in the control group to 17% in the group that received the most intensive teaching. The sample size was small for division into four groups and the results were not statistically significant; the findings are nonetheless suggestive and would certainly be clinically important if validated in a larger study.

Tagliacozzo and her colleagues (493) reported a longitudinal study of the impact of nurse teaching on compliance in 192 adults with chronic disease, mainly hypertension and diabetes. Subjects in the experimental group received a maximum of four teaching sessions while controls received none; all subjects were tested initially for knowledge of their disease and its treatment. Outcome measures included attendance at clinic and other medical appointments, disease knowledge, medication taking, and weight loss. Only 62 (34 experimental subjects, 28 controls) of 125 patients remained through the fourth visit/teaching session. There were essentially no differences between experimental and control subject outcomes, but within the experimental group those with higher education, income, initial disease knowledge, and lower dependence showed higher rates of compliance with medication (not statistically significant) than did those with the opposite characteristics.

Twenty-three hospitalized children between the ages of four and thirteen were instructed by nurses in dental hygiene twice a day for three days. Jeanes and Grant (1315) reported that brushing technique, nutritional knowledge and plaque control were taught directly to the children seven years and older, while mothers of younger children were included in the instruction. Interview and observation were used to assess knowledge and performance at three times: preinstruction, immediate postinstruction, and one to two months after hospital discharge. There was no control group. Children significantly improved in nutritional knowledge, plaque control, and brushing immediately following the teaching and, though they declined slightly one to two months later in all three areas, plaque control and brushing were still significantly higher than baseline levels.

The ultimate objective of health teaching, of course, is not only improved knowledge or even improved clinic attendance, but also control or prevention of disease. Unfortunately, the picture is not bright when health outcomes are examined. For example, Lowe, in a double blind experimental study of the effectiveness of teaching by public health nurses as measured by reported compliance during pregnancy (56 black primigravidas), found no difference between experimental and control subjects. She further found no association between reported compliance and pregnancy outcome as measured by infant birthweight, Apgar score, and maternal or infant complications (317, 318). In a study of diabetics, Williams and colleagues (1343) found no correlation between adherence to the prescribed regimen and actual control of the disease. Furthermore, there was actually a negative correlation between knowledge about diabetes and disease control. We know, of course, that many factors influence health outcomes and that medical care is only one of the these. We know, too, that our knowledge of how to treat certain chronic diseases is limited. Thus, the interpretation of studies such as this one is hampered by our inability to determine what part of the problem is due to poor compliance and what part is due to inadequate therapy.

Nevertheless, it is clear that transmitting information alone is not enough to overcome noncompliance. This notion is new to nursing and it is not broadly recognized. Powers and Ford (1329) have offered a possible explanation for this in their review of nurses' contributions to compliance: "the results of studies examining nursing interventions suggest that truly effective intervention must be based not only upon knowledge *per se* but also knowledge of the way the patient defines his situation." This observation leads to a review of a series of studies in an area that appears to be promising: patient participation.

Nursing Attempts to Facilitate Patient Participation.

Davies (1299) identified the problem of nursing attempts to facilitate patient participation as follows: "We have become experts in understanding cause and treatment for health problems, but we are novices in effectively obtaining the clients' participation in using the knowledge to increase his level of wellness.

Great technical knowledge may be irrelevant without commensurate under-standing of the client and who he is."

In a small, descriptive study, Sheridan and Smith (1332) drew upon a model of mutual participation to guide their evaluation of written family-nurse con-tracts by graduate students in community health nursing. Patients participating in the demonstration project said they felt cared for.

Written contracts were not part of Fink's study of public health nurses "tailoring" the care of children seen in an acute care clinic, but clearly the same notion of therapeutic alliance existed. The nursing role in this controlled trial was described as the "family health management specialist." Families in the study group met with the nurse to discuss health, the structure and functioning of the family and its experience and capacity for health behavior. In addition to "traditional clinic nursing services," general health education, counseling, and coordination of care of other family members were available. Compliance with medications, procedures, and appointment keeping, as well as "total" effectiveness, understanding, and total compliance were all significantly better among study than control families (165). Fink found that study families "re-ported increased feelings of personal worth, conviction of the interest and respect of the provider and institution toward the health status of the child and family, and a sense that the provider showed appreciation of individual family circumstances" (658). It is important to note that Fink conceptualized tailoring not so much as a set of tasks but more a relationship between patients and provider, a process.

Finally, we note a study, reported by Caplan and his colleagues (86), that was designed to enhance adherence to a treatment regimen for hypertension through the use of patient education and social support provided by nurse clinicians. Seventy adults with hypertension (in the longitudinal phase of the study) were allocated to either control (usual care) or one of two experimental groups (lecture or social support). The experimental interventions were performed by nurses. One study group attended a series of four weekly one-hour lectures on the nature of hypertension and its treatment. Members of the other study group attended (in groups of five to thirteen) a series of six, two-hour weekly classes which provided not only factual information but also social support designed to increase the patient's competence and motivation to adhere. After six to eight weeks systolic and diastolic blood pressures were compared for members of the three groups. The investigators concluded that both experimental groups were superior to the control treatment, and that there was essentially no dif-ference between lecture and social support groups. One interesting interpretation offered by Caplan and his colleagues is that the lecture group had been run in a very supportive manner, and therefore perhaps was not sufficiently different from the social support group. There are subtle and complex findings in this study to which we will refer indirectly as we make recommendations for practice and further research.

RECOMMENDATIONS FOR PRACTICE

A number of practical suggestions arise from the nature of nursing, the research reviewed above, and our own experience in helping people participate effectively in their health care. The suggestions should be particularly helpful in (but not limited to) the care of people with chronic disease. The complex nature of chronic illness (its long-term nature, uncertainty of course and prognosis, probability of involving multiple body systems, disproportionate intrusiveness on the lives of patients and their families, common requirement of services from several types of providers, and the ambiguity of social roles of the person who is neither sick nor well) lead to great challenges for providers, patients, and their families, all of whom are interested in compliance as a means toward the goal of optimum health (1302, 1306, 1339).

Think about the Regimen from the Patient's Point of View

If most of the treatment is administered at home by the patient and/or his family members, then it is crucial that the regimen be tailored to their operational framework. Here are some specific suggestions about how to approach the regimen from the patient's point of view.

Make the Prescribed Regimen Understandable.

Combs et al. (1298) and Egan (1301) suggest that in a helping relationship responsibility for the effectiveness of communication rests with the helper, not the recipient of help. Practitioners must use clear, nontechnical language whenever possible and should attempt to use the words and expressions the patient uses to express his understanding of his condition, its prognosis, and its treatment. The greater the socio-cultural distance between the patient and provider, the harder the provider must work to communicate effectively. The appropriateness of the language and the effectiveness of communication overall might be tested by immediate feedback from both the practitioner and patient: the patient describes what he has understood from the information presented, and the practitioner describes what she understands of the "definition of the situation" by the patient.

As a further aid to making the regimen understandable, specific goals should be developed by practitioner and patient, taking into account the categories of information described above. Caplan (86) reviewed studies that show the importance of specificity in contrast to vagueness in setting goals. Thus the goal "losing four pounds in one month" is superior to "losing weight." For further details, see Lawrence Green's chapter on patient education strategies (Chapter 10).

Help the Patient Feel Competent to Manage the Regimen.

Combs (1298) notes that "people feel challenged when confronted with problems that interest them and which they feel reasonably able to handle . . . . The difference between a threatening and a challenging situation lies in the degree of adequacy an individual perceives himself to possess." We have discussed setting specific goals based on provider knowledge of the disease and its course and on the patient's definition of his situation. To encourage the patient to take charge of his regimen, make decisions, and work toward set goals, Keith (1318) suggests that we encourage the patient's independence by reviewing with him his range of competency. German and Chwalow (1305) speak of "the need to evaluate the patient's capacities within the context of a specific situation in a specific setting in order to formulate the appropriate and potentially productive role for the patient," and Argyris (1291) indicates that people learn best under conditions of psychological success, that is, conditions of feeling they are competent and that they are making progress. Acknowledgement of competence builds the kind of self-esteem that helps people learn and change behaviors.

Acknowledge That the Medical Regimen Is Only
Part of the Life Regimen the Patient Must Manage.

The other social roles the patient must fill as a family member, worker or student, church member, etc. may lead to competing demands on the patient (1306, 1339). We may be more effective in helping patients attach some priority to their medical regimen if we understand their motives and demands.

Use the Power of Natural Support Systems

Repeatedly social isolation has been found associated with low compliance (405, 591, 694, 1314) and its converse, a supportive family, appears to promote high compliance (86, 384, 505, 604, 694, 1326). This suggests that compliance might be improved by harnessing and directing the energy of what Gerald Caplan (1296) has called the natural support system of family, friends, neighbors, and other lay people.

Social support has been described as both instrumental in nature (reminding the family member to wear a sling; providing transportation to a clinic) and expressive (acting as a buffer against the threat of uncertainty by providing emotional support, acceptance, or sanctuary) (1310, 1311). Although there is evidence that social support has its greatest impact in the presence of perceived threat or stress (1295), it is not yet known how social support works.

How can practitioners use support systems? We offer two ways.

Identify the Patient's Support System.

Ask who the key people are and how they (can) help. The mere identification of these supportive people may help the patient perceive a source of help and may encourage his "getting in touch." The suggestion here is not to *manufacture* supportive people. Indeed, there are lifelong isolates who have no perceived support system; they may be uncomfortable with too much closeness from either profesionals or lay people (1344). The intent of this suggestion is to facilitate the use of existing support systems.

Discuss the Regimen with Family Members.

Include a family member or other person identified by the patient as important to him in discussions of the regimen. Of course, this requires the patient's approval and often some additional planning. Davis (129), Stimson (820), and Twaddle (1341) in their reviews suggest that there must be agreement among health professionals, the patient, and his family and friends about the person's health status and the need for treatment if compliance is to occur. Such a strategy may increase the likelihood of concordance, thereby facilitating the sort of assistance through social support mentioned above.

Collaborate with Others Interested in the Patient's Progress

Finally, we suggest that practitioners form therapeutic alliances. Brill (1294), Horowitiz (1313), Katz et al. (1317), Leininger (1320), and Hogue (1312) have written of the benefits of teamwork when whole people and not just organ systems or diseases are the focus of care. We will not attempt to summarize those writings here, but will simply make two observations to support the suggestion for collaborative approaches.

Coordinated Team Approach.

A coordinated team approach may increase the quality of service available to the patient. If providers do not do the coordination, the patient has to do it.

Facilitating Teamwork.

A team approach does not necessarily demand a formally organized team; one person who understands the importance of coordination can reach out to others involved and facilitate the communication that is at the heart of teamwork.

In summary, we have made three suggestions to practitioners who wish to improve compliance: think about the regimen from the patient's point of view;

use the power of natural support systems; and collaborate with others interested in the patient's progress. As Fink (165) noted in his study of tailoring, these suggestions are for a series of interpersonal processes and enabling conditions, and are not a list of techniques.

PRIORITIES FOR FUTURE RESEARCH

Nursing research will make a greater contribution to health care if research designs include concepts and theories that guide nursing practice. This book is perhaps evidence of a trend toward interdisciplinary collaboration and research in the study of compliance. Sills noted that:

> Nursing needs to continue to develop and study what is within its boundaries and to study individually and collaboratively what is within the larger boundaries of health care. The promise for society in terms of the potential and the capacity of both areas of inquiry are too great to permit chauvinism of any ilk (1333).

With these thoughts in mind, and with attention to the research reviewed in this chapter and others, we suggest two areas for additional research. First, nurses can continue to increase our knowledge of how people cope with medical regimens. Finlayson and McEwan (1302), Gerson and Strauss (1306), Goffman (1307), Roth (1331), and Davis (1300) have extended the concept of career from its occupational source to chronic disease, emphasizing the processual nature of illness and its management. We might be able to offer better care if we understood the illness career of people with chronic disease. Vincent (505) has suggested that we learn why people cannot comply, and Green (1308) has asked if we can identify critical periods. The identification of critical periods might allow us to tailor interventions over time as well as over patient populations. Second, nurses should conduct and/or participate in more controlled trials of nursing interventions to enhance compliance. As a minimum, these studies should describe patient outcomes. Also of importance is, as Bloch (1293) notes, the systematic description of the process of care as well as the outcome.

CONCLUSION

Both in practice and through research, nurses have long displayed their concern about compliance problems. Indeed, nurses have always had the main responsibility for insuring as far as possible that hospital inpatients received their treatments. With the advent of efficacious treatments for chronic illnesses and the extension of the nursing role into ambulatory care, it seems only natural that nurses should take on compliance management as an important part of their responsibilities in this part of health care as well.

While the nurse has traditionally been instrumental in conveying to patients information about treatment, it appears that this necessary function is not the route to higher compliance. Therefore, nurses will have to rely less on this method in handling compliance problems than they have in the past. Other more effective interventions include promoting the patient's participation in his or her own care, reducing the barriers to compliance by tailoring the treatment and by identifying and helping to resolve any difficulties the patient may have that are interfering with compliance, and, finally, increasing the level of attention paid to patients who are having compliance difficulties by mobilizing professional and social support. The latter strategy appears to be particularly effective and is in harmony with the "expressive role" which is such an important part of the nursing process.

Improving low compliance is an exciting challenge with substantial rewards for patient and provider. Nurses can and are providing one of the keys to the humane and sensible solution of the problem.

16

The Clinical Pharmacy and Compliance

James M. McKenney

INTRODUCTION

It is logical that pharmacists be involved in measuring and improving patients' compliance with prescribed medications. They are already part of the normal delivery system for ambulatory patients, thus obviating the "creation" of yet another new health provider specializing in compliance management. Because pharmacists have frequent, repeated contact with patients they can routinely provide services designed to measure or improve compliance on a long-term basis. In addition, they have already established with prescribers the line of communication that is essential if compliance is to be attacked in a coordinated manner. Moreover, it should be noted that pharmacists dispense one of the products for which compliance is such a problem. Although pharmacists do not prescribe the regimen, it is in the pharmacist's jurisdiction that drugs and patients come together, thus providing a focus in the normal delivery of care where compliance can be measured and strategies to improve it can be provided. Finally, it is logical that pharmacists participate in the compliance issue because they are available. Since pharmaceutical manufacturers assume major responsibility for the "mixing and making" of drugs, the pharmacist often has been left with only the mechanical aspects of dispensing. He is thus unable to utilize his unique knowledge and professional training to the extent desired. However, as a result of the redirection of the professional role and the introduction of technical dispensing assistants, the pharmacist's considerable talents in drug therapy can be brought to bear on the compliance problem.

There are barriers to the participation of the pharmacist in the detection and management of patient noncompliance; the most obvious barriers are time and money. The time problem could be solved if the pharmacist relinquished some technical dispensing functions to pharmacy assistants. Although such a reorganization would enable pharmacists to address compliance problems, they might not be able to do so unless the redefinitions could be justified on an economic basis; the pharmacist must be able to receive financial reimbursement for services rendered. For example, an increased prescription volume (prompted by more compliant patients) and increased revenues from third party payers who recognize the health value and economic savings that could result from improved compliance would redress the economic imbalance that might otherwise result from adopting this new role.

Regardless of roles and revenue, what is needed in the day-to-day delivery of health care is a practical way of detecting noncompliant patients and of managing these problems on a continuous rather than sporadic basis. This chapter will present ways that pharmacists can address these problems.

THE MEASUREMENT OF COMPLIANCE IN THE PHARMACY

There are many methods for measuring compliance to prescribed drug therapy; these are reviewed in detail in Chapter 3. Ideally, the measurement used in the normal course of care should be practical, readily accessible, and of sufficient sensitivity to identify as many noncompliers as possible. Unfortunately, few available methods meet all of these criteria. For example, tracers or the "medication monitor" are valuable as research tools but are impractical in busy practice (364, 442). Conversely, drug histories or self reports by patients, although readily accessible and inexpensive, substantially underestimate noncompliance (199, 349, 392); it is only when the patient admits noncompliance that the provider can be reasonably assured of the accuracy of the history (392). Even the direct pill count, the method used in many compliance studies, is awkward to perform in most patient settings and, unless nonobtrusive and performed with discretion, can raise patients' suspicions to the point of causing them to dispose of unused tablets (107, 302, 329, 341, 449).

Blood, urine, or salivary levels of drugs are the most objective methods for measuring patient compliance (319, 1352). However, these methods are either unavailable for many commonly used drugs or tend to require sophisticated technology and take a long time to complete. Rapid advances are being made in this field and inexpensive, simple methods for rapid drug assays may soon be available for use in the physician's office or in the pharmacy. These developments are part of a major current thrust in pharmacy, the training of individuals who can interpret the results of drug assays in light of the absorption, distribution, metabolism, and elimination characteristics of a drug and translate them into clinical terms. This science, known as biopharmaceutics and pharmacokinetics, is currently taught in schools of pharmacy and is being applied increasingly by pharmacy graduates.

Until such assays become available to community practitioners, other methods of measuring compliance must be used. A major method builds on the fact that most pharmacists in ambulatory settings maintain records of medications dispensed to individual patients. These records, known as *patient medication profiles*, include each drug's name, dose, schedule, quantity, and the date each was dispensed to the patient. With this basic information, the pharmacist can project when patients should return for a given prescription refill and can compare the quantity of drugs dispensed with the quantity which should have been consumed according to the dosing schedule. Thus, the pharmacist has a readily accessible, noninvasive, inexpensive tool for estimating patient compliance and detecting patients who may be offered or would benefit from compliance-improving strategies. For example, Solomon and co-workers (1370) reported that the incidence of potential therapeutic problems pharmacists detected by using the medication profile was 5.8%, compared to a rate of only 0.1% detected without the profile. Furthermore, most of the problems concerned the overuse and underuse of drugs.

Unfortunately, the medication profile approach has limitations. Although it is valuable for measuring compliance with chronic therapy in which multiple prescription refills are required, it is of limited value for measuring compliance with single-prescription or other short-term therapy. In addition, its application assumes that all medications dispensed become medications consumed.

COMPLIANCE-IMPROVING STRATEGIES

Regardless of whether noncompliance is considered a patient or a practitioner problem, all health providers have a professional responsibility to offer services that adequately meet the needs of their patients, including those services that promote safe and appropriate drug use. For the pharmacist, this does not necessarily mean that specific strategies need to be pulled from a "bag of tricks" when a noncompliant patient is detected. Instead, the literature strongly suggests that certain basic, routine services which are considered a minimal part of any good pharmacy practice can have a dramatic impact on preventing a compliance problem. Some of the most important routine services are considered below.

Simplification of the Regimen

The complexity of a drug regimen appears to affect patient compliance. The greater the number of doses per day or the total number of drugs in the regimen, the less likely are patients to comply (63, 102, 256). Conversely, simplifying treatment regimens may improve compliance (1350). Thus, the pharmacist could foster patient compliance by insuring that drugs are used only when legitimately needed and that, when prescribed, they are scheduled in as convenient a regimen as possible.

One way in which the pharmacist can reduce the complexity of drug regimens is by referring to the patient's medication profile record. Because the pharmacist

TABLE 16.1. Comparison between patient satisfaction with pharmacy services and compliance.

Variables	Satellite pharmacy	Traditional pharmacy
Composite satisfaction		
Very unsatisfied to acceptable	0	7(18.4%)
Satisfied	16 (43.2%)	25(65.8%)
Very satisfied	21 (56.8%)	6 (15.8%)
Compliance		
Less than 25% deviation	15 (93.8%)	8 (47.1%)
Mean compliance	89%	70%

SOURCE: Ludy et al. 1977 (322).

is often the only health provider who can view the total drug regimens of patients, especially those with several physicians, the pharmacist can consult with prescribers when overly complex or otherwise problematic drug regimens are revealed.

The pharmacist can also help reduce the complexity of drug regimens by limiting the use of nonprescription drugs. Patients who medicate themselves with several drugs further complicate their regimens with what are often irrational, ineffective, or unnecessary agents (1371). The pharmacist is in an ideal position to monitor the use of these drugs and to provide key advice to patients on their nonprescription drug needs.

Modification of the Pharmacy Practice Setting

Frequently, today's pharmacists find themselves surrounded by a wide variety of nonpharmaceutical products in a large mercantile setting. There they must dispense hundreds of prescriptions each day, attempt simultaneously to get through physicians' office receptionists for prescription refill authorizations, complete one of a dozen or more third-party payment forms, and attempt to satisfy a public seeking the highest quality drugs for the lowest price with the shortest waiting time.

Does this practice setting and milieu discourage patient compliance? Recent work by Ludy and co-workers (322) suggests that it may affect both patients' satisfaction with pharmacy services and their compliance with prescribed therapy. As shown in Table 16.1, the percentage of patients taking 75% or more of their medications increased twofold when drug counseling services provided by a pharmacist were moved from the outpatient dispensing window to a private consultation room. Further, when patients were asked which setting they preferred, although nearly 70% of those being served through the open window had no preference, 80% of those receiving services in the private room preferred

TABLE 16.2. Comparison of patient comprehension and adherence with prescription label
            directions

Element	Prescription label	Comprehension	Adherence
Amount of doses	98.8%	91.3%	89.3%
Number of doses	92.7%	85.8%	63.8%
Timing	12.8%	70.5%	60.1%
Administration	98.2%	94.5%	98.1%
Purpose	15.3%	80.5%	97.2%

SOURCE: Boyd et al. 1974 (63).

the privacy. These findings suggest that changing the practice setting, in addition
to improving patient satisfaction and compliance, may also change what patients
expect from pharmacists.

The time taken to dispense medications is also important. Finnerty et al.
(168) reported that patients waited nearly two hours for their prescriptions in
his clinic. Even the hardiest of patients may be discouraged from having prescriptions filled or refilled as needed in such a setting. This time problem can be
largely solved with the employment of technical pharmacy assistants. Not only
does this speed the dispensing process, it also frees the pharmacist to provide
consultation and other compliance-improving services to patients.

Better Prescription Labels

There is general agreement that it is more important for patients to understand precisely how to take prescribed drugs and what to expect from them
than it is for them to learn interesting but ineffectual information about their
disease and its treatment (449, 612, 614, 616, 706, 772, 794, 813). The principal means of providing patients with this explicit "how-to" information is
through the prescription label; yet studies have shown repeatedly that labels
are often incomplete and misinterpreted by patients (239, 749, 1365). For
example, Mazzullo and co-workers (749) reported that none of 67 patients
uniformly interpreted the directions on ten prescription labels. Hermann (239)
reported that a third of 450 medication schedules were erroneously interpreted.
He also found that, as a direct result of their failure to comprehend the directions on their prescription labels, over 60% of 134 patients made administration
errors that precluded optimal response to therapy. Boyd et al. (63) reported
similar findings, as displayed in Table 16.2. If these studies accurately reflect
the situation for most patient groups, there is little wonder why compliance
is such a problem.

In most clinical settings, the prescription label is an exact replication of
the physician's written prescription. Thus, in order to improve the quality of

directions on these prescription labels, medical curricula must address prescription writing as a high priority. In addition, the pharmacist should assure that prescription label directions are complete and clear; at times, this will mean that these directions need to be expanded by the pharmacist. For example, if a physician indicates that a certain medication is to be taken twice daily, the pharmacist may choose to indicate specific times of day at which the medication is to be taken. The pharmacist should also be sure that the name of the medication, its strength, dosage form, and purpose are included in the directions for its use. These fairly simple approaches will enhance the explicitness of the directions for the patient substantially and thus describe more clearly the recommended behavior. In all of this, however, it is recognized that these changes should reinforce, not alter, the original intent of the prescribing physician.

Patient Education

Since compliance with prescribed therapy requires learning a new behavior, patients must first be taught how to take medications correctly. This cognitive stage of learning is very important, for without it compliance failure is inevitable. Thus, the cornerstone of compliance is patient education about the regimen. Many studies have confirmed that the education of patients by pharmacists has led to improved compliance (107, 136, 314, 329, 331, 341, 348, 349, 1357). Typical of these studies is the one by Cole and Emmanuel (107), which showed that 92% of 25 patients who consulted with a pharmacist at the time of discharge from a hospital were compliant with their therapy, whereas only 24% of 25 control patients not receiving these consultation services were compliant.

Although these studies have demonstrated an association between patient education and compliance, little attention has been given to the content of these educational messages. Just how much patients need to be taught is not at all clear. Recently, Sackett and co-workers reported (449) that patients who were given a "mastery learning" program learned a lot about hypertension but were no more likely than control patients to take their medications. While subjects in this study were instructed in some general principles on how to remember to take medications, the teaching format did not permit this information to be specific to the individual patient or to his prescribed regimen. It remains to be tested whether individualized instruction would improve long-term compliance. In any event, there is a great deal of evidence that patient education promotes compliance with short-term regimens (see below) and, while not sufficient for generalization to long-term treatment, it provides a useful starting point. Accordingly, the American Society of Hospital Pharmacists has stated that the pharmacist has the professional responsibility to inform patients properly about the following items for each medication in the patient's regimen (1375):

1. Drug name.
2. Intended use and expected action.
3. Route, dosage form, dosage, and administration schedule.
4. Special directions for preparation.
5. Special directions for administration.
6. Precautions to be observed during administration.
7. Common side effects that may be encountered, including their avoidance and action required if they occur.
8. Techniques for self-monitoring of drug therapy.
9. Proper storage.
10. Potential drug-drug or drug-food interactions or other therapeutic contraindications.
11. Prescription refill information.
12. Action to be taken in the event of a missed dose.
13. Information peculiar to a specific patient or drug.

This list represents what patients should be taught in order to administer their medications safely and appropriately. However, as shown in Table 16.3, patients may want to know even more. Joubert and Lasagna (1359) reported that, in addition to the foregoing information, at least 75% of the 137 patients they surveyed also wanted to know all possible risks of normal use (including rare but potentially lethal side effects), and important alternative uses other than the one for which the drug was prescribed.

Not only must patients be given specific instructions if they are to administer prescribed medications appropriately; they also must be motivated to accept this information and to translate it into behavioral change. This motivational stage is also an important step in the learning process, and the failure to motivate patients will result in noncompliance even if patients know how to take their medications correctly. Thus, while patient education is the cornerstone of compliance, motivation is a building block without which the structure cannot stand. Motivation to adopt a recommended behavior can be provided by a number of methods, including counseling, reinforcement, goal setting, tailoring, feedback, and adoption; these will be discussed in the next section of this paper. In addition to these, the Health Belief Model may provide a guide to the encouragement of patient motivation.

Work by Becker and others, described in Chapter 6 and elsewhere (34, 791, 1348, 1349), has helped us understand how health beliefs may affect patient behavior. Although its link to compliance is disputed (see D. Wayne Taylor's contribution to Chapter 6), the Health Belief Model suggests that patients will be more willing to comply if they: (1) perceive that they are susceptible to the disease; (2) perceive a threat from the disease; and (3) perceive that the benefits from prescribed therapy outweigh perceived barriers to compliance with it (for example, drug costs, side effects, and complex regimens). In attempting to moti-

TABLE 16.3. Drug information desired by patient

Name	97.1%
Specific use	93.4%
Common risks	89.1%
Risk of overdose	86.1%
Risk of underdose	80.3%
Risk of discontinuing	78.8%
All risks	76.6%
Other uses	74.5%

SOURCE: Joubert et al. 1975 (1359).

vate patients, therefore, counseling pharmacists might address each of these perceptions in the initial instructional process and provide reinforcement of this attention on a continuing basis. One component of the model in particular defines a remediable problem that pharmacists could tackle: barriers to drug taking. Strategies for reducing these barriers are discussed throughout this chapter.

Given the fact that patients deserve to be taught how to take their medications correctly and motivated to translate this knowledge into behavior, some consideration must be given as to how these educational messages may be delivered best. There are basically three choices: verbal consultation, audiovisual programs, and written material. Verbal consultation is clearly as effective as the other two choices in providing basic information (101, 331, 1373), and several studies have documented improved compliance after verbal consultations were used to instruct patients (348, 1357). In addition, patients appear to prefer verbal consultation from their physicians and pharmacists as their main source of information (1359). Perhaps the most important reasons for using this means of communication, however, are that it fosters rapport between health providers and patients and that it provides an opportunity to tailor the educational message to the individual patient's needs. Thus, verbal consultation should comprise a part of any attempt to instruct patients effectively.

However, when used alone, verbal consultation may not be the most effective or efficient method of either providing information or promoting compliance, and it clearly requires more of the health professional's time than do alternative methods (1373). In addition, work by Joyce et al. (715) and Ley and Spelman (1361) indicates that nearly half of the verbal information provided patients is rapidly forgotten. For these reasons, other means of communication need to be added to the verbal component in order to augment and reinforce its messages.

One method of augmenting verbal instruction is to use audio-visual aids (1364, 1369, 1373). For example, Welk and co-workers (1373) found that audio-visual instruction was at least as effective as verbal instruction in achieving patient recall of information, and it decreased by five-sixths the average professional time required to provide counseling. Although such audio-visual programs are effective and efficient, particularly in supplying general drug information, they provide only one-way communication, are not commercially available for many commonly used drugs, and may be prohibitively expensive. At this time, therefore, audio-visual strategies require further development and research before their full potential in improving patient compliance can be realized.

The most time-efficient and least expensive method of augmenting and reinforcing verbal information about drugs is the use of written instructions. Drug monographs have been developed by several groups (1356, 1367), have been tested in a number of practice settings (101, 341, 397, 460, 1346, 1353, 1354, 1355, 1358, 1359, 1360, 1374), and have recently been proposed for national distribution with some classes of drugs by the Food and Drug Administration in the USA (1376). The latter proposal is judged premature by some who question whether drug monographs will result in safer and more compliant drug use; how detailed need they be; what style, readership level, and design is best; will they change the liability of professionals or patients; and, if they are required by the Food and Drug Administration, who will develop, finance, and distribute them?

Preliminary evidence does suggest that written instructions are desired by patients (1359, 1360) and supported by the majority of practicing physicians and pharmacists (34, 101, 715, 791, 1346, 1354, 1356, 1359, 1360, 1361, 1364, 1367, 1369, 1373, 1374). Further, they appear effective in both increasing the patient's understanding of the correct use of drugs (1355, 1358) and promoting patient compliance (101, 341, 397, 460, 1353). Sharpe and Mikeal (460) reported 85% compliance in a group of patients receiving antibiotic therapy and written instruction as compared with 63% compliance in patients receiving only the usual prescription label. Mattar and co-workers (341) reported that 51% of 33 patients given both written and verbal instruction by pharmacists were fully compliant, while only 8.5% of 200 concurrent controls were compliant. Comparing verbal instruction with verbal instruction and written reinforcement, Paulson et al. (397) found that the latter was significantly more effective in presenting the proper way for patients to correct for missed doses, in describing the foods or drinks to be avoided while taking medications, in achieving an understanding of the purpose for the medication, and in developing the knowledge of how to refill the prescription. Parenthetically, this group also reported that informing patients about medication side effects did not lead to an increase in their occurence. Finally, Fleckenstein (1354), who studied a patient package insert currently included with oral contraceptives in the USA, reported that the majority of 828 women prescribed these drugs received the insert, read it, and found the information clear and useful. When their knowledge was tested, most of these women demonstrated that they had learned at least some of this information. These preliminary results are encouraging, for they suggest that written instructions such as drug monographs, when coupled with verbal counseling, can have a major impact on patient compliance.

Effective Communication

Since it is evident that patients require both information and motivation in order to comply, good communication between health providers and patients is vital. In fact, regardless of how complete the information provided the patient, noncompliance is likely to follow if communication is faulty (256, 1351, 1366). To the extent that the effectiveness of this communication is determined by the relationship established between patient and health provider, considerable attention must be given to the specific counseling techniques used by health professionals (130, 174, 1372). Too often, patient education is viewed as a lecture given to an attentive patient who understands the message and therefore adheres to the regimen. Nothing could be farther from the truth. Good counselors are interested not only in sending messages effectively but also in receiving them. They freely send and receive thoughts and feelings, both verbally and nonverbally. In this way they establish relationships with patients that engender trust and confidence and, therefore, foster patient compliance. Effective counselors specifically avoid confrontation, tension, attempts to control one another, or other factors known to impair the relationship (128, 670). Their communication is clear, explicit, and reinforcing. The basic attitude of the effective counselor is one of concern and compassion, with freely provided feedback to patients after the appropriate information has been solicited.

In an important recent study by Svarstad (490), these and other characteristics of the patient-provider relationship were assessed and related to patient compliance among 221 patient encounters with eight physicians in an urban health center located in a low socioeconomic area. Characteristics that were analyzed included (1) the amount of explicit instruction given regarding the use of medicatons; (2) the justification or rational appeal for the drug's use; (3) the friendliness or receptivity expressed by the provider toward the patient; (4) the exertion of medical authority; (5) the emphasis given on what was expected from the patient in medication taking; (6) the monitoring (questioning) by providers of previous medication-taking behavior; and (7) the responsiveness of providers to patients' complaints or admissions of noncompliance. The analysis of these characteristics and their relationship to patient compliance are displayed in Figures 16.1 and 16.2. Compliance was better when these characteristics were present to a high degree. Further, when all of these characteristics were present (depicted in the figures as "high motivation") and coupled with a major effort to instruct, patients were highly compliant with their regimens. This study strongly suggests—although it does not prove—that the manner of communication may be as important as the content of the communication, at least insofar as compliance is concerned.

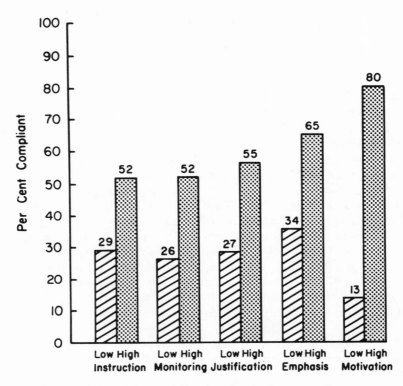

FIGURE 16.1. Association of characteristics of communication to compliance.

SOURCE: Adapted from Svarstad 1974 (490).

Monitoring and Feedback

Monitoring may be considered another aspect of communication. It involves inviting from patients feedback on problems they may have experienced in taking their medications and providing patients with appropriate strategies for solving the problems raised. Such a service can be provided on a continuous basis during follow-up visits, such as when patients return to pharmacies for prescription refills. Inviting feedback requires that the health provider be willing to listen to the patient. It also requires eliciting information about specific problems and allowing patients to describe their drug use problems and concerns fully. This aspect of monitoring is sometimes called "negative feedback," for it is principally concerned with uncovering problems that patients are having with the prescribed therapy—side effects, dose scheduling difficulties, administration problems. Soliciting feedback not only uncovers barriers to full compliance but also demonstrates inherent interest and concern on the part of the health provider.

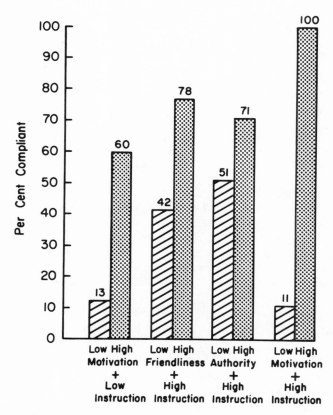

FIGURE 16.2. Association of characteristics of communication and instruction to compliance.

SOURCE: Adapted from Svarstad 1974 (490).

The work by Svarstad (490) suggests that health providers often do not encourage and may even discourage negative feedback from patients about side effects or problems with compliance. In her study, the usual method providers used to monitor compliance was simply to ask the question, "Did you take your medicine?" However, when the level of monitoring increased, a greater number of problems were detected, more compliance-improving strategies were initiated by providers, and the compliance levels of the patients inproved.

In our own work (348), patient monitoring proved an important element in enhancing patient compliance. In this study, pharmacists provided education and monitoring services to hypertensive patients when they returned to their community pharmacy each month for prescription refills; control patients did not receive these services. As shown in Table 16.4, most study patients were highly compliant and under good blood pressure control while receiving these

TABLE 16.4.   Effect of pharmacist counseling/monitoring services on compliance and therapeutic response

	Control Group			Study Group		
	Before	During	After	Before	During	After
Number of patients	24	24	21	24	24	24
Average consumption	63%	56%	60%	67%	92%	70%
Patients compliant	16%	17%	16%	25%	79%	25%
Normotensive	44%	20%	14%	20%	79%	42%

SOURCE: McKenney et al. 1973 (348).

services from their pharmacist. They were neither compliant nor controlled prior to the experimental period or after it was concluded; control patients remained hypertensive and noncompliant throughout these three periods. Because the general lack of knowledge about hypertension and its treatment did not diminish after contact with the pharmacist ceased, it was concluded that the following specific services accounted for the observed results:

1. Provision of verbal and written explicit instructions on how medications were to be taken.
2. Continuous measurement of patient compliance.
3. Continuous reinforcement of explicit instructions and motivation to comply.
4. Continuous soliciting of negative feedback and provision of appropriate responses to detected problems.
5. Contact with a provider who showed interest and care.

These services, if offered by pharmacists on a continuous basis in the normal delivery of care, should significantly improve the compliance of the majority of ambulatory patients.

Once problems have been uncovered through the feedback process, it is crucial that the health provider respond to them if patient compliance is to be improved or maintained. Indeed, even though it is not always possible to solve the compliance problem, the failure to offer help has an even worse effect. The responses that may be made, depending on the particular problem that has been detected, include tailoring, goal setting, further explanation, and referral.

Tailoring

Tailoring is particularly useful for patients who have difficulty in following a dose schedule (852). It involves selecting the dosage intervals and times that best coincide with the patient's daily lifestyle. In this way tailoring seeks to make drug taking as convenient, tolerable, and self-determined as possible. For example, the patient who has difficulty remembering to take his daily digitalis dose may be encouraged to use the time he brushes his teeth, has his morning meal, or performs other daily activities as cues for medication taking.

Goal Setting

Goal setting provides a method for patients to observe the results of compliance with therapy and may be of particular value for patients with asymptomatic diseases. The goals that are set should be readily measureable and interpretable by the patient; they should also demonstrate short-term results that can be used as a feedback mechanism to reinforce compliance. For example, the ultimate goal of drug therapy in hypertensive patients is to prevent cardiovascular and cerebrovascular complications of uncontrolled blood pressure. Attainment of this goal is neither readily measuable nor demonstrable from visit to visit. Instead, the patient could be given a blood pressure goal and allowed to follow his progress toward achieving and maintaining it, either during each visit, or by means of self-monitoring blood pressures at home.

Reassurance

Often there is no practical solution to the problem detected during the monitoring process. In this instance, the best approach involves simply acknowledging the legitimacy of the problem, explaining its origin or characteristics, clarifying misconceptions, and reassuring the patient of the benign or self-limiting nature of the problem. For example, the patient receiving a diuretic for the first time may complain of nocturia. After the pharmacist is assured that a dose is not being taken near bedtime, this patient could be told that diuresis is an expected action of the drug and that the problem, while bothersome, is not serious and will diminish as the drug is continued. Whenever possible, specific recommendations to correct the problem are preferred. For example, the patient who develops a bothersome dry mouth during methyldopa therapy should be reassured that the problem is not dangerous and that it can be relieved by sucking lozenges, chewing gum, or drinking liquids.

Referral

If the problem detected is potentially serious or requires evaluation and management by a physician, the pharmacist should refer the patient to the physician who initiated the regimen. In making such a referral, the pharmacist needs to avoid undue anxiety while emphasizing the importance of the referral.

ADDITIONAL COMPLIANCE-IMPROVING STRATEGIES

Even if the foregoing strategies are made available routinely by pharmacists, there will remain a group of patients who continue to be noncompliant with prescribed regimens. The reasons for this noncompliance will vary from forgetfulness to deliberate rejection of the regimen and therapy. Once pharmacists

TABLE 16.5.   Effect of drug packaging on patient compliance

Package	Percentage of doses consumed	Percentage of patients taking ± 10% of doses
Vial, label	73.3	28.0
Vial, label calendar, instruction card	83.9	37.5
Unit doses, instruction card	92.5	61.9
Dial Pack, instruction card	97.3	88.5

SOURCE: Linkewich et al. 1974 (314).

have detected noncompliant patients (through the use of medication profiles or other measurement systems) and are convinced that patients will not respond to routine compliance-improving strategies, they need to examine the patients more closely in order to detect specific reasons for noncompliant behavior and to offer other compliance-improving services. These adjunct compliance-improving strategies include medication calendars, drug packaging devices, group encounters, family support, contracts, and reward systems.

Medication Calendars

A number of investigators have reported that medication calendars are helpful in improving patient compliance (365, 1362). Moulding (365), for example, reported a threefold increase in the percentage of patients who took 90% or more of their medications when a medication calendar was used.

Patients with the most to benefit from medication calendars are those who are noncompliant because they have particularly difficult regimens to follow. For example, patients on decreasing corticosteroid regimens, alternating doses of anticoagulants, or multiple drug therapy of any sort may find a medication calendar invaluable in achieving high compliance. In addition, such calendars may be valuable to the forgetful patient. In either case, the pharamacist who initiates this strategy may find that it can be discontinued once correct pill-taking behavior has been learned.

Special Drug Packaging

The use of specialized drug packaging has also been shown to improve compliance (147, 314, 419, 1363). Linkewich and co-workers (314), as shown in Table 16.5, tested four compliance-improving strategies and found that the most compliant behavior was achieved when a pharmacist provided both verbal and written instructions for medications that were dispensed in a dial pack. Eighty-eight percent of the patients receiving this strategy were considered compliant, whereas only 28% of patients receiving the traditional vial and label without counseling were compliant. Likewise, Rehder and co-workers (419) found that nearly 90% of patients were compliant when a Dosett® dispensing device was used, but only 50% of patients in the control group were compliant.

As with medication calendars, special drug packaging devices may be of particular value in facilitating the compliance of patients who forget doses or confuse difficult regimens. However, since many of these devices are both expensive and difficult to use, further development and testing is needed before their full potential in patient compliance can be realized.

Group Discussions

Some patients are noncompliant because they dislike taking medications, fear their consequences, or are not convinced of their efficacy despite extensive instruction. Although such patients may need continuous support and encouragement in order to comply, they may not accept this from a health provider. For this group of patients, discussions with other patients with similar medical problems may encourage compliance (438, 1347). For example, Avery and co-workers (1347) reported that significantly fewer asthmatic patients participating in discussion groups required visits to the emergency room than did control patients who were not placed in these groups. He concluded that the difference was due to better compliance.

In spite of encouraging reports such as this, discussion groups are often difficult to initiate and maintain. It appears that discussion groups are more likely to be successful if: (1) there is a common ground for participation (i.e. similar medical problems or therapy); (2) there is a structure similar to other club organizations (i.e. officers, scheduled meetings, and programed activities); (3) meetings are held in a group member's home; and (4) health providers participate only as advisors and refrain from lecturing to or directing the group.

Family Support

When the family becomes involved in the care of the patient, by providing either support or supervision, compliance often improves (165, 475). This strategy may be of particular value in improving the compliance of patients who are pessimistic about either their prognosis or the efficacy of their therapy, are "tarzan types" who ignore their own vulnerability to disease, or deny therapy to punish themselves or to gain attention. In these and similar instances, when there are no ethical or professional barriers, pharmacists may improve compliance by describing the nature of the medical problem and its treatment to other family members who are in a position to help the patient with the compliance problem.

Contracts

A written or verbal contract between the health provider and the patient has been successful in modifying compliance (337, 1368). In applying this strategy, a description is provided both of what is expected of the patient and of the services or rewards the patient would receive if the specified level of compliance were achieved. Contracting has the advantages of emphasizing that the patient is responsible for a portion of his care and, to the extent that the contract is negotiated, that he is an active participant in his overall management. While more experience with and testing of patient contracts is needed, the use of this strategy to improve compliance may warrant a trial for the capricious noncomplier, the uncooperative patient, or the patient who fails to understand his responsibility despite being informed through more traditional means.

Rewards

In a strategy closely related to contracting, other reward systems may be substituted in an effort to encourage compliance among patients who do not respond to traditional health-related motivation techniques (228). For example, rebates, theater tickets, trips, or other "prizes" may be awarded to patients who are found compliant or who are under defined therapeutic control because of good compliance. Conversely, penalty systems, analogous to those imposed on members who gain weight in the Weight Watcher's Club, may provide a stimulus for compliance. Once patients have learned to take prescribed drugs appropriately as a result of this reward/penalty system, other positive systems of motivation, more closely related to the goals of therapy, should be substituted.

CONCLUSION

This chapter has reviewed the ways in which pharmacists may be involved in measuring and improving the compliance of patients with prescribed drug therapy. It is suggested that many of the strategies for measuring and improving compliance reported in the literature can be offered as a routine service to patients in the normal delivery of care in the pharmacy. Further, if these services are provided on a continuous basis, the compliance of the majority of ambulatory patients would be improved significantly. Fruitful areas of further research have been identified, among them drug monographs, communication techniques, and patient monitoring.

In conclusion, noncompliance is a complex behavioral problem that, if not caused by, is at least strongly influenced by a complicated, sometimes unresponsive and impersonal, busy health delivery system. The problem is not a simple function of the regimen, the patient, the illness, or any other single component. Accordingly, it is naive to suggest that changing a single aspect of the system, such as the practice of pharmacy, would solve the compliance problem. It would be equally naive to suggest that a similar change in physician services or a simplification of treatment would solve the problem. What is needed ultimately is a mutual recognition of and response to the compliance problem by all health providers, each of whom must be sensitive to the needs of patients. What is needed is a concerted effort to offer quality health services.

17

Compliance
and the
Organization
of Health Services

Edward S. Gibson

INTRODUCTION

From one perspective, compliance with preventive and therapeutic regimens can be considered a problem in logistics or organization. Individuals seeking or requiring care for potential or actual illness must hurdle a number of organizational barriers before appropriate treatment is offered. Previous chapters have described the effect on compliance of isolated organizational factors such as waiting time, the method of clinic scheduling, and the level of clinical supervision. It is the purpose of this chapter to bring these factors together. In doing so, attention shifts from individual noncompliers (with which most of this book is concerned) to focus on the facilities, organizations, and people whose purpose it is to provide health services.

As will be seen, there is evidence that organizational change can prevent or reduce compliance problems, often without the need for investigating the compliance of individual patients, altering provider workloads, or increasing budgets. In addition, such organizatonal changes can also enhance "treater" or provider compliance with optimum treatment.

It is also important to recognize that many of the organizational changes proposed here are not unique inventions; they simply institutionalize compliance maneuvers that previously have been successful on an ad hoc basis. The need for institutionalization in this context is derived from the frequency of the noncompliance problem. For example, it may be possible to accommodate a few noncompliers without any major organizational change, simply by making special appointments at odd hours or by guaranteeing quick services for this subgroup. If such maneuvers do indeed enhance compliance, then the frequency with which such special arrangements are required should be considered. At some point the proportion of patients requiring special accommodation may be sufficient to make it more economical and easier to provide a regular evening or weekend clinic routinely or to change the routine method of scheduling so as to avoid waiting room delay. Such organizational changes are less flexible than individualized solutions, but they can greatly enhance the overall efficiency of dealing with common problems; compliance thus demands the consideration of organizational change in the delivery of health services. However, wholesale reorganization is not advocated here. The foundations of such change should be compliance-improving strategies that are of *established* efficacy for compliance problems of *sufficient frequency* to merit institutional alterations.

ORGANIZATIONAL STEPS TO THE EFFECTIVE MANAGEMENT OF COMPLIANCE PROBLEMS

In order to identify areas in which organizational change might improve compliance a model used by Sackett et al. (1390) to designate the steps required for effective hypertension control will be used as a framework. The steps in this model are, in order, detection, linkage, clinical evaluation, initiation of the regimen, compliance with the regimen, and long-term follow-up and care. In this chain, compliance refers to the individual patient's compliance with prescribed antihypertensive medications. However, for our purposes noncompliance at any stage in the process, by either provider or patient, merits attention to organizational considerations, because such noncompliance results in failure to achieve health benefits.

Detection

Management of any health problem begins with its recognition or detection. Factors preventing this detection include a lack of patient awareness of the condition, lack of access to health care, and inadequate detection maneuvers themselves. Of these factors, we are only concerned here with noncompliance with the recommendation to seek health care.

When the health problem poses a threat to public safety (as with venereal disease, "open" tuberculosis, or violent emotional disorder) the health care system, sometimes with assistance from the legal system, can impose compliance upon even the most unwilling citizen (117, 118, 273). It might therefore be tempting to employ these same maneuvers throughout the organizational approach to improving compliance, since the success of such methods in promoting detection is beyond doubt (see Chapter 8). However, the infringements on liberty inherent in such tactics are unacceptable when the condition being detected is a threat only to the affected individual. Beyond informing the public of the availability of detection facilities for relevant disorders, the current concensus holds that it is inappropriate to force the use of detection services for conditions whose danger is restricted to the affected individual. Even this low key approach may be going too far. The justification for offering detection services to people who do not present themselves voluntarily to the health care system can only come from studies showing that such a detection maneuver ultimately results in more good than harm for those who use the service. Since it cannot be assumed a priori that a treatment for a given disease is efficacious (that is, that it does more good than harm to those who take it), attempts to detect the disease among asymptomatic individuals cannot proceed in the absence of proof of benefit. This is especially important in view of recent evidence that telling persons that they have a disease such as hypertension ("labeling") leads to increased absenteeism and decreased psychosocial function, whether or not treatment is initiated (1381, 1382, 1384, 1385). Furthermore, these disadvantages are particularly prominent in noncompliers (1382). Until and unless compliance with efficacious treatments can be assured, it is not justified to promote compliance with detection programs for presymptomatic disease. It is of interest in this regard that a recent review of screening for presymptomatic disease found few conditions for which such detection could be justified on any grounds (1391).

Linkage to a Source of Care

Linkage becomes an important issue whenever referral for definitive care is required. For example, Finnerty et al. (169) described a major problem of linkage in community screening for hypertension. Initially, 50% of the hypertensives who screened positive failed to link to care by keeping a verification appointment. This could be reduced to 29% if a personal contact were made with each subject. However, by instituting an organizational change, a more effective, less costly strategy was derived: by scheduling the verification appointment for within 48 hours of the initial screen the linkage noncompliance was reduced to less than 5%.

Here we see an excellent example of the benefits gained from changing the organization of health services to deal with a frequent compliance problem. Another dramatic demonstration occurred in our own work. In an industrial cohort (1379), initial attempts to refer patients with two or more cardiovascular risk factors to family physicians by means of the traditional personal letter were successful in only 14% of cases. However, in a subsequent program based at the same plant the detection staff prepared brief clinical summaries of each subject who tested positive and sent these to the subjects' family physicians after telephoning for an appointment; linkage was achieved for 100%. In addition, however, the family physicians in the latter study had received general information about the associated investigation so that it was not possible to assess the individual contribution of each of the components (appointment making, clinical assessment, and study publicity). Similarly, Curry (117) achieved increased compliance with posthospital outpatient appointment keeping by scheduling the first clinic appointment prior to discharge and by having the physician in charge of this follow-up review the case prior to discharge. Again, however, the individual contribution of the separate strategies could not be assessed.

Similar problems in linkage arise whenever the hospital care for a patient is provided by a specialist without continuing involvement of the family practictioner. The possible negative effects of this arrangement on compliance with postdischarge regimens needs to be identified, since it might induce those responsible for the organization of these health care services to develop and test strategies that would involve the physician responsible for follow-up prior to discharge.

One way to avoid linkage problems is simply to discontinue community-based screening programs; this is not as unrealistic a solution as it appears. Most individuals in any community (at least here in North America) have family physicians and visit them at reasonably frequent intervals. For example, the Harris Poll (1381) found that 83% of a population sample had seen a doctor within the previous two years. If these visits, for whatever purpose, were also utilized to detect treatable disorders such as hypertension, then the vast majority of the public could be screened at no extra expense and within a reasonable time span, and the problem of linkage could be eliminated (1388, 1390). Indeed, utilizing this case-finding approach would actually decrease the amount of organization required for the community control of several common disorders.

But what if recalcitrant individuals who achieve linkage only after strenuous efforts are destined to be less compliant at subsequent steps than are those who enter the system without special assistance? Such a result would suggest that the additional effort was wasted. However, the findings of Craig and Huffine (113) are reassuring. In an investigation of inner city clients of a mental health clinic, they discovered that those patients who were most difficult to get into the system exhibited the same compliance as did easily linked individuals once they were brought under care. This finding is reinforced by additional data on health care utilization and compliance reported previously by Haynes (694).

Clinical Evaluation

We will broaden the term clinical evaluation to encompass the entire clinic process, including attendance at appointments. Unfortunately, most of the relevant literature deals with the 20% of doctor-patient encounters that occur in hospitals and very little with those that take place in the community. Furthermore, most of the relevant articles deal with appointment keeping only; accordingly, the generalizability of the resulting conclusions is suspect and caution is warranted in their interpretation.

There do appear to be a number of organizational strategies that increase appointment keeping. Fletcher et al. (173) found that a follow-up clerk in the emergency department could improve attendance of patients referred to a follow-up hypertension clinic. Shepard and Moseley (461) demonstrated that a simple mail reminder was nearly as effective as a telephone reminder yet only half as costly. It has also been shown that appointment-scheduling systems that decrease waiting time are associated with increased compliance (1377). However, the power of waiting time as a determinent is apparently overshadowed by other, nonorganizational factors such as patients' perceptions of the effectiveness of the treatment and of the physician, as found by Kirscht et al. (1383).

Curry (117), studying tuberculosis follow-up clinics in San Francisco, demonstrated a marked increase in compliance with appointment keeping when clinic convenience was tailored to three specific groups of problem patients. However, augumented convenience in a Canadian industrial setting (449) (treatment at the job site on company time) did not affect medication compliance despite the fact that substantially more individuals were brought under active care than was the case in a community control group. The latter study both demonstrated the inappropriateness of utilizing attendance as a surrogate for medication compliance and also illustrated that although organizational changes may help keep patients under surveillance, they are not sufficient by themselves to insure that the medication is consumed. An exception to the latter point occurs when the treatment is actually administered at the visit. In Curry's study, cited above (117), antituberculosis therapy was given under supervision at the time of the visit. Attendance in this situation was thus a perfect measure of compliance. The organizational lesson to be learned in this case is that when a disease is serious enough to warrant close supervision and when there is a long-acting treatment that can be administered at the time of a visit, low compliance can be obviated by setting up clinics that deliver such treatment directly and have sufficient staff to retrieve or make home visits to nonattenders. This lesson has already been learned by those who care for individuals with several types of psychiatric illnesses (273), with tuberculosis (117, 255, 387), or who are susceptibile to recurrences of rheumatic fever (159, 160).

Initiation of the Regimen

Regimens are often divided into three categories: those for "cure" (for example the treatment of active tuberculosis); those for "secondary prevention" (for example rheumatic fever prophylaxis); and those for "primary prevention" (such as the use of automobile seat belts). It appears likely that these three types of regimens are accompanied by different levels of compliance. Unfortunately, however, there is very little information available to assess this relationship, and it is often not possible to separate the effect of the treatment category from the provider's decision to initiate treatment.

There are some data available on the latter point, however. In our work in an industrial setting (1387), men with sustained blood pressure elevations were randomly allocated to referral to community physicians or to industrial physicians. Overall, treatment was initiated in only 57% of these men. An analysis of baseline data revealed that the doctor's decision to initiate therapy was influenced both by clinically, relevant findings such as baseline diastolic blood pressure and by nonclinical factors such as the year of medical school graduation of the physician. Two organizational factors influenced these physicians' compliance with recommended care. First, industrial-based physicians, who had organized themselves so as to take on this area of therapy, were statistically significantly more likely to treat patients. Second, both community and industrial physicians were more likely to initiate therapy when they were told that their patients would be receiving an educational program on hypertension. These rather provocative findings may be interpreted in several ways; they nonetheless raise the possibility that the organization of health services may influence the vigor of therapeutic interventon in that the physician's perceptions of both the patient's willingness to accept therapy and the patient's knowledge of the disease appear to influence the decision to prescribe treatment. We need to explore this possibility further.

Apart from regimens initiated within the health care system, there exists another major set of orthodox lifestyle or *class regimens*. The past few years have witnessed the emergence of "consumerism," and the accompanying legal phenomenon of "class action" in the form of legal proceedings against manufacturers and providers of services. In a similar way, citizens, government, and the media have projected regimens (usually primary prevention) for several conditions, and these regimens have become known to and are frequently followed by large segments of the general population outside the traditional health care system. Included in this category would be regular strenuous exercise, smoking withdrawal, seat belt use, and alcohol restriction. Such regimens might be called class regimens.

We know very little about why apparently healthy individuals diet, stop smoking, begin exercising, and fasten their seat belts. Indeed, it is possible that the current downward trend in cardiovascular disease mortality in North America is due to compliance with a class regimen rather than to direct intervention by the health care system. A promising approach to the explanation of this phenomenon is the Health Belief Model as outlined in Chapter 6. It remains to be validated, however, whether health attitudes can be changed by organized efforts and whether this will lead to altered health behavior. Encouraging preliminary results in the modification of community-wide health behavior through mass media have been reported by Farquhar et al. (156), but at the same time the dismal results of vigorous promotional tactics to effect seat belt use described by A. Benjamin Kelley in Chapter 12 are enough to discourage many a public health campaigner.

Compliance with Long-Term Follow-up and Care

As noted earlier, *compliance* in this context concerns the individual patient's adherence to a prescribed regimen and assumes that the prior barriers to detection, linkage, and clinical evaluation have been surmounted and that a decision has been made to initiate therapy. Craig and Huffine (113), in their investigation of inner city clients of a mental health clinic, have reported evidence that resources allocated at the regimen compliance step can also help overcome barriers at the prior steps. They found, for example, that once in the system, patients who had been the most difficult to get into the system showed the same degree of compliance as did other patients. This finding led these investigators to shift their emphasis from crisis-oriented services (which were instituted on the assumption that most patients would drop out) to long-term therapeutic programs which promised to be much more effective.

Increased supervision appears the most potent and generally applicable strategy to improve compliance with therapy and, as described in Chapters 8, 15, and 16, this can be achieved by a number of means, including hospitalization, home visits, special nursing care, and special pharmacy services. Thus far, these strategies have been applied on an ad hoc basis or as part of formal research projects. It is important that real world versions of these strategies be instituted and evaluated, perhaps even going as far as implementing the "compliance service" previously suggested by Sackett (796).

Another organizational arrangement of importance concerns the development of laboratory services that can provide quick results of drug level measurements in body fluids. This strategy would provide a highly accurate approach to detecting compliance problems and would permit an immediate opportunity for remedial action.

Finally, the incorporation of specialists in educational and behavioral modification techniques into the health care team will be warranted in situations in which there are sufficient numbers of patients with compliance problems amenable to these approaches. These programs can be expensive, however, and may be difficult to apply to heterogeneous patient groups.

SUMMARY

The strategies described here have, for the most part, been subjected to formal evaluation and appear genuinely worthwhile. However, little of this evaluation has taken place out in the community where, in North America at least, 80% of patient care takes place (1383). Unfortunately, the effective compliance-improving strategies that have emerged from these studies incorporate the organizational features of research hospitals and may not apply in solo or small group practice. Many of them require special staffing and funding and are appropriate only for larger groups of patients with common conditions and treatments. The "compliance service" suggested earlier may be a solution, but no such service has yet been evaluated. Furthermore, the nature of traditional private medical care in North America often mediates against active, outreach programs of follow-up. The attitude often prevails (and perhaps rightly so) that once the prescription has been given it is solely the patient's right to accept or reject it. The advent of efficacious treatments for common chronic conditions such as hypertension is changing our attitudes in this area but it remains to be seen whether private medicine will or can make the organizational changes required to provide long-term follow-up services to enhance compliance.

The recognition of compliance as a problem, and the identification of worthwhile intervention strategies, also raise the issue of whether the system can afford to provide compliance detection and treatment services. Stason and Weinstein (1388) in their model for the community control of hypertension concluded that a strategy that increased compliance with referral and long-term treatment by more than 10% would bring more hypertensives under control at less expense than could be achieved by a maximum screening effort. Thus, the decision is no longer whether but which of these strategies should be implemented in the private as well as the public sector of health care. The available data suggest a number of organizational approaches that can maintain and improve compliance, and it is high time that we got on with the task.

18

A Compliance Practicum for the Busy Practitioner

David L. Sackett

INTRODUCTION

The other chapters in this book (including mine!) are mostly "ivory tower" in their origins and are either irrelevant to clinical practice or difficult to apply in the busy places where most patients receive their care. Accordingly, this chapter will translate the various findings of compliance research into practical suggestions that can be applied readily in the "front lines." In doing so, it will be brief, will synthesize rather than analyze, and will for the most part cite other chapters rather than references since the latter are not usually at hand for the busy practitioner.

CLINICAL PREREQUISITES

Before any attempt is made to find and help the patient with low compliance, the practitioner must answer these questions:

1. Have I made the correct diagnosis?
2. Has the preventive or therapeutic regimen I have prescribed been proven to do more good than harm?
3. Is the patient a free, informed, consenting participant in this intervention?

If the answer to any of these questions is *no*, the search for a solution to the problem of low compliance should be abandoned. If the diagnosis is wrong or the regimen worthless, improved compliance wastes money and increases the patient's risk of side effects and toxicity with no prospect of benefit. Similarly, because compliance-improving strategies are therapeutic maneuvers (with costs and side effects of their own) and because most of them require active cooperation, the practitioner must inform the patient and seek his consent.

286

STEPS IN THE DETECTION AND
IMPROVEMENT OF LOW COMPLIANCE

The steps are five:
1. Identify patients who have dropped out of treatment.
2. Identify patients who, despite treatment, have not reached the treatment goal.
3. Be sure that the regimen prescribed is vigorous enough to achieve the treatment goal if the patients were compliant.
4. Find the subgroup of patients with low compliance.
5. Apply the compliance-improving strategies in sequence.

These five steps can be executed quickly and without extensive detective work, confrontation, or despotism, as we shall now discover.

1. Identify Patients Who Have Dropped Out of Treatment

The commonest form of noncompliance, especially with long-term regimens, is dropping out of care altogether. Unless you have an effective system for keeping track of your patients you will miss this group. One way to keep track of them is always to schedule the next appointment before they leave (even if it's several months away). Then, if you keep a "day sheet" or pull charts at the start of the day you will know at the end of the day that these patients have not shown up and you can call them back. Because they have failed to keep a scheduled appointment, it is ethical (with all of the disciplinary bodies we have contacted) to contact them without running the risk of "soliciting."

2. Identify Patients Who, Despite Treatment,
Have Not Reached the Treatment Goal

Since it is usually much easier to tell whether patients have, for example, reached goal blood pressure or symptomatic relief than whether they are consistently taking their thiazides or aspirin, the quick and practical approach is to identify those patients who have not reached the treatment goal. Table 18.1 illustrates this point.

The targets for compliance-improving strategies are problem patients in cell D who have not reached the treatment goal and whose compliance is low or zero. Patients who have reached the treatment goal are either highly compliant (cell A) or have reached the goal despite low compliance (cell C) and require no immediate attention.*

---

*Of course, if the regimen is expensive or causes clinically significant side effects or toxicity, the practitioner should identify patients in cell C and "step down" their regimens, but that is outside the focus of this discussion.

TABLE 18.1. Compliance and the treatment goal

Compliance	Treatment goal	
	Reached	Not reached
High	A: Fine	B: Lacks vigor?
Low or zero	C: Overprescribing?	D: Target

3. Be Sure that the Regimen Prescribed Is Vigorous Enough to Achieve the Treatment Goal if the Patients Were Compliant

As Table 18.2 shows, of a group of hypertensives we studied during their sixth month of treatment, roughly half of those who were not at goal blood pressure were, in fact, taking most or all of their medicine (cell B); they needed bigger doses and/or multiple or alternative drugs, not compliance-improving strategies. Thus, before concluding that the failure to reach the treatment goal is the result of low compliance, the practitioner should be sure that the regimen is vigorous enough to do the job among compliant patients.

4. Find the Subgroup of Patients with Low Compliance

Suggestions for finding the noncompliant patient fall into seven categories: clinical judgement; failure to achieve the treatment goal; the absence of pharmacologic effects or side effects; low compliance with previous or related recommendations; body fluid analyses; measurement of remaining medication; and asking the patient. The first approach does not work; those in the middle are often insensitive, expensive, or time consuming; and the last approach has been shown to be remarkably useful. These approaches are described in considerable detail in Chapter 3 and will only be summarized here.

Clinical Judgement.

Every time the ability of clinicians to predict the future compliance of their patients has been put to a rigorous test, clinicians have failed to outperform the toss of a coin. Furthermore, although more seasoned clinicians are progressively less optimistic about their patients' future compliance, their misjudgment continues; clinical experience generates cynicism, not accuracy, and this approach is included here only in order to be discouraged.

Failure to Achieve the Treatment Goal.

In those instances in which the regimen and the treatment goal are synonymous, this approach works (e.g., have this tooth filled or these eyeglasses made; have this mole excised).

TABLE 18.2. Compliance with antihypertensive drugs and goal blood pressure

Compliance by pill count	Diastolic blood pressure <90 mm Hg	
	Reached	Not Reached
Taking 80% or more of medications	A: 23%	B: 34%
Taking less than 80% of medications	C: 12%	D: 31%

SOURCE: Adapted from Sackett et al. 1976 (1392).

For other regimens, the link between compliance and achievement of the treatment goal may be strong but is not assured (the fat man who loses weight after being prescribed a 1,000-calorie diet is probably compliant, but he may have continued to eat as before and taken up jogging, contracted tuberculosis, or developed an enterocolic fistula). For still other regimens, as illustrated in Table 18.2., the relation between achievement of the treatment goal and compliance, although real, is too variable for the former to be used as an accurate index of the latter. This last situation probably applies to most regimens, and the failure of patients to reach treatment goals should be used to narrow, but not to conclude, the search for low compliance.

The Absence of Pharmacologic Effects or Side Effects.

Some regimens produce clear-cut pharmacologic effects or side effects, the absence of which suggests low compliance (e.g., urinary frequency with diuretics, dry mouth with anticholinergics, dark stool with oral iron). However, the link between these effects and the treatment goal may be tenuous (postural hypotension from antihypertensive drugs can occur without reaching goal blood pressure, and vice versa) and, as seen in cell *B* of Table 18.2, high compliance with an inadequate regimen (or with an oral medication that is poorly absorbed) will result in neither side effects nor achievement of the treatment goal. Moreover, as documented in Chapter 4, many side effects appear to result from the act of being medicated rather than from the medication itself. Accordingly, this approach has the same limitations as the previous one, plus the additional disadvantage that it is not coterminus with the treatment goal.

Low Compliance with Previous or Related Recommendations.

Patients with previously documented low compliance are at high risk of repeating such behavior. As emphasized earlier, patients who miss appointments or have dropped out of follow-up have often stopped their regimens as well. Similarly, those patients who exhibit low compliance with one component of a diet-plus-exercise-plus-medication regimen are likely to manifest low adherance to other components as well. Finally, patients cannot take their medicine if they have not (re)filled their prescriptions. However, these associations are not perfect; patients may keep appointments but not diets, and they may fill prescriptions but not take their pills. Once again, therefore, this approach is best used for raising the possibility of low compliance rather than confirming it.

Body Fluid Analyses.

One sure way to tell whether a medicine has been taken is to analyze the appropriate body fluid for the drug or its metabolites. Indeed, this is acknowledged to be the "hardest" evidence that can be obtained about compliance with medications. Moreover, telling the patient the results of these analyses has been shown to lead to improved compliance with drugs like digoxin and diphenylhydantoin. However, this approach has major drawbacks. First, the availability of drug analysis is sharply limited by geography, cost, and technology; as a result, this approach is simply not available to most practitioners for most drugs. Second, because of the rates of metabolism and excretion of most drugs, body fluid analyses reveal compliance behavior for only the previous few hours. Finally, the results of these analyses are not usually available during the clinical encounter, when they would be the most helpful. Nonetheless, if these drawbacks can be overcome, body fluid analysis can become the major approach to detecting low compliance.

Measurement of Remaining Medication.

In this approach the amount of medication left in the bottle is compared with the amount expected if the patient had followed the regimen exactly. Such "pill counts" can be useful, but are impossible when patients fail to bring all of their remaining medication with them to the practitioner's office, and are confusing when medicines are not begun on the day the prescription is filled or renewed and when medications are shared with others. Accordingly, the measurement of remaining medication is usually impractical in busy clinical practice.

Asking the Patient.

When patients are asked, in a nonthreatening fashion, whether they are taking their medicine* the results are striking, as shown in Table 18.3.

Because when patients deny any problems with low compliance (cells *C* and *D*) we do not know whether they are telling the truth, we forget that when they admit that they have a compliance problem (cells *A* and *B*) they are virtually

---

*The author uses the following wording with his hypertensive patients: "Most people have trouble remembering to take their medicine. Do you have trouble remembering to take yours?"

TABLE 18.3.   Comparison of clinical interviews and pill counts in hypertensive patients

Compliance by clinical interview	Compliance by pill count	
	Less than 80% of medications taken	80% or more of medications taken
Admit taking less than 80% of medications	A: 20%	B: 2%
Deny any problem with low compliance	C: 30%	D: 48%

SOURCE: Adapted from Sackett et al. 1976 (1392).

always telling the truth! Moreover, it is precisely that group of patients who admit low compliance (cell *A*) who show the greatest response to compliance-improving strategies (in terms of reaching treatment goals). Thus, it is possible for the busy practitioner, by performing a simple clinical interview, to identify those patients who will benefit most from compliance-improving strategies without having to resort to pill counts, body fluid analyses, or other detective work.

In summary, there are several ways to find the patient with low compliance; at our current state of knowledge and technology the nonthreatening clinical interview will detect roughly one-half of patients with low compliance and has the advantages of simplicity, immediate results, and the identification of precisely those patients who will respond most positively to compliance-improving strategies.

5. Apply the Compliance-Improving Strategies in Sequence

Detailed explorations of the validity of the individual compliance-improving strategies appear at several places in this book. They are reviewed in general in Chapter 8; other chapters deal with pharmacologic (Chapter 9), educational (Chapter 10), behavioral (Chapter 11), and organizational (Chapter 17) strategies, with strategies for helping problem smokers (Chapter 13) and problem drinkers (Chapter 14), and with the roles that nurses (Chapter 15) and pharmacists (Chapter 16) can play in assisting patients with low compliance. Accordingly, the present chapter will simply summarize those strategies that appear best suited for application by a busy practitioner. The clinical reader can track them through the index or Table 12 in Appendix I for more detailed discussions.

It makes sense to begin with those compliance-improving strategies that are the easiest to apply. Table 18.4 lists them in order of increasing cost and complexity.

Increased Attention and Supervision.

The easiest way to begin helping patients with low compliance is to pay more attention to them. This can be done in several ways. Patients who miss

TABLE 18.4.   Compliance-improving strategies for use by the busy practitioner

Easiest	Increased attention and supervision

	Modification of the regimen
	    injectables
	    simplification
	    tailoring
	    calendar dispenser

	Referral for help
	    office personnel
	    pharmacists
	    public health unit
	    employee health service

Most complex	Behavioral strategies

appointments should be contacted promptly to arrange a new appointment. Repeated breaking of appointments should lead to direct contact by the clinician in order to identify and try to solve the problems that are interfering with compliance.

Patients who keep their appointments but whose low compliance interferes with their achievement of the treatment goal should be given more frequent appointments, such as every one or two weeks, until their compliance and therapeutic responses improve. It is important to make the reasons for these extra visits plain; the more attention that is focused specifically on compliance and on achievement of the treatment goal the better. The actual visits may be brief, but their cumulative effect permits frequent compliance checks to be carried out, barriers to high compliance to be identified and corrected, and patients to be convinced that the practitioner is both concerned and ready to help.

Modification of the Regimen.

If the foregoing strategy fails, the practitioner can experiment with the treatment regimen itself. If a medication is involved, can it be given in a long-acting injectable form? If so, compliance with appointment keeping will become synonymous with compliance with the regimen.

Can the regimen be simplified in other ways? Can a q.i.d. schedule be reduced to a b.i.d. schedule at twice the dose (the q.i.d. schedule is often more justified by tradition than by pharmacokinetics)? Can the taking of medications or the performance of other regimens be tailored to coincide with the performance of daily habits or rituals such as awakening to the alarm clock, brushing one's teeth, or drinking the inevitable 10:00 a.m. cup of coffee or tea?

Finally, if the regimen involves several medications per dose and multiple doses per day, the practitioner may recommend that the patient obtain one of

VI
RESEARCH APPLICATIONS
AND FUTURE RESEARCH

19

The Effect of
Compliance Distributions
on Therapeutic Trials

Charles H. Goldsmith

INTRODUCTION

Compliance with therapy is seldom discussed in the reports of clinical trials that appear in the literature. Indeed, even when compliance is considered, few articles describe the measure of compliance used or report any portion of the compliance distribution.

The purposes of this chapter are to propose a measure of compliance, to present some possible compliance distributions, and then to study the effect of these differing distributions on the conduct and outcome of clinical trials. In particular, the effect on the number of patients required to study a new therapeutic intervention will be explored. The chapter will close with two suggestions for incorporating compliance information into the statistical analysis of clinical trials.

A MEASURE OF COMPLIANCE

Although there are few adequate techniques for measuring compliance that are acceptable to every therapeutic regimen, for the purpose of this chapter a working measure of compliance will be defined.

The *measure of compliance*, denoted by C, is defined as the ratio of the number of prescribed "doses" of the therapy taken by the patient to the number of "doses" prescribed for the patient, and expressed as a percentage, i.e.,

$$C = \frac{\text{number of prescribed doses taken by the patient}}{\text{number of doses prescribed for the patient}} \times 100 \quad [1]$$

Expressed in this form, the measure of compliance, C, would ordinarily take on values between 0% and 100%, i.e.,

$$0\% \leqslant C \leqslant 100\% \quad [2]$$

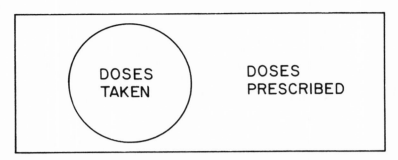

FIGURE 19.1. Compliance Venn diagram.

Although this measure of compliance is useful, it should be recognized that it does not allow for the possibility of net overconsumption of therapy (i.e., the taking of doses that were not prescribed), nor does it distinguish among the different patterns in which the patient may have consumed the number of "doses taken."

The ingredients of this compliance measure [1] can be expressed pictorially with the Venn diagram shown in Figure 19.1.

The rectangular box in Figure 19.1 represents the set of possible doses prescribed for the patient, while the circle represents the set of times that the prescribed dose was adhered to by the patient. Clearly, from this representation the set of prescribed doses taken is a subset of the doses prescribed, so that the bounds stated for the compliance measure in [2] are indeed reasonable.

Various modifications of the definition [1] have been employed in the literature. Gordis et al. (199), when studying compliance with oral prophylactic penicillin therapy in children with prior rheumatic fever, used as their compliance measure

$$C = \frac{\text{urine tests positive}}{\text{urine tests done}} \times 100\%$$

In this case, the number of urine tests done was a substitute for the number of doses prescribed, and the positive urine test served as an indication that the prescribed penicillin therapy had been taken. Although no individual measures of compliance were given for their sample of 103 children, the authors did state that their mean compliance was 49%.

Roth et al. (442), when studying compliance with antacid therapy in peptic ulcer prophylaxis used as their compliance measure

$$C = \frac{\text{bottles of antacid consumed}}{\text{bottles of antacid prescribed}} \times 100\%$$

Here the number of bottles consumed was analogous to the pill count that has been used in other studies. Again, although no individual measures of com-

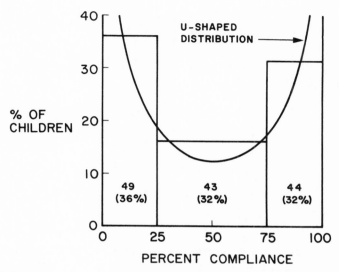

FIGURE 19.2.

pliance were given for their sample of 105 patients, the authors did state that the mean compliance was 54%.

COMPLIANCE DISTRIBUTIONS

Once a measure of individual compliance has been developed, it becomes possible to begin understanding the impact that compliance has upon a therapeutic trial by combining these individual measurements into a distribution of compliance. Although, as we shall see, the shape of this distribution has profound effects upon the design and analysis of these trials, very few studies have reported compliance distributions. (This may be more a reflection upon journal space and editors than upon authors.) Nonetheless, we still may be able to postulate some possible compliance distributions from the data that are available.

Gordis et al. (198), reported that 49 (36%) of the 136 children in their rheumatic fever prophylaxis study were noncompliers ($0\% \leqslant C \leqslant 25\%$), while 43 (32%) of the children were intermediate compliers ($26\% \leqslant C \leqslant 74\%$), and 44 (32%) were said to be compliers ($75\% \leqslant C \leqslant 100\%$). Even though the individual compliance values were not given, it would appear from these date that the compliance distribution is U-shaped.* This postulation is represented in Figure 19.2.

---

*A subsequent personal communication from Leon Gordis to the Editors provided an even finer partition of these data into deciles, and the compliance distribution was confirmed as being U-shaped.

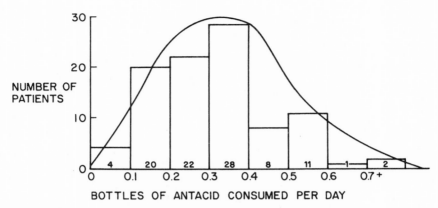

FIGURE 19.3.

Other sets of data may suggest other possible forms for compliance distributions. For example, Roth et al. (442), in a study of antacid therapy in patients with peptic ulcers, provided enough information to permit the construction of a compliance distribution. Using as the compliance measure the ratio of bottles of antacid consumed to bottles of antacid prescribed, a bell-shaped distribution (slightly skewed to the right) results, as shown in Figure 19.3. The mean consumption for the 96 patients who completed follow-up was 0.31 bottles per day, somewhat less than the prescribed 0.57 bottles per day.

Still other compliance distributions are suggested in the remaining literature. For example, the tuberculosis chemotherapy study of Ireland (265), and the psychopharmacological rehospitalization study of Mason et al. (338), suggest compliance distributions for INH and phenothiazines that are nearly uniform over the compliance interval, as displayed in Figure 19.4.

From these examples, it is clear that there are an enormous number of possible shapes for compliance distributions; in this brief survey we have a U-shaped curve, a uniform curve, and a roughly bell-shaped curve. The compliance distributions in these specific studies varied with the nature of the therapy, the type of patients, the type of compliance measures chosen to study, and possibly with several other factors as well. Clearly, more information is needed in order to sort out the determinants of these distributions and to determine whether one shape predominates.

There are at least three major ramifications of this inquiry. The first concerns attempts to improve compliance by means such as shifting an entire compliance distribution to the right. If the compliance distribution in question were bell-shaped, such a shift might produce a dramatic increase in the number of compliant patients. If, on the other hand, the compliance distribution were U-shaped, all that might be produced would be a dramatic increase in overmedicated patients.

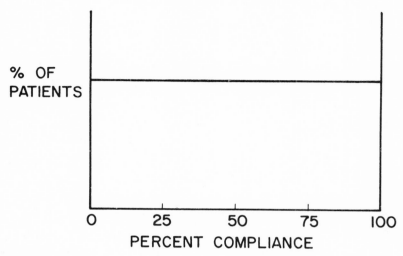

FIGURE 19.4.

The other two ramifications of the definition of compliance distributions concern their effects upon interpretations of the dose-response curve and upon the calculation of sample size requirements in clinical trials. The remainder of this chapter will deal with these issues.

THE EFFECT OF COMPLIANCE UPON THE INTERPRETATION OF DOSE-RESPONSE CURVES

As with compliance distributions, dose-response curves may have many possible forms. However, the most common dose-response curve is sigmoid-shaped, like the one displayed in Figure 19.5. In this case, as the dose increases the response increases, although not in a linear fashion. Suppose there is a dose, denoted by A, below which the response is of no therapeutic value. Also suppose there is a dose, denoted by B ($B>A$), above which the patient becomes toxic from the drug. The dosage interval, A to B, is known as the therapeutic dose and the interval J to K on the response axis denotes the interval within which a therapeutic effect will take place. Consequently, for any drug-outcome combination, the prescribing clinician should have a knowledge of the therapeutic range and should prescribe corresponding doses of drugs for his or her patients.

The actual amount of a drug available to the patient can be influenced both by the compliance of the patient and by the bioavailability of the drug. While not wishing to ignore the importance of the latter, we shall assume in the following example that it is constant and high.

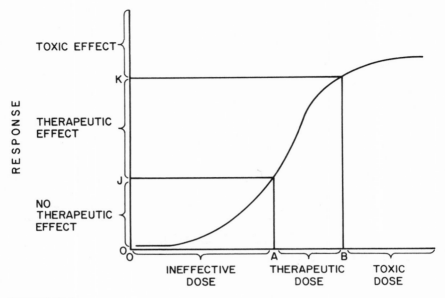

FIGURE 19.5.

Let us assume a set of patients, each of whom has been prescribed a thera-peutic dose R of the same drug, in an effort to achieve the corresponding thera-peutic effect F. Furthermore, let us assume an S-shaped dose-response curve R. This results in the situation shown in Figure 19.6. If we know the form of the compliance distribution and we know the form of the dose-response curve, how do we combine these two to determine the effect of compliance on the thera-peutic response?

Consider the conceptual equation

Response = f (compliance, dose response) [3]

where f is a particular function that combines the dose-response curve and the compliance distribution to predict the therapeutic response. Although the func-tion f may have many forms, the most intuitively attractive one is the one that multiplies the two factors, dose-response and compliance. Conceptually, then, the multiplicative function causes [3] to reduce to

Response = compliance X dose response.

If we consider a uniform compliance distribution (as in Figure 19.4) acting on the S-shaped dose-response curve, then the mean compliance will be a constant by which the dose-response curve is multiplied; the effect of this is illustrated in

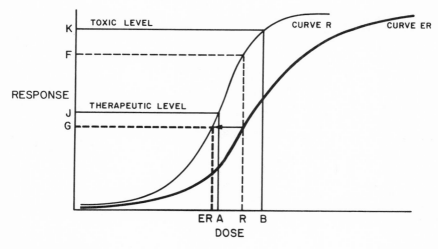

FIGURE 19.6.

Figure 19.6. (The other compliance distributions shown in Figures 19.2 and 19.3 will have different effects through the multiplicative function.)

Here, a therapeutic dosage lies in the interval A to B. Suppose the physician prescribed the dose R, which is in the therapeutic interval A to B, but the patient did not comply totally with the therapy. Suppose the patient's compliance measure was C (as the proportion and not as a percentage), and the relationship between the compliance distribution and the dose-response curve was multiplicative. Then, the effective dosage denoted by ER is computed by

$$ER = C \times R$$

Instead of the dosage R having the desired therapeutic effect F (obtained by projecting the dosage R vertically to the dose-response, denoted by curve R, and then horizontally to the outcome axis to get F), the patient gets an effective dose ER that yields a subtherapeutic effect G. An alternative view of this problem is povided by constructing an effective dose-response curve, denoted by curve ER, by moving the outcome of the effective dosage ER horizontally to the right to the prescribed dosage R position (to complete this alternative view, we would have to relocate A and B, the limits for the therapeutic dosage).

A study of Figure 19.6 reveals two other points worth noting. First, as long as the effective dosage remains within the therapeutic interval, noncompliance is not a problem. However, whenever the clinician routinely prescribes a dosage level higher than B, the toxic level, in an effort to counteract general lack of high compliance, those patients who do comply with the therapy will be exposed to the toxic effects of the drug.

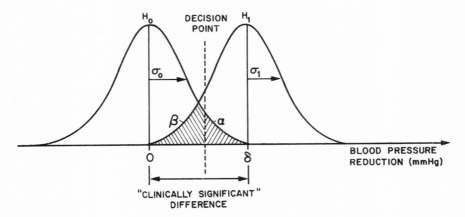

FIGURE 19.7.

EFFECT OF COMPLIANCE ON SAMPLE SIZE

How can we use this information to plan therapeutic trials? One of the common planning considerations in a therapeutic trial is the problem of determining the number of patients needed.

Suppose we are studying blood pressure reduction in hypertensive patients, and preliminary inpatient trials with a new drug on closely monitored patients have established a dose level (R) at which the blood pressure falls nicely (F) and the side effects are at a tolerable level. Here the definitive trial would be planned to see if this specific test drug lowers the blood pressure of ambulatory hypertensive patients. Suppose that design considerations dictate two samples, one treated and one control, and that the outcome (blood pressure reduction) was to be evaluated by means of a one-tailed, two-sample Student's t-test (1394). Suppose, in addition, that the blood pressure reductions produced by the test drug are independently normally distributed. The null hypothesis, denoted by H_0, would be that the test drug had no effect, so that differences between the treated and control groups would have a distribution whose mean was zero. This is displayed as the left-hand distribution (labeled H_0) in Figure 19.7. These differences between the treated and untreated subjects would have a true standard deviation σ_0, which is usually estimated by the pooled standard deviation obtained from the study subjects.

By statistical convention, we limit the probability of concluding that the test drug has an effect when, in fact, it really does not lower blood pressure. This probability, denoted by a, is commonly called the level of statistical significance. Since we are going to use a one-tailed test, the area a is placed in the right-hand tail of the left-hand distribution curve and thus specifies the decision point. If the difference in mean blood pressures between the treated and control groups lies to the left of this decision point, we will conclude that the test drug has no effect on reducing blood pressure. The same mean falling to the right of this decision point causes us to conclude that the therapy is effective in reducing blood pressure for this kind of hypertensive patient.

Returning to Figure 19.7, suppose that it is possible to specify a blood pressure reduction, δ (viz., 10 mm Hg), that is the minimum reduction needed before the test drug will be considered to have an effect of clinical importance. This clinically significant difference is specified as the alternative hypothesis and is denoted by H_1, with true standard deviation σ_1. In the remaining part of this discussion we will assume that $\sigma_0 = \sigma_1 = \sigma$. The distribution of means of differences between the treated and control groups is represented by the right-hand bell-shaped curve in Figure 19.7, and the means have a mean of δ. Now note that the area under the right-hand curve but to the left of the decision point is denoted by β. This is the probability that the data from our study will give rise to the conclusion that the test drug causes no reduction in blood pressure, when, in fact, it produces a real fall in blood pressure at least as large as δ. To maximize the validity of any therapeutic trial, α and β should be made as small as is feasible.

Let us now turn to consideration of the number of hypertensive patients we will require if we are to demonstrate this clinically significant difference (δ) in blood pressure between the treated and control groups.

Actually, the required sample size n depends on α, β, δ, and σ, as well as the kind of test statistic employed in the trial (here, a one-tailed, two-sample Student's t-test). What we must realize, however, is that the compliance of patients with the test drug treatment protocol has a profound effect on both sample size and our interpretation of the study. This can be seen by integrating Figure 19.6 and Figure 19.7 into Figure 19.8.

In this ambulatory trial, we are prescribing the test drug in a dose R to the treatment group in the hope that it will produce the effect F, resulting in the clinically significant difference in blood pressure δ projected in the lower portion of Figure 19.8 as the curve H_1. If these ambulatory patients take all of their medicine and we retain our decision point as before, it is possible to calculate the sample size required to demonstrate a difference of, say, one standard deviation (if this is the size of our clinically significant difference), at given levels of α and β, using a one-tailed, two-sample Student's t-test (for example, 23 patients are required in each of the treated and control groups to show this difference when compliance is complete and the levels selected for α and β are both 0.05).

However, what if our ambulatory patients fail to take all of their prescribed drug? The effect of this lowered compliance can be traced in Figure 19.8. Suppose that the dose of the test drug that is actually taken, ER, is lower than prescribed. Its effect, G, can be projected to show the resulting distribution of

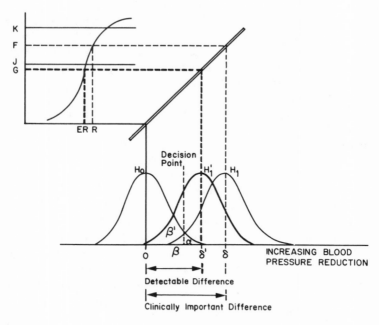

FIGURE 19.8.

blood pressure differences (curve H_2) with a mean difference of δ'. Using the same decision point, note the dramatic increase in β to β'; we are now much more likely to conclude that the test drug is worthless. Conversely, even if we are satisfied with accepting a smaller blood pressure reduction as being clinically significant, we will require many more patients in our trial in order to control a and β at the same level. The magnitude of this effect is shown in Table 19.1 and illustrated in the following example.

Suppose we wanted to plan a blood pressure reduction trial in mild ambulatory hypertensive patients, where the standard deviation of blood pressure reductions was 10 mm Hg (σ), the minimum clinically significant reduction in mean blood pressure was 10 mm Hg (δ), and we have selected $a = 0.05$ and $\beta = 0.05$. If compliance were 100%, the required sample size would be $n = 23$ (see Table 19.1) for each of the treatment and control groups. However, if compliance were only 50%, the required sample size to conclude any real effect would be $n = 88$ for each group. This example shows that the sample size required to detect the clinically significant difference of 10 mm Hg is nearly four times as large at 50% compliance as it would be at 100% compliance.

It is presumed that a similar situation holds when other statistical tests are employed. Indeed, whether less than complete compliance implies an increased sample size in other analytic situations needs to be investigated. Nonetheless,

TABLE 19.1. Required sample sizes (for each group)*

Mean percentage compliance	$a =$	0.05		0.01	
	$\beta =$	0.05	0.10	0.05	0.10
100		23	18	33	28
90		28	22	41	34
80		35	28	51	43
70		45	36	66	55
60		61	49	90	74
50		88	70	–	106
40		–	180	–	–

*Values were derived from Table E in Davies (1396).
The dashes indicate that the sample sizes were not available.

it can be seen that incomplete compliance can have a devastating effect, both upon the sample size requirements for showing real differences between treatment and control groups and upon the ability to conclude that treatments have clinically significant effects.

ANALYSIS OF THERAPEUTIC TRIALS

If one has gone to the trouble of measuring compliance in a therapeutic trial, then one should take that compliance measure into account when the data from the trial are being analyzed. Two alternative approaches should be considered.

If it can be assumed that the level of compliance is the same for the test drug and the placebo, then the compliance measurement can be considered as concomitant information and, hence, included in the analysis of the trial by the procedures of analysis of covariance. Readers unfamiliar with this procedure may wish to refer to Cox (1395) for an excellent discussion or to Armitage (1394) for computational details and examples. It should be recognized that covariance analysis requires that the compliance data be measured on an interval or ratio scale.

In many studies, however, differences in side effects between the active treatment and placebo groups may lead to different rates of compliance and so violate the assumption needed for covariance analysis. If one is concerned about the therapy affecting compliance or if the compliance data are at most ordinal, then the form of prognostic stratification suggested by Feinstein (1397) would be more appropriate. The paucity of compliance data in the published literature makes it impossible to give reasonable examples of these analytic techniques.

PRIORITIES FOR FUTURE RESEARCH

As a result of the considerations arising in the preparation of this chapter, the author offers the following suggestions for further research:

1. Encourage the precise definition and measurement of compliance in therapeutic trials as a matter of course.

2. Encourage the reporting of compliance distributions in therapeutic trials.

3. Reanalyze completed therapeutic trials, taking compliance into account.

4. Statistically simulate the compliance/dose-response-outcome chain for the common design models used in therapeutic trials.

5. If needed, develop new statistical procedures for incorporating compliance in the planning and analysis of therapeutic trials.

20

"Compliance Bias" and the Interpretation of Therapeutic Trials

Alvan R. Feinstein

Most discussions of compliance are concerned with a patient's maintenance of an assigned therapeutic regimen. Since no drug, diet, or other agent of therapy can work unless it is taken, one of the main clinical reasons for studying compliance is to increase it. By finding out why patients fail to comply and how we can encourage compliance, we hope to develop better ways of implementing a presumably beneficial therapeutic regimen. With these goals in mind, we may investigate the various clinical, social, and behavioral features that are determinants of compliance and the educational, communicational, and packaging features that may enhance it.

In trying to achieve or increase compliance with a therapeutic regimen, we begin with the basic assumption that the therapy is desirable —that it is safe, effective, and worth using. Once these virtues have been established, the regimen will warrant the efforts by both medical personnel and patients to ensure that it is maintained as prescribed. On the other hand, the complex spectrum of compliance has effects that can alter the basic data analyzed to determine the virtues of a regimen. These ramifications of compliance are the focus of discussion in this essay. Unless suitable biostatistical attention is given to the diverse patterns and effects of compliance, it can act as a source of confusion and distortion in the original therapeutic data. If various forms of compliance bias are not properly recognized and adjusted, a valuable therapeutic regimen may be dismissed as worthless or an ineffectual treatment may be promulgated as good.

I should like to discuss here six features of compliance that can affect the biostatistical data and interpretations. These features relate to issues in regimen

The text of this chapter, which appeared as installment 30 (December 1974) of the "Clinical Biostatistics" series published in *Clinical Pharmacology and Therapeutics*, is reprinted here by courtesy of the C. V. Mosby Co., publisher, and Walter Modell, editor, of that journal.

compliance, the evaluation of compliance, the control of noncompliance, protocol compliance, the compliance sample, and the compliance-confounded cohort.

Regimen Compliance

The first point to be considered is the way that the results of a therapeutic regimen can be distorted by the compliance it receives. Let us assume that an index of success has been established in a randomized, double-blind therapeutic trial, comparing drug A versus drug B. Let us further assume that the two drugs are equally effective. Despite this equivalence in efficacy, compliance bias can alter the results of the trial so that a major difference can occur falsely in the success rates of the two drugs. The observed success rate might be 50% for drug A and 66% for drug B.

A false difference of this magnitude could occur as follows. Suppose that the condition under treatment had a 70% remission rate when either drug A or drug B was maintained faithfully and a 30% remission rate when either drug was abandoned. Now suppose that drug A has an unappealing taste, appearance, or schedule of administration, so that it is faithfully maintained by only 50% of the patients to which it is assigned, whereas drug B receives excellent compliance by 90% of the patients. With these distinctions, if 200 patients were assigned drug A, 100 patients would maintain the drug faithfully and 70 of these 100 would have a successful outcome. Of the 100 patients who abandon the drug, 30 would be successful. The net result for drug A would be 100 successes per 200 patients—an overall success rate of 50%. With drug B, 180 of the 200 assigned patients would maintain excellent compliance and 126 (70%) of them would have a successful outcome. Of the 20 patients who abandon the drug, 6 (30%) would be successful. The total success rate for drug B would thus be 132/200, or 66%.

The difference between the two success rates would be large enough (16%) to be clinically significant and the magnitude of the sample sizes cited here would also make the difference statistically significant at $P < .005$ ($X^2 = 10.5$). If we had not attempted to investigate and analyze compliance, however, we would be unaware of its role in causing the difference. We would then conclude erroneously that drug B is pharmacologically more effective than drug A, although the actual cause of the difference is a matter of compliance, rather than pharmacologic efficacy.

The effect of compliance bias in the situation just described was to cause a false difference in the apparent efficacy of two drugs that actually had equal pharmacologic action. An analogous set of problems might work in the opposite direction to produce a false difference in the adverse reaction rates of two drugs with equal toxicity.

The Evaluation of Compliance

Since distinctions in compliance can affect the appraisal of a therapeutic regimen's efficacy and safety, the evaluation of compliance is an important, although often neglected, aspect of clinical biostatistics. Probably the main reason for this neglect is that compliance is an entirely subjective and human phenomenon. Its data are extremely "soft." The degree of compliance is determined by the patient; the act of compliance usually occurs in circumstances where it cannot be observed directly by the investigator; and its appraisal depends on what the patient decides to do and on what he reports. In an era devoted to the analysis of hard data, compliance is a variable that lacks scientific appeal, no matter how important the phenomenon may be.

The prejudice against this type of information has been well summarized by the recent Nobel laureate, Konrad Lorenz:

> If the subject of investigation happens to be human, he or she is being literally dehumanized by being prevented from showing any response which a guinea pig or pigeon might not show as well (in fact, the same experimental set-up is often applicable to animal and human subjects). Worse, in that kind of experimentation, the experimenter himself is not permitted to be quite human, as he is strictly prevented from using most of the cognitive mechanisms with which nature endowed our species. . . . The worst of this widespread contempt for description is that it discourages people from even trying to analyze really complicated systems (1403).

Types of Data.

For investigators who are willing to cope with complicated human systems, three different methods can be used for getting data to describe and evaluate compliance.* Perhaps the most objective technique is to measure the presence of the drug (or one of its metabolic products) in the urine. The main disadvantage of this method is that it pertains only to the one specimen for which the test was made. The result does not indicate the patient's compliance during the remaining time when no urine tests were performed. Furthermore, the single urine test may not be able to indicate whether the drug was taken correctly even on the day of the test.

A second quantitative technique is based on dosage unit counts. At each visit, the patient is given a fixed number of doses to be counted at the next visit. This technique provides quantitative data, but it will fail if the patient forgets to bring the container. Furthermore, the pill count cannot demonstrate whether the medication was taken in the desired pattern or disposed in various unprescribed manners.

---

*The measurement of compliance is discussed in detail in Chapter 3.

The best way of finding out what a patient has done is to ask the patient directly. From the reply, an investigator can learn the qualitative and quantitative information that is not provided by the other two techniques. For getting the totality of data needed to evaluate compliance, a well-constructed interview technique cannot be replaced by any of the available objective procedures.

The interview technique, however, is patently subjective. It depends completely on the patient's recall and reliability and also on the skill of the interviewer. An interviewer who is punitive or whose manner is otherwise unacceptable to the patient may not elicit accurate data. For these reasons, the interview technique is often used as the prime source of compliance data, but one of the objective techniques is added to verify the patient's reliability. A patient would be regarded as truly compliant only if the information stated in the interview is consistent with the results of the objective test.

Types of Rating.

Regardless of the method used for assembling data about compliance, the results must be cited in a manner that allows the data to be analyzed. Since compliance cannot be expressed readily in dimensional terms (which might be used for such variables as height or serum cholesterol), the investigator must choose a scale that provides a rating. The scale that is chosen can be a dichotomous partition (such as "good" and "not good") or a set of ordinal ranks containing such categories as "poor," "fair," "good," and "excellent." For many analytic purposes, a dichotomous partition will suffice, since the investigator may want to engage in only a simple comparison in which the outcomes of the "good" group or "not good" group are contrasted against all others.

The choice of criteria for these ratings will obviously be affected by the type of regimen under study and the purpose for which it has been prescribed. For example, the criteria for good compliance may differ if a daily antibiotic is being taken to prevent rather than to eradicate an infection. To illustrate this distinction, I shall list here two sets of criteria used during investigations (158, 159, 160) of daily oral antibiotics in the prevention of Group A streptococcal infections and rheumatic recurrences in a population of children and adolescents who had all had at least one previous episode of acute rheumatic fever:

Dose of drug	Oral penicillin G, 200,000 units daily	Oral penicillin G, 400,000 units three times daily for ten days
Purpose of regimen	Continuous prophylaxis against streptococcal infection	Eradication of streptococcal infection
Criterion of "good" compliance	Reliable history and no more than five days missed per month and no two days missed consecutively	Reliable history and no more than one dose missed during the ten days

Regardless of whether the reader agrees or disagrees with the details of these criteria, they demonstrate the fact that different types of therapeutic regimens will require different criteria for ratings of compliance.

The Noncompliance Control

Although the scientific prejudice against talking to patients is one of the main reasons that compliance has been so neglected as an important variable in statistical analysis, another type of prejudice has caused clinical investigators to lose other valuable data related to compliance. This prejudice is the tendency of doctors to dismiss patients who reject their recommendations.

In ordinary clinical practice, a patient who fails to carry out the doctor's recommendations is performing an important experiment that the doctor was unwilling to undertake. The patient has decided, in effect, to test a counter-hypothesis. If the experiment fails, the failure helps support the propriety of the doctor's original therapeutic decision. If the experiment succeeds, the doctor has learned that success does not always require the original plan of action. Consequently, a patient who refuses to comply with an offered treatment becomes a type of control whose results can be compared with those of patients who received the treatment.

Nevertheless, in ordinary clinical practice, a patient who appears to reject the doctor's recommendations is often rejected by the doctor. Because the patient may then be urged actively or passively to seek medical attention elsewhere, the doctor may miss the opportunity to learn the results of the counter-experiment. This type of loss may be a necessary event in circumstances where a busy practitioner wants to use his time "efficiently" and has no intention of ever tabulating his therapeutic results. The loss is highly undesirable, however, if the practitioner's data ever become biostatistics.

An illustration of the problem has appeared regularly in surveys reporting the outcome of therapy for cancer. In such surveys, the results of surgically treated patients have generally been compared with those of patients who received radiotherapy or chemotherapy. This comparison is unfair because the nonsurgical patients were not an operable group; they were usually deemed inoperable and referred for other modes of treatment. For an unbiased comparison, those in the group of operable patients who received surgery should be contrasted with those in a group of operable patients who received some other treatment.

This type of contrast would be arranged deliberately in a randomized therapeutic trial, but very few such trials have been conducted for operable patients. Consequently, the only source of operable nonsurgical patients in ordinary clinical practice is the patients who were deemed operable and who refused the offered surgical treatment. These noncompliant patients would be a reasonable control group for the surgically treated patients; but the noncompliant patients are usually rejected by their surgeons and seldom receive follow-up examinations at which their outcomes could be noted, recorded, and analyzed.

Noncompliant patients can also serve as an important control group in circumstances where the results of placebo therapy are not available. For example, when several antibacterial agents were receiving randomized clinical trials in order to compare their value in preventing streptococcal infections, ethical considerations militated against the examination of results in groups treated with placebo. In the absence of a placebo-treated group, however, major problems arose when two of the active drugs were found to yield essentially similar results. Was either drug really more effective than the placebo? The issue was resolved when the streptococcal attack rate in compliant patients (who maintained good prophylaxis) was found to be substantially lower than in patients who failed to comply.

Another opportunity to make analytic use of compliance distinctions occurred during an investigation of the role that tonsil size might play in predisposing rheumatic children and adolescents to streptococcal infections (157). Among the patients who maintained good continuity of antibiotic prophylaxis, the attack rate of streptococcal infections was unaffected by tonsil size. Among patients who did not maintain good prophylaxis, the streptococcal attack rate increased with the increasing size of the tonsils.

Protocol Compliance

In all the issues discussed so far, the idea of compliance referred only to the patient's acceptance or maintenance of an assigned therapeutic regimen. Another important aspect of compliance refers to the maintenance of a research protocol. During the course of a therapeutic trial or other investigation, many planned procedures must be carried out by both investigator and patient. The compliance or noncompliance given to these protocol procedures can affect the results of the research.

Compliance by the Investigator.

The likelihood of violating a research protocol is particularly high when multiple investigators are collaborating. The violations usually arise because of poor communication among the collaborators or inadequate attention by individual investigators. One frequent violation occurs in the criteria for admission to the trial. For example, in the UGDP cooperative study of therapy for diabetes mellitus, 95 of the admitted patients did not fulfill the minimum standards of glucose intolerance that had been established as diagnostic criteria for diabetes mellitus. Aside from the ethical problems produced by this type of protocol violation, it can create a major statistical problem if the results in the ineligible and eligible patients are substantially different (1404).

Another type of violation, which is often inadvertent, is the investigator's development of the ability to discern the identities of the drugs being studied in a double-blind trial. This unmasking is particularly likely to occur if the active drug can be recognized from a physiological side effect such as the bradycardia that often occurs with beta-blocking agents. The consequence of this type of protocol violation is the delusion that symptoms and other subjective data have been determined with the presumptive objectivity of an effectively maintained double-blind technique. If doctors (or patients) become able to differentiate successfully the active drug from the placebo, the clinical trial is converted into a pseudo-double-blind exercise, having all the logistical disadvantages of double-blind research and none of the scientific advantages.

A third protocol problem in therapeutic trials is the need to exclude supplementary drugs that might affect the results of the main drug under investigation. The violation of this specification of a protocol is often overlooked if the violations have occurred with equal frequency in each group of patients receiving the compared therapeutic regimens. Since the qualitative characteristics of the "ineligible" medications may not be equivalent for each group of patients, the differences may be responsible for distinctions that erroneously become attributed to the principal therapeutic agents.

Of the many other potential issues in investigator noncompliance, the only one to be cited here is the problem of preserving the letter of a research protocol, while ignoring its spirit. For example, suppose we are conducting a therapeutic trial to determine whether the maintenance of normoglycemia will prevent vascular complications in adults with diabetes mellitus. If we prescribe a fixed dosage of an oral hypoglycemic drug and determine whether the patient complies with the prescribed regimen, we have adhered to the specifications of the protocol. On the other hand, if we fail to check whether the patient's blood sugar is actually being maintained in a normal range, or if we fail to adjust the dose of the drug so that it produces normoglycemia, we have not complied with the basic idea of the research.

There are many other ways in which an investigator's noncompliance with protocol can distort the research data. Nevertheless, the published reports of a research project often contain no indication of efforts made to check whether protocol compliance has occurred. An interesting aspect of the peculiar double standard used on the current research scene is that pharmaceutical companies are expected to monitor the compliance of clinical investigators who perform trials of new drugs, but an analogous monitoring may not be demanded when a federal agency sponsors a multicenter therapeutic trial involving investigators at academic institutions.

Compliance by the Patient.

While complying with the prescribed medication, a patient may violate the prescribed protocol in several different ways. One violation consists of breaking the double-blind code. A recent example of this problem was provided by

Chalmers (1398). He described the way in which a sophisticated group of patients (employees of the National Institutes of Health), who were participating in a double-blind clinical trial, tested the contents of the capsules to distinguish vitamin C from the placebo. According to Chalmers, the rates of the outcome event in the trial were substantially different for patients who did or did not identify their medication correctly.

Another important form of patient noncompliance is improper attendance for repeated examinations after treatment is initiated. If a patient scheduled to have a particular test done at four weeks and at eight weeks after treatment appears only at six weeks, where are the results of the six-week test counted? Suppose the patient does not appear often enough to have all the periodic tests that are needed to rule out episodic events, such as asymptomatic streptococcal infections or anicteric hepatitis. How are the incomplete data to be analyzed? There are no simple statistical answers to these questions. Each decision requires subtle judgments according to the particular circumstances that are involved.

The ultimate act of noncompliance, of course, is the patient's decision to drop out of a study altogether. Except for one issue, to be cited later, the problems of analyzing data for dropout patients are beyond the scope of this discussion. The problems are difficult, complex, and not always well managed by the actuarial ("life-table") analysis that is usually proposed as a solution.

The "Compliance Sample"

A different type of biostatistical problem arises when a therapeutic trial is conducted with a "compliance sample" of patients. Such a sample arises in the following way. Before admission to the trial, patients who are otherwise eligible are screened to determine their ability and willingness to comply with both the protocol and the therapeutic regimens under investigation. Patients whom the investigator regards as noncompliant are then excluded from admission, so that the trial is conducted with the group of seemingly cooperative patients who constitute the compliance sample. A clue to the existence of such a sample can be noted from an account of the criteria used for excluding patients from a trial. These criteria customarily depend on various features of diagnosis, prognosis, co-morbidity, or co-medication. If the criteria also include a statement about willingness to cooperate, the investigators have used a compliance sample. To choose patients in this way seems perfectly reasonable. After all, in conducting a therapeutic trial, the investigators do not wish to expend major amounts of time and vigorous research efforts on patients who are not likely to maintain the proposed medication or appear for the proposed examination procedures. By screening out the noncompliant patients, the investigators would eliminate wasted energy and increase the efficiency of the research activities.

In attaining this efficiency, however, the investigators take a substantial risk. The risk is that the compliant patients may not be representative of the people who have the condition under treatment. The risk is minute if the excluded non-compliant patients constitute only a small proportion of the total group of otherwise eligible patients. If the excluded group occupies a large fraction of eligible cases, however, the results of the trial may be pertinent for compliant but not for other patients with the same clinical condition.

An example of this type of problem occurred in the recent Veterans Administration Cooperative Study (1405) of the treatment of hypertension. Because the results provided hard (randomized) evidence of the value of treating patients with asymptomatic hypertension, the trial has received much justified praise for the excellence with which it was designed and conducted. Nevertheless, the group under study contained a highly restricted compliance sample of hypertensive patients. The selection procedures were described as follows (1401):

> Since an appreciable number of dropouts would jeopardize the study, we wished to minimize their occurrence as much as possible. "Skid row" alcoholics, vagrants, psychopaths, antagonistic personalities, mentally incompetent persons who are not properly cared for at home, and all those who for one reason or another could not return to clinic regularly are therefore excluded from the trial. In addition, the prerandomization trial period serves to eliminate other potential dropouts that are missed during the initial evaluation."

The VA investigators have not published data on the number of otherwise eligible patients whose anticipated (or demonstrated) noncompliance kept them from being admitted to the trial. It has been estimated* that between one-half and two-thirds of the patients with eligible blood pressures were excluded from entry. The exclusion of this large proportion of patients would not affect the results found in the compliant patients who were treated in the trial, but it would impair the ability to draw general conclusions about the treatment of other patients with hypertension. The vascular systems of docile hypertensive patients who were willing to comply in such a trial may have benefited from therapeutic agents that lower blood pressure; but these agents may not have worked as well on the many nondocile hypertensives who were rejected as noncompliant.

As public campaigns are mounted to deliver appropriate treatment to all patients with hypertension, the results (if noted and evaluated) may be somewhat disappointing. If the rate of vascular complications is not reduced as much as was expected, the disparity may arise from the unresponsiveness of the noncompliant patients whose therapeutic refractoriness had not been discovered previously.

---

*E. D. Freis, personal communication.

The "Compliance-Confounded Cohort"

The last problem to be cited here is particularly subtle and complex. It can arise if the ability to comply with a therapeutic regimen is also related to the event that is to be noted as the main outcome of treatment. If compliance ability and outcome event are closely related, the results will be distorted by a confounding variable. Regardless of treatment, the cohort of people who can comply with treatment will be destined to have an outcome event rate that differs substantially from the corresponding rate in the people who do not maintain compliance. Consequently, an ineffectual regimen may falsely appear to be distinctly beneficial (or detrimental) to the patients who maintain it.

To illustrate this point, suppose that people who have a high degree of the particular kind of inner drive or stress that might be called psychic tension are more likely to develop cardiovascular disease than are people who are not psychically tense. Let us now suppose that an unappealing and difficult to maintain new diet has been proposed as an agent that prevents cardiovascular disease. Let us further assume that the diet is actually ineffectual. Finally, let us assume that the tense people have great difficulty in complying with this new diet, whereas nontense people are much better able to comply. Under these conditions, when the diet is prescribed for a large population, the rate of cardiovascular disease will be lower in people who maintain the diet than in people who do not. The false conclusion may then be that the diet effectively prevents cardiovascular disease.

Since this type of problem may arise in the multiple risk factor intervention trial (MRFIT) now being executed (1402) throughout the United States, I shall cite some contrived numerical data to illustrate the possibilities.

Let us assume that we can identify a tense group of people who will also have a 30% rate of cardiovascular events during the interval under study. In nontense people, the corresponding rate is 5%. Let us further assume that the population under study consists of 70% nontense people and 30% tense people. If nothing were done to this population, we would expect the overall rate of cardiovascular events to be

$$(.70)(.05) + (.30)(.30) = .035 + .09 = .125 = 12.5\%.$$

Now suppose that the entire population enters a randomized clinical trial in which the action of a special new diet is being tested. Half the population is assigned this new diet and the other half continues to maintain its usual dietary pattern.

The compliance problem might now occur as follows. For the people who are not receiving a special diet, there is no difficult regimen acting as provocation to drop out. The only dropout incentive is the nuisance of participating in the clinical trial itself. Consequently, the dropout rates in the control group would be the usual attrition to be expected in any trial, and the rates would be similar in the tense and nontense patients. Let us assume that these dropout rates are 5% in each group. The remaining population in the control cohort will thus be composed of 95% of the starting members of each psychic group and will be 95% of its original size. [This figure can be verified as $(.95)(.70) + (.95)(.30) = .665 + .285 = .950 = 95\%$.]

For the patients in the cohort assigned to receive the special diet, the difficulties of maintaining the diet will create a strong stimulus toward dropping out. Among nontense patients, let us assume that the dropout rate is 10%, twice as high as the rate in similar patients not receiving the diet. Among tense patients, the problems of maintaining the special diet are formidable, so that 80% of these patients drop out. The total group of people who maintain the special diet will thus be reduced to 69% of the original cohort. [This figure can be verified as $(.70)(.90) + (.30)(.20) = .63 + .06 = .69 = 69\%$.] This rate of compliance will not seem unusually low, because a relatively high dropout rate would be anticipated for people assigned to the special diet.

Now let us consider what will be observed as the outcome rates for cardiovascular events in this study. For the cohort of people who continued to participate in the control group, the event rate would be 5% in the 66.5% of nontense people and 30% in the 28.5% of tense people. The total event rate would be $(.05)(.6) + (.30)(.285) = (.03325) + (.0855) = .11875$. When adjusted for the population of no-diet people who actually completed the trial, this rate would be $(.11875) / (.95) = .125 = 12.5\%$. For the cohort of people who continued to maintain the special diet, the event rate would be 5% in the 63% of nontense people and 30% in the 6% of tense people. The total event rate for the special diet group will therefore be $(.05)(.63) + (.30)(.06) = .0315 + .018 = .0495 = 4.95\%$. When adjusted for the special-diet people who actually completed the trial, this rate would be $(.0495) / (.69) = .072 = 7.2\%$.

If we knew nothing about the relationship of personality, compliance, and cardiovascular rates in tense versus nontense people, we would observe only the outcome rates. Without a stratification for psychic state, we would not be aware of the differential dropout distinctions that had produced the differences in outcome, and we might draw conclusions based only on the gross outcomes. Thus, in a randomized clinical trial comparing a special diet versus no diet, we would have noted that the people who maintained the special diet had a cardiovascular event rate of 7.2% and the people who maintained no special diet had a corresponding rate of 12.5%. The special diet would appear to have reduced the cardiovascular event rate by $(12.5 - 7.2)/12.5 = 5.3/12.5 = 42.4\%$. This magnitude of reduction would obviously seem clinically significant; and furthermore, with the large number of patients in the trial, the difference would also be statistically significant.*

*With calculations that are too extensive to be repeated here, it can be shown that this difference in the two groups of compliant patients will have a P value below .05 (by χ^2 test) if as few as 636 patients are initially enrolled in the trial.

The obvious conclusion would seem to be that the special diet had reduced the rate of cardiovascular disease by more than 40%—and yet the conclusion would be totally wrong. The apparent benefits of the diet, which we know was actually ineffectual, would have arisen only from the fact that it received compliance mainly from people destined to have a low rate of cardiovascular events.

At this point in the discussion, a student of clinical trials would note immediately that the analysis presented thus far is incomplete. We have not yet looked at the results of the dropout patients. Under the conditions noted earlier, we should note a substantial difference in cardiovascular rates in the two groups of patients who dropped out. These rates would be 12.5% in the control group and 24.4% in the special-diet group. The explanatory calculations are as follows. In the control group, the nontense dropouts would contain $(.70)(.50) = .35$ and the tense dropouts would contain $(.30)(.05) = .015$ of the original population. The cardiovascular rate in this group of dropouts would be $[(.035) (.05) + (.015)(.30)] / .050 = [.00175 + .00450] / .050 = .00625 / .05 = .125 = 12.5\%$. In the special-diet group, the nontense dropouts would contain $(.70) (.10) = .07$ and the tense dropouts would contain $(.30)(.80) = .24$ of the original population. The cardiovascular rate in this group of dropouts would be $[(.70) (.05) + (.24)(.30)] / .31 = [.0035 + .072] / .31 = .0755 / .31 = .244 = 24.4\%$. The finding that one dropout group had a cardiovascular rate twice as high as the other dropout group immediately should alert our suspicions that something extremely peculiar has happened.

Furthermore, if we look at the results of all patients who were randomized, regardless of those who dropped out, we would find that the cardiovascular rates are the same. In the control group, the rate would be $[(.11875) + (.00625)] / [(.95) + (.05)] = [.12500] / 1.00 = 12.5\%$. In the special-diet group, the rate would be $[(.0495) + (.0755)] / [(.69) + (.31)] = [.1250] / [1.00] = 12.5\%$. This similarity in cardiovascular rates for the two randomized groups, regardless of dropouts, would help confirm the existence of some strange phenomenon among the dropout cases.

To obtain all this additional information, however, would require that the therapeutic trial be conducted with an extraordinary passion for obtaining complete, detailed follow-up data for all patients who have dropped out. This intensity of follow-up surveillance almost never occurs in a therapeutic trial. If the outcome event is death, the investigators can usually learn about its occurrence in dropout patients who have been lost to follow-up previously, but if the outcome event is a nonfatal cardiovascular event (such as angina pectoris, myocardial infarction, intermittent claudication, or stroke) the occurrence or nonoccurrence of this event is difficult to document in a standardized manner for living patients who have been lost to follow-up. Because of these difficulties in the follow-up of dropout patients, the investigators may be tempted to confine their main analysis to the patients who, having complied with the research protocol, continued under observation. If this temptation is accepted, the investigators will reach the erroneous conclusion described earlier.

The possibility of this type of error is a major hazard in the work of the MRFIT study. Abundant evidence has now been assembled to suggest that a distinctive relationship exists between certain personality types (or psychic states) and subsequent cardiovascular disease. The main issue is no longer whether such a relationship exists, but how to identify it—by which particular psychological test or other psychiatric examining instrument can we best discern the people who are especially susceptible to cardiovascular disease. Another reasonable belief is that the people who have a particular psychic constitution may be unwilling or unable to maintain the forms of special dieting or other interventions that are prescribed as active therapy in the MRFIT trial. Since the control group will receive no diet, rather than an equally unpalatable but standard diet, the MRFIT investigation thus possesses all the ingredients needed for a major scientific error in the interpretation of results.

The most cogent way of avoiding this error is for the patient's psychic condition to be examined using test procedures that are as thorough as those used for examining the condition of serum lipids. With such data, the investigators could identify the different degrees of psychic risk, and they could use the results for the analysis needed to demonstrate that compliance bias is absent. This approach may not be scientifically appealing, however, because the questionnaire and other written instruments used for examining psychic status have not received intensive attention from epidemiologists. The ideological belief of most contemporary epidemiologists has been that risk factors arise from nurture but not from nature, i.e., from such environmental features as food, water, tobacco smoking, and exercise; but not from such constitutional features as heredity and psychic status. Because of this ideological belief, both heredity and psyche generally have been ignored in epidemiologic research, and suitable scientific instruments have not been developed or applied for obtaining the necessary data in large cohort studies.

In the absence of suitable psychic examinations and correlated data analysis, another way of trying to avoid the cited error is for all the MRFIT patients to continue to receive intensive medical surveillance, even if they drop out, so that the detection of cardiovascular events is performed equally for everyone, regardless of regimen compliance. If the cardiovascular rates are different for noncompliant patients in the several therapeutic regimens, the investigators will have received a major signal that their basic data may be distorted by a compliance-confounded cohort. Equality of diagnostic surveillance may not be achievable, however, because the dropout patients may be unwilling to continue returning to the MRFIT clinics for the necessary examinations. To cope with this problem, the investigators may need to arrange night clinics, home visits, or other special procedures that will allow dropout patients to receive suitable follow-up examinations for detecting cardiovascular events.

CONCLUSIONS

These six features of compliance should suffice to indicate its intricacies and its potential for creating major biostatistical delusions. Compliance bias can be added to selection bias (1399), detection bias (1399), and chronology bias (1400) as another major source of the confounding variables that produce fundamental errors in biostatistical analysis. Confounding variables in biostatistics are like counterhypotheses in any other form of scientific research. If the investigator does not contemplate and rule out the counterhypotheses, they may vitiate his chosen hypothesis and invalidate his research. Like the biases due to inequities in selection, detection, and chronology, compliance bias will not disappear because an investigator hopes that it does not exist. It also will not disappear if the data analyst tries to adjust for bias by using age, race, sex, or other variables that are conveniently available, instead of concentrating on the "inconvenient" variables that create the confounding.

To acquire the data needed for analyzing compliance and ruling out the existence of compliance bias, investigators will have to restore attention to a traditional activity of clinical medicine: talking to the patient. The investigators who have neglected or abandoned this information because it is scientifically "soft" have created the hazard of a clinical science that is "hard" but often irrelevant or erroneous. By perpetuating a restricted focus on hard data while ignoring important soft data that are obtained by direct conversation with patients, biostatisticians have abetted the malefaction. In addition to the cited scientific defects, however, therapeutic investigations that depend only on hard data create an important humanistic hazard. The idea may be established that biostatistical analysis is unable to distinguish between an act of patient care and an exercise of veterinary medicine.

21

Methods for Compliance Research

David L. Sackett

INTRODUCTION

The rules of scientific evidence are universal, and the research strategies that they engender cut across all branches of science. It is not the intent of this chapter to review the basic strategies that comprise that "potentiation of common sense, exercised with a specially firm determination not to persist in error" known as the scientific method (1414).

However, when these general strategies are converted into specific tactics for compliance research, they warrant a detailed discussion of their properties and usefulness. This chapter will deal with that series of methodologic issues that confronts those who undertake compliance research. The solutions proposed here are derived from the preceding chapters in this book, from our review of the compliance literature, from leading publications concerned with the execution of clinical research (1409, 1412, 1413), and from personal work in the methodology of clinical epidemiology (1416-1421).

Methodologic issues of concern in any compliance research are discussed first. This is followed by the discussion of a second series of methodologic issues that also must be confronted when performing randomized trials of compliance-improving strategies.

**METHODOLOGIC ISSUES OF
IMPORTANCE IN ANY COMPLIANCE RESEARCH**

For many readers, particularly those from the clinical disciplines, a compliance investigation may represent the first attempt at health research. When this is the case, the study of this chapter should be coupled with the reading of more general works on health research methods. Other works that best combine basic methodology with highly practical advice include the books of Mainland (1413), Hill (1412), Murphy (1415), and Feinstein (1409), plus the latter author's continuing "Clinical Biostatistics" series which appears in *Clinical Pharmacology and Therapeutics*. A portion of the series is now available in book form (1410).

Although individual compliance investigations present unique methodologic problems to be solved, seven issues recur in all compliance research, and these must be considered before embarking upon any study.

Defining Compliance

The definition of compliance must be precise, unambiguous, and appropriate both to the research question and to the research setting; this has been introduced in Chapter 1 and is stressed repeatedly in succeeding chapters. It appears once again in the methodologic standards presented in Appendix I, where its key property is identified as replicability by the reader.

Investigators should ask themselves questions such as: Have I defined what I mean by compliance in terms so clear that someone who reads of my work will know precisely what I mean and be able to replicate my work? If compliance is defined as keeping appointments with the clinician, does this mean just initial appointments arranged by the patient, follow-up appointments arranged by the clinician, or both? Is the patient still considered compliant when a previously arranged appointment is canceled by the clinician or when the patient is trapped in a snowstorm on the way to the clinician's office?

Those who feel that the previous passage belabors the obvious should refer to Appendix I, where they will learn that a substantial number of compliance investigators have failed to provide a proper definition of the object of their research. Incidentally, this need for a clear and replicable definition is in no way obviated by the decision to use alternative technical jargon terms for compliance in an effort to minimize any unfavorable connotations of this word.

Selecting and Describing the Sample

The selection and description of the sample of patients studied in an investigation of compliance demands considerable thought and, in reports of the investigation, full disclosure. If the results of the study are to be applied to ambulatory patients in the community at large, the study should be executed in that setting or in a closely similar one. Once again, the issues of concern are discussed in earlier chapters and in Appendix I. They can be summarized in the question: To which patients does the investigator wish to generalize the research results? Although the answer to this question usually is stated as, to all patients who are prescribed regimen A for the disease X, the methodologic demands imposed by this intention are rarely considered, much less met. These methodologic demands include asking several additional questions.

For example, one must ask if it is not essential to utilize "inception" cohorts (Chapter 2). If the failure of patients to comply with therapy is a central issue in the investigation, surely the sample must include all patients who were initially prescribed regimen A for disease X (including those who quit and dropped out along the way), and not simply those patients who could be found in a clinic or other facility at some later date. Early dropouts from treatment are frequent, and their omission will invalidate conclusions about the magnitude of compliance, its determinants, and the effectiveness of strategies for its improvement.

This is not to say that the start of a compliance research project must coincide in calendar time with the initiation of therapy; as long as an accurate registry is available for all eligible patients who were placed on therapy, this "inception cohort" registry can be used as the sampling frame for studying the phenomenon of compliance, its determinants, or strategies for its improvement. Although the pretreatment evaluation of these patients may not be sufficiently thorough, standardized, and documented to make them an appropriate sample, the time saved by this shortcut warrants the exploitation of suitable opportunities when they do arise.

Secondly, investigators must ask whether the study population is biased in other ways that can distort conclusions drawn about compliance. The selective factors that influence the generation of clinical samples of patients such as those found in referral centers are not widely appreciated (1416, 1417, 1420). Thus, investigators must consider whether potential study populations are biased with respect to the ascertainment of their illness (1407), the stage in their disease and its treatment (1408), and, indeed, their level of compliance itself. As a result of these selective factors, compliance studies performed at tertiary referral centers are often more likely to characterize the institution where they were executed than the condition under scrutiny.

The need to consider this issue when assessing educational strategies has been stressed earlier, and references dealing with sampling bias should be reviewed in the design stages of any compliance research. Although the generation of study groups from industrial or general populations or from a series of primary care practices presents formidable operational hurdles, no other approach can provide a valid representation of compliance at the community level.

Defining the Disease and the Therapeutic Regimen

The definition of the disease and the therapeutic regimen must be precise. If the study concerns compliance with antibiotics among patients with urinary tract infections, how are patients determined to be eligible? Is asymptomatic bacteriuria sufficient, or must the patients have symptoms of infection? If so, which ones? What inclusion and exclusion criteria will be used to accept or reject patients?

With respect to the regimen, which drugs will be studied, in what forms and doses will they be prescribed and for what duration of time? What is the cost and convenience of filling prescriptions for this group of patients, and what side effects can they be expected to experience?

Once again, at issue are the replicability of the criteria by other investigators and the generalizability of the research results; the methodologic standards in Appendix I will provide a model for addressing this issue.

When selecting a research topic from the array of possible diseases and regimens, it should be borne in mind that the disease or syndrome selected should be an important cause of disability or untimely death, and one for which there exists a therapeutic regimen of demonstrated efficacy; if low compliance with the associated regimen is widespread, it follows that unsatisfactory clinical outcomes will result.

Selecting Compliance Measures

The choice of compliance measures must be appropriate both to the individual investigation and to the wider goals of pooling and of comparison with the results obtained by other investigators in other settings. As discussed in Chapter 3, it is important to select compliance measures that are appropriate for the setting, illness, regimen, and purpose of the investigation (whether for gaining new research knowledge or for improving an existing clinical program). Whenever possible, investigators should apply multiple measures of compliance. The methodologic standards that appear in Appendix I will serve as a supplement to Leon Gordis's listing of measures in Chapter 3.

In making these measurements it should be borne in mind that dropouts, the bane of pharmacologic trials, represent endpoints in compliance studies and should be assessed systematically. Did patients drop out because of dissatisfaction with the care they received or because of the compliance-improving strategy? In doing so, did they stop taking their medicine as well? The need for unobtrusive compliance measures (and the effect of inappropriate interpretations of informed consent upon this measurement) are discussed elsewhere in this chapter and in Chapter 3.

Correlating Compliance with the Treatment Goal

Reintroducing a theme from Chapter 18 (depicted graphically in Figure 18.1), compliance should be correlated with the treatment goal in applied investigations. The necessity for this approach becomes clear when one considers the following examples.

When patients who consume only 60% of their medicine still achieve the therapeutic goal, why subject them to behavioral modification maneuvers in an effort to raise their compliance to 90%? When compliant and noncompliant patients are equally likely to achieve the treatment goal, the issue is one of efficacy, not compliance. In addition to identifying patients who require no intervention (i.e., those who have achieved the treatment goal, regardless of their compliance status) correlation of compliance with the treatment goal identifies two other groups of patients that may benefit from further study. In the upper right cell of Figure 18.1 we find patients who, although they comply, have not achieved the therapeutic goal. How are they to be handled in the analysis? Do they constitute improperly diagnosed patients who should never have been in the study in the first place? If they are simply underprescribed for by their clinicians, would their high compliance have persisted when they were exposed to full doses of medications? Rules for handling such cases, sensibly derived and consistently applied, will enhance both the scientific merit and the clinical credibility of the research report.

The other group of patients identified by the correlation of compliance with the treatment goal resides in the lower right cell of Figure 18.1; they are neither compliant nor at the treatment goal. The size of this cell, relative to the others, provides a direct estimate of the clinical implications of low compliance and is of major interest to all those who care for patients.

Identification of the latter group of patients is also of potential tactical importance in the performance of compliance research. Studies of potential predictors of compliance can focus upon the attributes of this group in order to determine whether they possess unique characteristics or "markers" that could have identified them at the inception of therapy. Furthermore, randomized trials of compliance-improving strategies may wish to use this lower right cell as a sampling frame for an experiment involving strategies that are particularly expensive or complex.*

Basic research into the nature of compliance as a phenomenon need not undertake the additional task of quantifying and analyzing the achievement of the treatment goal; however, the above examples demonstrate the need to include the treatment goal in any compliance investigation that is to be used as the basis for recommending changes in the care of patients.

Ethical Issues

While the planning and execution of any research must involve the consideration of ethical issues, compliance investigations pose two unique ethical dilemmas. The first of these can arise both in descriptive and in analytic studies of

---

*This advantage arises from the observation that a portion (usually about one-third) of patients placed on almost any therapeutic regimen will exhibit high, prolonged compliance without any additional expenditure of effort by their clinicians. Accordingly, the application of the compliance-improving strategy to this already compliant subgroup may be wasteful in both economic and statistical terms. Although compliant patients must be followed with the rest of the study subjects, investigators may choose to apply a more complex compliance-improving strategy to only a random sample of those who both fail to comply and fail to achieve the treatment goal, thereby concentrating the strategy where it can show its beneficial effects, if any.

Our randomized trial of strategies for improving compliance with antihypertensive medication combined both approaches (228, 449). In Phase I, relatively simple and inexpensive strategies were applied to random samples of all patients who were beginning treatment. In Phase II, more complex and potentially more expensive strategies were applied to a random 50% of patients who neither complied nor achieved goal blood pressures by the end of Phase I.

compliance as a phenomenon and in randomized trials of compliance-improving strategies. If carried to its illogical extreme, the doctrine of informed consent can require the investigator to explain every component of every maneuver executed at every encounter with the study subject. In compliance research, this interpretation could compel the investigator to tell the study subject that one of the reasons for taking a given specimen of urine is the measurement of whether medications are being taken as prescribed. As pointed out in Chapter 3 by Leon Gordis, forewarning the study subject that a compliance check will be made on a given day is quite likely to change that subject's compliance on that day, thus rendering this measurement a poor reflection of the subject's usual degree of compliance. Thus, adherence to the picayune letter, rather than the laudable spirit, of ethical regulation in some centers in the United States may cripple compliance research by rendering the measurement of compliance highly biased.

The second relatively unique ethical problem in performing compliance research stems from the fact that the strategies for improving compliance that undergo testing in randomized trials are clearly designed to alter human behavior. Their effectiveness in improving compliance may depend upon (or at least be closely linked with) modification of the way that patients feel about themselves, about their healthiness, and, for example, about their dependence upon medications.

Concern about this ethical issue is expressed at several other points in this book, especially in Chapter 7, and may be summarized in the following methodologic recommendations:

1. Trials of strategies for altering compliance should include measurements of patients' self-perceptions and of their social and emotional function, both before and after they undergo the experimental maneuver. Any deteriorations in these indexes should be weighed against the improvements, if any, in the achievement of favorable clinical outcomes.

2. These trials should only be carried out among patients who have been correctly diagnosed as having nontrivial disorders, the treatment of which has been shown to do more good than harm.*

3. Informed consent must encompass the possible side-effects and toxicity of the compliance-modifying strategy as well as those of the therapeutic regimen.

The Need for Collaborative Efforts

The number of academic disciplines and health professions that have contributed to this book underscores the need for multidisciplinary collaboration

---

*If the regimen lacks efficacy, the trial becomes subverted to one in which the successful compliance-improving strategy only serves to increase patients' explosure to the deleterious effects of the medications or of other regimen components.

in the design, execution, analysis, and interpretation of compliance research. Anyone who has worked by this maxim can attest to its substantial productivity and frequent delight; if these testimonies are candid, they will also identify the exasperation that results from the occasional conflict between, and cross-sterilization of, disciplines.

Nonetheless, it is clear that no single discipline can provide the expertise in human biology, statistics, educational theory, pharmacology, epidemiology, behavior, social psychology, clinical management, biochemistry, nursing, pharmacy, economics, administration, and health care systems that is necessary for the execution of sophisticated and relevant research into compliance. It is also clear that the sequestrating of both the research and the educational functions of these disciplines into separate departments and faculties renders multi-disciplinary collaboration more difficult.

METHODOLOGIC ISSUES OF
PARTICULAR IMPORTANCE IN RANDOMIZED TRIALS

Although we are slow to learn, even from our own mistakes, the frequency with which proper experiments have shattered our prior conclusions about the value of a host of established preventive, therapeutic, and rehabilitative maneuvers has convinced all but closed minds of the need to validate new clinical and health care proposals rigorously. Accordingly (and because they possess the same potentials for benefit and harm as do other therapeutic maneuvers), compliance-improving strategies must undergo experimental validation in proper randomized trials.

General discussions of the methodology of randomized clinical trials appear in the sources previously cited (1409, 1412, 1413, 1416, 1418, 1419). The following discussion provides a supplement to the foregoing section and introduces six additional tactics of importance in the performance of randomized trials of compliance-improving strategies.

Further Points on the Selection and Specification of the Clinical Problem

When planning randomized trials of compliance-improving strategies, investigators should consider two additional points regarding the clinical problem selected for study. First, an estimate of the compliance distribution for the therapy of interest should be obtained (readers who are unfamiliar with the term *compliance distribution* should refer to Figures 19.2 through 19.4 and the accompanying text), and the prevailing explanations for poor compliance should be scrutinized. This will permit a more appropriate matching between the compliance-improving strategy and the clinical problem it is intended to solve.

The second additional item of information that should be sought at this stage is the quantitative relation between compliance and achievement of the treatment goal; that is, how many doses can the patient omit and still derive the desired benefit? This information is crucial in setting the criterion of satisfactory compliance and it will also aid in the selection of an appropriate compliance-improving strategy, if the zone of the compliance distribution where the latter is most influential is known.* This is but one of several stages in the planning and execution of compliance trials where the active collaboration of those who deal directly with the clinical problem is vital; ideally, such clinicians should be co-investigators.

Definition of the Precise Experimental Maneuver

The compliance-improving strategy, once selected, must be defined with precision. Who will do what to which patients, for what reasons, where, how often, with what expenditure of time and effort, and with what feedback to whom? This detailed specification serves four purposes.

First, it will force the investigator to specify the active principle and to avoid the confounding of multiple strategies. If, for example, the strategy of interest is based on a specific behavioral modification technique, the process of precise definition should indicate the inappropriateness of providing the experimental group (but not the controls) with an automated appointment call-back system if subsequent effects on compliance are to be attributed entirely to behavior modification.

Second, the definition of the precise experimental maneuver provides an exact picture of the strategy for those who wish to replicate the trial or to apply its results in clinical practice. Third, it provokes a more careful selection of the compliance agent who is to carry out the strategy; such a review will often result in the realization that a less expensive therapist can execute the strategy. Finally, the detailed specification of the compliance-improving strategy greatly aids in setting up appropriate control groups. For example, if the execution of the strategy results in the agent spending a substantial amount of additional time with the patient, the investigator may wish to apply an "attention placebo" to the control group.

Random Allocation

Random allocation is a keystone to experimental research that is acknowledged more frequently than it is actually executed. It thus deserves emphasis

---

*This admonition may be premature, for information of this nature is still rare. Nevertheless, the careful analysis of successful trials should indicate which strategies can improve compliance from 0% to 30%, which from 70% to 95%, etc. It can thus provide a useful information base for later randomized trials.

here. Investigators who wish to execute this task correctly will study key references on the topic (1406, 1411) and will rely upon random number tables or established computer programs for random number generation. Random allocation is not achieved when study subjects are assigned to experimental and control groups on an alternative or rotating basis, or on the basis of the calendar, the patient registration number, or the like; the codes for these nonrandom allocation systems have the additional fatal disadvantage of being broken easily.

If the investigator has prior information that the likelihood of achieving either high compliance or the treatment goal is substantially affected by some patient characteristic that can be identified prior to the randomization, study subjects should be stratified with respect to these characteristics before random allocation occurs; the objective here is to guarantee the comparability of the experimental and control groups with respect to these prognostic characteristics, rather than to leave this comparability to the "luck of the draw." A comprehensive discussion of prognostic stratification has been published elsewhere by Alvan Feinstein (1410).

Avoiding Contamination, Co-intervention, and "Mistaken Identity"

The ability to demonstrate the maximum specific effect of a compliance-improving strategy depends to a considerable extent on whether the investigators avoid a series of pitfalls as well as execute a series of correct procedures. Three of these pitfalls warrant attention here. First, when members of the control group inadvertently receive the compliance-improving strategy the resulting contamination will tend to diminish the observed differences in compliance between the experimental and control groups. Clinical collaborators caring for control patients must adhere to the protocol and treat them as controls, and investigators must monitor this adherence.

Second, patients in the experimental group must not undergo any additional diagnostic or therapeutic maneuvers that are not also applied to the control patients (unless these maneuvers are part of the compliance strategy). Bias arises when this co-intervention has an independent effect upon either compliance or the achievement of the treatment goal that spuriously increases or decreases the apparent effect of the compliance strategy being tested. In view of the possibility that simply spending time with patients increases their compliance, investigators must recognize co-interventions that have this property and treat the comparison groups accordingly. Contamination and co-intervention are discussed in greater detail elsewhere (1416).

The third source of bias has been labeled "mistaken identity." I have selected this term to represent the situation in which application of a compliance-improving strategy affects the achievement of the treatment goal, but has no effect upon compliance. This apparent paradox can arise when the strategy affects not the patients in the trial but the clinicians looking after them, thus causing the latter to change their prescribing habits. For example, if clinicans believe that their therapeutic skills are being tested in the trial, they unconsciously may prescribe more vigorously and give higher doses of drugs to experimental patients. A similar result may occur if study patients are aware of their progress toward the treatment goal, because they may place pressure on the treating clinician to increase the vigor of their treatment (228). If this occurs, experimental patients who comply with a constant relative portion of an increasing regimen will become more likely to achieve the therapeutic goal, and an ineffective strategy may masquerade as a useful one.

The converse can also occur. Clinicians prescribing regimens in which even slight overdoses carry high risks of toxicity may shy away from prescribing full doses to patients in the experimental group. In this case, an effective compliance-improving strategy may go undetected. Accordingly, the analysis of a trial should test for this bias by comparing the doses, potency, or other indicators of the vigor of treatment between the experimental and control groups and adjust for any differences detected.

It must be emphasized that the "mistaken identity" bias refers to the results of a mechanism that is at least quantitatively different from the "Hawthorne" phenomenon, in which the mere act of being measured leads to changes in clinician behavior; indeed, in properly designed compliance trials, the Hawthorne phenomenon should operate in the management of both experimental and control patients.

Determination of Side Effects and Toxicity

The analogy with the pharmacologic trial is again useful, for randomized trials of compliance-improving strategies should include the search for potential harm caused patients by these strategies.* Does the compliance-improving strategy cause patients to become preoccupied with their infirmities and to adopt the "sick role," and do the benefits of the regimen outweigh the damage done in gaining compliance with it? The overall social and emotional function of patients in compliance trials, as well as more specific indexes suggested by the individual strategies, should be assessed at entry and again after suitable intervals in an effort to determine their side effects and toxicity.

Unfortunately, the measurement of social and emotional function is not well developed, and current indexes may be insensitive (1422). Furthermore, as in the case of new drugs, some serious side effects of compliance-improving strategies may be so subtle or so rare that they will not be noticed until after the strategies are in general use.

---

*If compliance is generally low at the start of the trial, the investigators should also monitor for increasing side effects and for toxicity of the therapeutic regimen itself, since these will increase if the compliance-improving strategy is effective.

Compliance trials should also look for another potential side effect in the form of progressively more health conscious patients who make increasing demands for unnecessary and nonbeneficial health services. By monitoring for this type of side effect one may discover additional, hidden costs of the compliance-improving strategy.

Monitoring for Decay

In order to determine whether and how much compliance decays when patients are on their own, the measurement of compliance should extend well past the time that the compliance-improving strategy is withdrawn. The proper duration of this follow-up period will become clear as we learn more about the "natural history" of compliance. Monitoring for decay is of greater importance when the compliance-improving strategy is time consuming or otherwise costly to apply.

CONCLUSIONS

The methodologic standards set down in this chapter can serve two different sorts of users. First, they can help new compliance research workers design and execute studies from which valid conclusions can be drawn; of particular value to this group are the identification of methodologic pitfalls into which those of us who preceded them have fallen. In addition, to the extent that following these standards results in compatible data, sensible comparisons between study results will become increasingly possible.

The second group that may find these methodologic standards useful encompasses those who, rather than generating new knowledge about compliance, seek to apply what is already known in the detection and alleviation of compliance problems among their patients or clients. These standards can help in assessing evidence and in deciding, for example, whether the claims of those who champion the latest compliance-improving strategy should be accepted or ignored. Indeed, the use of these methodologic standards for such purposes might lead to an almost unique situation in clinical and health care: the acceptance or rejection of new information on the basis of its scientific merit, rather than on the extent to which it agrees or disagrees with the beholder's prior opinion (or public statements) of the nature of man or the value of a clinical maneuver!

VII
REFERENCE MATERIALS

Appendix I:

Annotated and Indexed Bibliography on Compliance with Therapeutic and Preventive Regimens

R. Brian Haynes, D. Wayne Taylor,
John C. Snow, David L. Sackett

in collaboration with:
Peter J. Tugwell, Margaret Walsh,
Brenda C. Hackett, and Jayanti Mukherjee

INTRODUCTION

This appendix serves several functions:

1. It is a common reservoir for compliance references cited repeatedly in this book. Citations 1 through 853 are listed here (citations 854 onward are located in Appendix II).

2. It is a freestanding, annotated bibliography on compliance with therapeutic and preventive regimens.

3. It provides a detailed description of a system for assessing and scoring the methodologic adequacy of compliance research reports and applies this system to each of the original articles in the bibliography.

4. The bibliography is followed by a series of 13 tables which index the contents of the bibliographic entries, including determinants of compliance evaluated, measurement methods used, intervention strategies investigated, and the clinical condition being treated. The index tables are the key to optimum use of the bibliography.

Although we have included many recent articles on "bad habits" and lifestyle problems such as smoking and alcoholism, the main focus of the bibliography is

The preparation of this annotated bibliography was supported by the Sun Life Assurance Company of Canada and the National Health Grant of Health and Welfare Canada.

the compliance of patients with therapeutic regimens for medical illnesses. It is not possible to claim that the collection exhausts the supply of published articles on therapeutic regimen compliance. We have done our best, however, to collect and collate newly published and soon-to-be published studies into the bibliography that was first published in our previous book on compliance (693), more than trebling its size. This process is ongoing and has been facilitated by computerizing the entries (if only the computer would review the articles too!).

The articles in the bibliography are listed alphabetically by first author and are numbered consecutively in three sections entitled: Original Articles on Compliance; Special Articles on Measurement; and Reviews, Commentaries, and Editorials. A brief notation follows each citation. Beneath the notation for each original article are the numbers of subjects studied and a methodologic profile derived as described below.

METHODOLOGIC STANDARDS FOR COMPLIANCE RESEARCH REPORTS

Important differences in the ability of investigators to recognize and control essential features in the design and execution of their research have led to substantial variation in the certainty of their conclusions. Since it was important to temper the claims of published reports with a consideration of the adequacy of the methods that produced them, it was necessary to establish a series of relevant methodologic standards that could be used to assess the reports in an objective, reproducible fashion. Through a process of repeated refinement and assessment for multiple observer agreement, the following standards and scores were developed.

1. Study Design

Points

4	randomized trial
3	quasi-experimental design (before-after; alternate treatments assigned by investigator, but by nonrandom means)
2	analytic (case-comparison; cohort)
1	descriptive (e.g., single patient group studied at a point in time, and comparisons made between compliers and noncompliers)
1 bonus	for all categories
	—indication that sample is an "inception cohort," i.e., studied from the beginning of the disease or its therapy

Notes:

a) If two studies are reported in a single article, rate each study separately in the order that the studies were done chronologically.
b) Rate the design only as it relates to compliance. Thus, if compliance is of only peripheral interest in the study and does not enjoy the advantages of the central study design, then it should be rated according to the design considerations that apply to it.

2. Selection and Specification of the Study Sample

Points

3	random population sample*
or	three or more hospitals/clinics in a geographical area*
or	regional program/referral center*
2	same as for 3, but inadequate demographic description
1	grab sample or single clinic, including adequate description of demographic features* of sample
0	same as for 1, but inadequate demographic description
1 bonus	for all categories

—indication that sample is an "inception cohort" i.e., studied from the beginning of their disease or its therapy

—indication of the proportion of patients excluded

—indication of "consecutive admissions" or "all patients" during a stated time period or of a "random sample" of a single clinic population with at least 80% follow-up

*Criterion includes descriptions of four of the following: age, sex, race, socioeconomic status, marital/family status.

3. Specification of the Illness or Condition

Points

3	replicable diagnostic criteria stated with inclusion/exclusion criteria
2	diagnostic criteria stated
1	diagnoses only
0	no diagnosis or diagnosis can only be inferred (e.g., visiting the dentist)
1 bonus	for all categories

—if co-morbidity is described

Note:

If article deals with preventive health behavior (e.g., exercise, immunization, dental prophylaxis) do no attempt to score under "Illness."

4. Compliance Measures
(Rate only the measure scoring highest.)

	Points	Pills	Attendance	Habits
Objective *direct* measures longitudinal	4	Tracer substances Physiology Immediate direct measures when applied on at least 3 separate occasions for at least 80% of subjects		Physiological change Anatomical change Behavioral changes
Immediate *direct*	3	Blood level of drug Urine tracer Short-term physiological effects	Only when treatment is guaranteed for all who show up (e.g. injection)	Direct observation
Objective *indirect* measure	2	Pill count R_X refill	When attendance is the only measure of compliance (and 3 point standard is not met)	
Subjective measures	1	Interview of patient, patient's family, clinician (or chart examination in the case of pills and habits)		
Not stated	0			
Bonus A	1	For codes 1, 2, and 3 in the case of pills and habits random (as opposed to scheduled) determination when patient unaware of purpose of determination For codes 2 and 3 in the case of attendance		
Bonus B	1	when follow-up period of measuring attendance is six months or more For each compliance measure utilized in addition to the measure scoring highest		

5. Description of the Therapeutic Regimen

Points

2	complete description that would permit the reader to replicate the regimen with precision
1	incomplete description
0	no description or regimen can only be inferred
1 bonus	for all categories
	—if co-intervention with a second regimen is precluded by study design or is noted when it occurs

Examples of Complete Description:

Drug features (at least five of the following six features): (1) name, (2) dose schedule, (3) cost/convenience of filling prescription, (4) duration, (5) form, (6) side effects.
Diet: (1) calories or intended effect upon body mass, (2) composition (low fat, etc.).
Exercise: (1) activity to be undertaken, (2) frequency.
Rest: (1) activity to be avoided, (2) duration.

6. Definition of Compliance

Points

2	replicable by reader in own setting
1	vague definition
0	no definition

Beneath the annotation for each of the original articles appear the number of study subjects in the investigation and the scores the study received for each of the methodologic standards. The resulting methodologic profile may be useful in several different types of inquiry. First, the total score for an article gives a crude estimate of the validity of its conclusion (the median total score for all articles is 9). Furthermore, individual scoring categories provide a description of the methods used. For example, all studies with a score of 4 following *design* are randomized experiments, whereas those with a score of 1 are descriptive in nature. As a second example, those articles with a score of 2 or more in the *measurement* category utilized objective methods of measuring compliance. Thus, anyone who wishes to review methods of measurement or desires objective estimates of the magnitude of noncompliance can readily select the appropriate articles.

One final note: the methodologic scores recorded here will not, of course, reflect the very strenuous efforts of many of the authors to overcome the problems in feasibility, financing, and cooperation which continuously hamper the search for new knowledge. Accordingly, these scores are often lowered by factors beyond the control of the investigators.

Categorical Tables

The contents of all articles in the bibliography have been reviewed and categorized. The results of this process appear in a set of tables following the bibliography. *Familiarity with the index tables facilitates optimal use of the bibliography.* We use the tables constantly in our own reviews and in helping others find material pertinent to their own interests and questions.

Some words of warning though: the headings in the tables are necessarily somewhat arbitrary, both in terms of the descriptors used and in the position of descriptors within the tables. Thus, for example, *education* appears in the tables as a sociodemographic characteristic (Table 6) whereas *knowledge of therapy/disease* appears in Table 5 on general patient characteristics. If the user wishes to know what bearing education, intelligence, and specific knowledge have on compliance then it is most appropriate to browse through the tables to pick out all the relevant descriptors. Another caveat: not all the contents of all the articles are indexed. Some of the ideas and findings reported by investigators and reviewers cannot be classified with simple descriptors; some were uninterpretable (by us); some were undoubtedly omitted through our own error. Finally, the index tables do classify the nature of conclusions for the so-called determinants of compliance (for example, articles reporting a statistically significant positive association between age and compliance are noted under the appropriate column in Table 6). However, they are not a substitute for reading the original articles, because the descriptors for classification are often somewhat broad. Thus, the index heading *age* in Table 6 includes all ages but what might apply in the age range of one to five years might not obtain for twenty-five to seventy-five years of age. Anyone who is seriously interested in a given factor is encouraged to review the identified references rather than to accept the highly summarized chart entries at face value.

ORIGINAL ARTICLES ON COMPLIANCE

1. Abernethy JD: The problem of noncompliance in long-term antihypertensive
   therapy. *Drugs* 11:86-90, 1976
   Withdrawal rates in the Australian national hypertension study.
   N=1,593
   Design=4+1 Sample=2+1 Illness=1 Regimen=1 Measure=0 Definition=1
2. Adamson JD, Fostakowsky RT, Chebib FS: Measures associated with outcome on one year follow-up of male alcoholics. *Br J Addict* 69:325-337, 1974
   Attitudinal and life history variables measured during treatment were
   correlated with drinking status one year later.
   N=52

Design=2+1 Sample-1+1 Illness=1 Regimen=1 Measure=0 Definition=0
3. Adler LM, Goin M, Yamamoto J: Failed psychiatric clinic appointments.
   Calif Med 99:388-392, 1963
   Consecutive new applicants to a county psychiatric OPD were surveyed for
     sociodemographic features and observed for attendance at an initial
     appointment after application.
   N=199
Design=2 Sample=0+1 Illness=0 Regimen=0 Measure=2 Definition=1
4. Alderman M, Schoenbaum E: Detection and treatment of hypertension at the
   work site. *N Engl J Med* 293:65-68, 1975
   Program results for a hypertension project linking detection and treatment
     for employees of a large department store.
   N=121
Design=1 Sample=0+1 Illness=3 Regimen=2 Measure=2 Definition=1
5. Allen D, Bergman A: Social learning approaches to health education: utiliza-
   tion of infant auto restraint devices. *Pediatrics* 58:323-328, 1976
   An evaluation of three behaviorally oriented learning approaches, applied
     in a maternity ward, to increase purchase and use of infant car
     restraints.
   N=202
Design=3 Sample=1+1 Illness=NA Regimen=1 Measure=1 Definition=2
6. Allen EA, Stewart M, Jeney P: The efficiency of post-sanatorium manage-
   ment of tuberculosis. *Can J Public Health* 55:323-333, 1964
   Adherence to post-sanatorium chemotherapy was studied in an extensive
     sample of tuberculosis patients.
   N=1,000
Design=1+1 Sample=3+1 Illness=1 Regimen=1 Measure=3+2 Definition=1
7. Alpert JJ: Broken appointments. *Pediatrics* 34: 127-132, 1964
   Chart and interview survey of "breakers" and "attenders" at a general
     medical OPD clinic at a children's hospital.
   N=1,588
Design=1 Sample=0 Illness=0 Regimen=0 Measure=1+1 Definition=2
8. Anderson FP, Rowe DS, Dean VC, Arbisser A: An approach to the problem
   of noncompliance in a pediatric outpatient clinic. *Am J Dis Child* 122:
   142-143, 1971
   Dropout families of a pediatric outpatient department were traced and re-
     trieved by two nonmedical undergraduate students.
   N=95
Design=3 Sample=0 Illness=0 Regimen=0 Measure=2+1 Definition=1
9. Antonovsky A, Anson O: Factors related to preventive health behavior,
   pp 35-43, in Cullen JW, Fox B, Isom R (eds): *Cancer: The Behavioral
   Dimensions*. New York, Raven Press, 1976
   The study presents two analyses of breast cancer examination data gathered
     by interviews.
   N=98
Design=2 Sample=0+1 Illness=1 Regimen=1 Measure=1 Definition=2

10. Anwar R, Roberts J, Wagner D: The continuing emergency care clinic: Improving patient compliance with follow-up care. *J Am Coll Emerg Phys* 6:251-253, 1977
A report on patient compliance to follow-up appointments after initial treatments at a continuing emergency care clinic.
N=798
Design=1 Sample=0+1 Illness=1 Regimen=1 Measure=2 Definition=2

11. Archer M, Rinzler S, Christakis G: Social factors affecting participation in a study of diet and coronary heart disease. *J Health Soc Behav* 8:22-31, 1967
Differences are described between active and inactive subjects who had initially joined the anticoronary club in New York.
N=757
Design=1 Sample=1+1 Illness=1 Regimen=1 Measure=3 Definition=2

12. Arnhold RG, Adebonojo FO, Callas ER, Callas J, Carte E, Stein RC: Patients and prescriptions: Comprehension and compliance with medical instructions in a suburban pediatric practice. *Clin Pediatr* 9:648-651, 1970
Home interview study of compliance and compliance characteristics among pediatric patients and their parents.
N=104
Design=1 Sample=1 Illness=0 Regimen=1 Measure=2+1 Definition=2

13. Arnhold RG, Pike MC: Patients and prescriptions: Understanding medical instructions. *J Trop Pediatr* 14:10-14, 1968
Study of level of understanding of dispensing instructions by mothers of pediatric patients at a free government clinic in Uganda where 32% were illiterate. No data on compliance per se.
N-variable
Design=4 Sample=0 Illness=0 Regimen=1 Measure=1 Definition=1

14. Aron W, Daily D: Graduates and splitees from therapeutic community drug treatment programs: A comparison. *Int J Addict* 11:1-18, 1976
The interaction of several social and psychological factors was studied for graduates and dropouts from two community drug treatment centers.
N=286
Design=1 Sample=1+1 Illness=1 Regimen=1 Measure=1 Definition=2

15. Atkinson RM: AMA and AWOL discharges: A six-year comparative study. *Hosp Community Psychiatry* 22:17-20, 1971
Retrospective six-year chart survey analysis of all "against medical advice" (AMA) and "absent without leave" (AWOL) discharges of first-time admissions to an acute care neuropsychiatric institute.
N=223 AMA, 89 AWOL
Design=1 Sample=0+1 Illness=0 Regimen=0 Measure=1 Definition=2

16. Azrin NH, Powell J: Behavioral engineering: The use of response priming to improve prescribed self-medication. *J Appl Behav Anal* 2:39-42, 1969
Two types of timer-alarm pill containers were compared with regular pill

containers in the compliance of healthy volunteers with a half-hourly placebo pill schedule.
N=6
Design=3 Sample=0 Illness=NA Regimen=2 Measure=3 Definition=2

17. Badgley RF, Furnal MA: Appointment breaking in a pediatric clinic. *Yale J Biol Med* 34:117-123, 1961
Interview study of reasons for breaking appointments at a pediatric OPD.
N=77
Design=1 Sample=0 Illness=1 Regimen=0 Measure=1 Definition=2

18. Baekeland F, Lundwall LK: Effects of discontinuity of medication on the results of a double-blind study in outpatient alcoholics. *J Stud Alcohol* 36:1268-1272, 1975
A study emphasizing the necessity for considering compliance information in interpreting the results of clinical trials.
N=196
Design=4 Sample=1 Illness=1 Regimen=2 Measure=1+1 Definition=1

19. Baekeland F, Lundwall L, Shanahan TJ: Correlates of patient attrition in the outpatient treatment of alcoholism. *J Nerv Ment Dis* 157:99-107, 1973
Admission characteristics of patients admitted to an alcoholic clinic were correlated with those of dropouts at differing time intervals from immediate to six months.
N=143
Design=1+1 Sample=0+1 Illness=1 Regimen=1 Measure=2+1 Definition=2

20. Baker PG, Read AE: Continuing gluten ingestion and its detection in treated coeliac patients. *Gut* 15:827, 1974
Study among coeliac patients of failure to comply with gluten-free diet and its correlation with the presence of villous atrophy on biopsy and with circulating gluten antibodies.
N=51
Design=1 Sample=0 Illness=1 Regimen=1 Measure=4+1 Definition=1

21. Bakker CB, Dightman CR: Psychological factors in fertility control. *Fertil Steril* 15:559-567, 1964
Volunteers and referrals taking oral contraceptives and "highly motivated" to continue were given a battery of psychological tests to detemine any factors associated with reported forgetting of medication.
N=72
Design=1 Sample=0 Illness=NA Regimen=0 Measure=1 Definition=1

22. Ballinger BR, Ramsay AC, Stewart MJ: Methods of assessment of drug administration in a psychiatric hospital. *Br J Psychiatr* 127:494-498, 1975
Hospitalized psychiatric patients receiving phenothiazines, imipramine, amitriptyline, phenobarbitone, primidone, phenytoin, chloral compounds, benzodiazepines, paracetamol, and salicylates were assessed for compliance by urine tracers and by direct observation.
N=64
Design=1 Sample=0 Illness=0 Regimen=1 Measure=4+1 Definition=2

23. Ballweg JA, Maccorquodale DW: Family planning method change and
    dropouts in the Philippines. *Soc Biol* 21:88-95, 1974
    Interview study of determinants for continuing use of contraceptive
    methods by clients of family planning clinics.
    N=1,321
    Design=1 Sample=2+1 Illness=NA Regimen=1 Measure=1 Definition=1
24. Bar A: Decreasing the no-show rate in an urban speech and hearing clinic.
    J Am Speech Hearing Assoc 17:455-456, 1975
    Description of methods undertaken to improve attendance at a speech and
    hearing clinic.
    N=NA
    Design=3 Sample=0+1 Illness=1 Regimen=0 Measure=2 Definition=1
25. Barkin S, Barkin R, Roth M: Immunization status. *Clin Pediatr* 16:840-
    842, 1977
    Immunization status was used as a measure of the delivery of good preven-
    tive medical services to young infants.
    N=141
    Design=1+1 Sample=0+1 Illness=NA Regimen=1 Measure=1 Definition=2
26. Barnes KE, Gunther D, Jordan I, Gray AS: The effects of various persuasive
    communications on community health: A pilot study. *Can J Public
    Health* 62:105-110, 1971
    Parents of children requiring dental care were sent messages containing
    different levels of fear-arousing content with subsequent compliance
    with recommendations as the dependent variable.
    N=80
    Design=4 Sample=2 Illness=NA Regimen=1 Measure=2 Definition=2
27. Barnum JF: Outlook for treating patients with self-destructive habits.
    Ann Intern Med 81:387-393, 1974
    Damaging habits with associated diseases and compliance with treatment
    advice were studied in consecutive unselected patients in a general
    internal medicine private practice.
    N=1,000
    Design=3 Sample=0+1 Illness=1 Regimen=1 Measure=1+1 Definition=2
28. Barrett TJ, Sachs LB: Test of the classical conditioning explanation of
    covert sensitization. *Psychol Rep* 34:1312-1314, 1974
    Evaluation of several variations of the covert sensitization procedure to
    reduce smoking in university students.
    N=46
    Design=3 Sample=0+1 Illness=NA Regimen=1+1 Measure=1 Definition=2
29. Barton AK: Following up on aftercare: Show versus no-show rates in North
    Carolina. *Hosp Community Psychiatry* 28:545-546, 1977
    A brief retrospective study of follow-up care for psychiatric outpatients.
    N=78
    Design=1 Sample=0+1 Illness=0 Regimen=1 Measure=2 Definition=2
30. Bass LW, Wilson TR: The pediatrician's influence in private practice
    measured by a controlled seat belt study. *Pediatrics* 33:700-704, 1964

To induce parents of pediatric patients to buy car seat belts, several tactics (including face-to-face confrontation plus personal letter from physician, personal letter alone, letter from local safety council alone, no letter or confrontation) were used on subsets of three private pediatric practice populations.

N=1,423

Design=3 Sample=2 Illness=NA Regimen=2 Measure=1 Definition=2

31. Beck E, Blaichman S, Scriver CR, Clow CL: Advocacy and compliance in genetic screening: Behaviour of physicians and clients in a voluntary program of testing for the Tay-Sachs gene. *N Eng J Med* 291:1165-1170, 1974

Relation between advocacy and compliance was evaluated in a voluntary testing program to identify carriers of the Tay-Sachs gene.

N=30,000

Design=2 Sample=3+1 Illness=NA Regimen=2 Measure=3 Definition=2

32. Becker MH, Drachman RH, Kirscht JP: Motivations as predictors of health behavior. *Health Serv Rep* 87:852-861, 1972

Prospective study of the "health belief model" with certain modifications, used to predict compliance among pediatric outpatients with otitis media through interview of their mothers prior to initiation of treatment.

N=125

Design=1 Sample=0+1 Illness=2 Regimen=1 Measure=3+1 Definition=2

33. _____: Predicting mothers' compliance with pediatric medical regimens. *J Pediatr* 81:843-854, 1972

Health beliefs and demographic factors were assessed among families with children presenting with acute otitis media to a pediatric outpatient department; results were compared with compliance.

N=125

Design=1 Sample=0+1 Illness=1 Regimen=1 Measure=3+2 Definition=2

34. _____: A new approach to explaining sick-role behavior in low income populations. *Am J Public Health* 64:205-216, 1974

Health beliefs of mothers were tested as predictors of compliance with an oral antibiotic regimen for children with otitis media.

N=116

Design=1 Sample=1+1 Illness=1 Regimen=1 Measure=3+1 Definition=1

35. _____: A field experiment to evaluate various outcomes of continuity of physician care. *Am J Public Health* 64:1062-1070, 1974

A conventional pediatric clinic and a continuous panel team were compared through interviews with mothers and through appointment-keeping ratios.

N=250

Design=4+1 Sample=0+1 Illness=0 Regimen=0 Measure=1 Definition=1

36. Becker MH, Kaback MM, Rosenstock IM, Ruth MV: Some influences on public participation in a genetic screening program. *J Community Health* 1:3-14, 1975

A comparison of health perceptions among participants and nonparticipants in a genetic screening program for Tay-Sachs disease.
N=432 participants, 318 nonparticipants
Design=2 Sample=3 Illness=NA Regimen=0 Measure=2 Definition=2

37. Becker MH, Maiman L, Kirscht JP, Haefner D, Drachman RH: The health belief model and prediction of dietary compliance: A field experiment. *J Health Soc Behav* 18:348-365, 1977

Three groups of mothers of obese children received high, low, or no health-threat message and follow-up adherence to diet and to appointmnt-keeping was measured. Correlations between health beliefs and compliance were also reported.
N=182
Design=4 Sample=0+1 Illness=1 Regimen=1 Measure=3+1 Definition=1

38. Bellack AS: A comparison of self-reinforcement and self-monitoring in a weight reduction program. *Behav Ther* 7:68-75, 1976

Self-monitoring of food intake was compared with self-reinforcement of eating behavior in a weight reduction program.
N=38
Design=4 Sample=0+1 Illness=3 Regimen=1 Measure=3+1 Definition=2

39. Bender A, Bender D:Maintenance of weight loss in obese subjects. *Br J Prev Soc Med* 30:60-65, 1976

Successful "weight watchers" who had then become staff of the organization were studied to determine pattern of initial weight loss.
N=215
Design=1 Sample=0+1 Illness=2 Regimen=1 Measure=4 Definition=2

40. Bender KJ: An exploratory study of one community pharmicist as a dispenser of drug education. Unpublished Master's thesis, Graduate School of Human Behavior, United States International University, 1972

Study of chronic ambulatory patients on multiple drug regimens with respect to acceptance of a single community pharmacist as a source of drug information and the effect of this on drug knowledge and compliance.
N=20
Design=3 Sample=0 Illness=0 Regimen=1 Measure=2 Definition=1

41. Berglund G, Andersson O, Wilhelmsen L: Treatment of hypertension in the community. *Acta Med Scand (suppl)*606:11-17, 1976

A comparison of morbidity and mortality between a group of hypertensive men under treatment and a control group over a period of seven years in Sweden.
N=330 control, 696 treatment
Design=2 Sample=2+1 Illness=2 Regimen=1 Measure=4 Definition=2

42. Bergman AB, Werner RJ: Failure of children to receive penicillin by mouth. *N Engl J Med* 268:1334-1338, 1963

Compliance with oral penicillin at several time intervals after the initiation of therapy was assessed among children with suspected acute streptococcal infections.

N=59
Design=1 Sample=1+1 Illness=2 Regimen=2 Measure=3+2 Definition=2

43. Berkowitz NH, Malone MF, Klein MW, Eaton A: Patient follow-through in the outpatient department. *Nurs Res* 12: 16-22, 1963
Physicians in 55 OPD clinics of 7 urban hospitals were asked to assess the compliance of their patients with (1) treatment other than medications, (2) medications, (3) attendance, (4) referral appointments, (5) tests ordered, (6) restrictions. The validity of assessments of 3, 4 and 5 was checked by chart survey and clinic-specific error-scores were derived; validation was not possible for 1, 2, and 6 and scores were analyzed at face value.
N=variable
Design=1 Sample=2 Illness=1 Regimen=0 Measure=1 Definition=1

44. Bernard HS, Efran JS: Eliminating versus reducing smoking using pocket timers. *Behav Res Ther* 10:399-401, 1972
The buzz of a pocket timer was tested as a strategy to reduce or eliminate smoking in psychology students.
N=30
Design=3 Sample=0+1 Illness=NA Regimen=1 Measure=1 Definition=2

45. Berry D, Ross A, Huempfner H, Deuschle K: Self-medication behavior as measured by urine chemical tests in domiciliary tuberculous patients. *Am Rev Respir Dis* 86:1-7, 1962
Tuberculous outpatients were visited at home without warning on up to eight separate occasions to assess compliance with INH and PAS and the effect of time from discharge.
N=26
Design=2 Sample=0+1 Illness=1 Regimen=1 Measure=4+1 Definition=2

46. Berry D, Ross A, Deuschle K: Tuberculous patients treated at home. *Am Rev Resp Dis* 88:769-772, 1963
Home visits to posthospital tuberculous patients were used to separate compliers from noncompliers; determinants of compliance were assessed.
N=26
Design=2 Sample=1+1 Illness=1 Regimen=1 Measure=4+1 Definition=2

47. Best JA, Bass F, Owen LE: Mode of service delivery in a smoking cessation programme for public health. *Can J Public Health* 68:469-473, 1977
Study of the effects of group size and telephone support in the success of smoking cessation programs.
N=72
Design=3+1 Sample=0+1 Illness=1 Regimen=2 Measure=1 Definition=1

48. Best JA, Owen LE, Trentadue L: Comparison of satiation and rapid smoking on success in quitting smoking. *Addict Behav*, in press
Study of the effect of two strategies, satiation and rapid smoking, on success in quitting smoking.
N=82
Design=3+1 Sample=0+1 Illness=1 Regimen=2 Measure=1+1 Definition=2

49. Best JA: Tailoring smoking withdrawal procedures to personality and motivational differences. *J Consult Clin Psychol* 43:1-8, 1975
Factorial evaluation of a variety of ancillary maneuvers designed to improve the effect of an aversive antismoking program.
N=89
Design=4 Sample=0+1 Illness=1 Regimen=2 Measure=1+1 Definition=2

50. Bewley B, Bland J: Academic performance and social factors related to cigarette smoking by school children. *Br J Prev Soc Med* 31:18-24, 1977
Factors were studied that may influence children aged ten to twelve years to start smoking.
N=491
Design=2 Sample=3+1 Illness=NA Regimen=NA Measure=1 Definition=2

51. Biener KJ: The influence of health education on the use of alcohol and tobacco in adolescence. *Prev Med* 4:252-257, 1975
An intensive health program among adolescent male apprentices in a machine factory led to improved measures of physical fitness and exercise, smoking and alcohol consumption habits compared with those of control apprentices over a four year period.
N=60 experimental, 60 control
Design=3 Sample=1 Illness=NA Regimen=1 Measure=4+5 Definition=2

52. Bierenbaum ML, Fleischman AI, Raichelson RI, Hayton T, Watson PB: Ten-year experience of modified-fat diets on younger men with coronary heart disease. *Lancet* 1:1404-1407, 1973
Men with confirmed coronary-artery disease and past myocardial infarction were placed on a low fat diet after weight reduction and followed over ten years along with a subsequently matched control group. Compliance was a peripheral issue,but proportion achieving and maintaining ideal weight is given.
N=100
Design=3 Sample=0 Illness=3 Regimen=2 Measure=3+2 Definition=0

53. Bigger JF: A comparison of patient compliance in treated vs untreated ocular hypertension. *Trans Am Acad Ophthalmol Otolaryngol* 81:277-285, 1976
Differences in dropout rates were studied between treated and untreated patients with asymptomatic ocular hypertension in a twelve to twenty month follow-up period.
N=89
Design=1 Sample=0+1 Illness=3 Regimen=0 Measure=3+1 Definition=2

54. Bille DA: The role of body images in patient compliance and education. *Heart Lung* 6:143-148, 1977
Myocardial infarction patients who reported more positive body images during hospitalization, reported greater compliance with post-hospitalization medical advice.
N=24
Design=2 Sample=0 Illness=1 Regimen=0 Measure=1 Definition=2

55. Blackburn SL: Dietary compliance of chronic hemodialysis patients. *J Am Diet Assoc* 70:31-37, 1977

The effect of several variables on the dietary compliance of hemodialysis patients was studied.

N=53

Design=1 Sample=1+1 Illness=3 Regimen=2 Measure=4+2 Definition=2

56. Bloch S, Rosenthal A, Friedman L, Caldarolla P: Patient compliance in glaucoma. *Br J Ophthalmol* 61:531-534, 1977

A report on the effect of some psychosocial and demographic variables on compliance with treatment for glaucoma.

N=40

Design=2 Sample=1+1 Illness=2 Regimen=1 Measure=1 Definition=2

57. Bonnar J, Goldberg A, Smith JA: Do pregnant women take their iron? *Lancet* 1:457-458, 1969

Antenatal iron medication compliance was assessed among patients randomly assigned to receive their pills free at the clinic or at usual cost through prescriptions.

N=60

Design=4 Sample=0+1 Illness=1 Regimen=2 Measure=4+1 Definition=2

58. Borkman T: Hemodialysis compliance: The relationship of staff estimates of patients' intelligence and understanding to compliance. *Soc Sci Med* 10:385-392, 1976

An analysis of the consistency among staff attitudes towards patients' intelligence, understanding of restrictions, and perceived compliance in hemodialysis programs.

N=661

Design=1 Sample=3+1 Illness=1 Regimen=1 Measure=1 Definition=2

59. Borofsky LG, Louis S, Kutt H, Roginsky M: Diphenylhydantoin: Efficacy, toxicity and dose-serum level relationships in children. *Pediatr Pharm Ther* 81:995-1002, 1972

Dose-serum levels and therapeutic efficacy of diphenylhydantoin were studied among ambulatory pediatric epileptics. Those who exhibited low serum levels and poor seizure control were confronted regarding their compliance and the serum level response was monitored.

N=53

Design=1 Sample=0 Illness=1 Regimen=1 Measure=3+1 Definition=1

60. Bourne PG, Alford J, Bowcock J: Treatment of skid row alcoholics with disulfiram. *Q J Stud Alcohol* 27:42-48, 1966

Alcohol abstinence was assessed among voluntary and among legally referred alcoholics prescribed disulfiram.

N=64 volunteers, 132 court referrals

Design=2 Sample=0+1 Illness=1 Regimen=2 Measure=0 Definition=1

61. Bowen RG, Rich R, Schlotfeldt RM: Effects of organized instruction for patients with the diagnosis of diabetes mellitus. *Nurs Res* 10:151-159, 1961

Controlled trial of special lectures on diabetes for insulin-dependent diabetic outpatients.

N=23 study, 28 control

Design=3 Sample=0+1 Illness=1 Regimen=1 Measure=3+2 Definition=2

62. Bowen WT, Soskin RA, Chotlos JW: Lysergic acid diethylamide as a variable in the hospital treatment of alcoholism. *J Nerv Ment Dis* 150:111 118, 1970

Two studies assessing the relative efficacy of LSD in the long-term management of alcoholism.

A. N=99

Design=3+1 Sample=0+1 Illness=1 Regimen=2 Measure=1 Definition=2

B. N=57

Design=4+1 Sample=0+1 Illness=1 Regimen=2 Measure=1 Definition=2

63. Boyd J, Covington T, Stanaszek W, Coussons R: Drug defaulting Part II: Analysis of noncompliance patterns. *Am J Hosp Pharm* 31:485-494, 1974

A study investigating the interrelationship among several variables affecting drug defaulting and comprehension in outpatients of a teaching hospital.

N=380 prescriptions

Design=1 Sample=0+1 Illness=1 Regimen=1 Measure=2+1 Definition=1

64. Bracken MB: The Jamaican family planning programme: Clinic services and social support as factors in dropping out. *Int J Health Educ* 20:126-135, 1977

Report of descriptive data from a study of several variables in a sample of women who had dropped out of a family planning program.

N=299

Design=1 Sample=2+1 Illness=NA Regimen=0 Measure=2 Definition=2

65. Brand F, Smith R, Brand P: Effect of economic barriers to medical care on patients' noncompliance. *Public Health Rep* 92:72-78, 1977

Patients were interviewed at home six months after hospital discharge to determine compliance; the relationship of financial status, amount of drugs prescribed, and frequency of dosage to compliance was assessed.

N=299

Design=2 Sample=1+1 Illness=0 Regimen=1+1 Measure=1+1 Definition=1

66. Brand F, Smith R: Medical care and compliance among the elderly after hospitalization. *Int J Aging Hum Dev* 5:331-346, 1974

The association of demographic and therapeutic variables with compliance to medical treatment was reported for a group of chronically ill elderly patients.

N=114

Design=1 Sample=1+1 Illness=1 Regimen=1 Measure=1+1 Definition=2

67. Brechner K, Shippee G, Obitz F: Compliance techniques to increase mailed questionnaire return rates from alcoholics. *J Stud Alcohol* 37:995-996, 1976

The effects of three compliance techniques were examined.

N=202
Design=4 Sample=0 Illness=1 Regimen=1 Measure=3 Definition=2

68. Briggs WA, Lowenthal DT, Cirksena WJ, Price WE, Gibson TP, Flamenbaum W: Propranolol in hypertensive dialysis patients: Efficacy and compliance. *Clin Pharmacol Ther* 18:606-612, 1975
Descriptive comparison of compliance measured by serum propranolol with blood pressure control and blood renin, in hypertensive dialysis patients.
N=35
Design=1 Sample=0 Illness=2+1 Regimen=1 Measure=3 Definition=2

69. Brook RH, Appel FA, Avery C, Orman M, Stevenson RL: Effectiveness of inpatient follow-up care. *N Engl J Med* 285:1509-1514, 1971
Follow-up care including patient compliance with medication and clinic appointments was assessed six months following hospital discharge from general medical wards.
N=403
Design=2 Sample=1+1 Illness=1 Regimen=1 Measure=2+1 Definition=2

70. Brooks PM, Mason DI, McNeil R, Anderson JA, Buchanan WW: An assessment of the therapeutic potential of azapropazone in rheumatoid arthritis. *Curr Med Res Opin* 4:50-57, 1976
Reasons for withdrawing prematurely from a controlled study of azapropazone versus aspirin.
N=108
Design=1 Sample=0 Illness=2 Regimen=2+1 Measure=1 Definition=1

71. Brown BS, Brewster GW: A comparison of addict-clients retained and lost to treatment. *Int J Addict* 8:421-426, 1973
Descriptive study comparing concepts of real and ideal selves in compliers and noncompliers.
N=110
Design=1 Sample=1+1 Illness=1 Regimen=1 Measure=2+1 Definition=2

72. Brown EM, Benante J, Greenberg M, MacArthur M: Study of methadone terminations. *Br J Addict* 70:83-88, 1975
Descriptive study of reasons for dropping out of a methadone program.
N=101
Design=1 Sample=2+1 Illness=1 Regimen=1 Measure=2 Definition=2

73. Brown HB, Meredith AP, Page IH: Serum cholesterol reduction in patients; response, adherence and rebound measured by a quantitative diet test. *Am J Med* 33:753-762, 1962
As part of a lipid research dietary program, adherence to two diets was measured by nutritionists through interview technique and, on a subset, by comparison of blood lipids while at home and while on a hospital-based dietary "test." The results of the two assessment methods are compared.
N=variable
Design=3 Sample=0 Illness=2+1 Regimen=2+1 Measure=3+1 Definition=1

74. Bruce EH, Frederick R, Bruce RA, Fisher LD: Comparison of active partici-
    pants and dropouts in Capri cardiopulmonary rehabilitation programs.
    Am J Cardiol 37:53-60, 1976
    Descriptive study of case records to look for predictive factors of dropouts
    from an exercise program.
    N=603
    Design=1 Sample=0 Illness=1 Regimen=1 Measure=2+1 Definition=2
75. Buchanan N, Mashigo S: Problems in prescribing for ambulatory black
    children. *S Afr Med J* 52:227-229, 1977
    A brief report of a study assessing patient, pharmacist, and physician
    features of noncompliance in a group of black children.
    N=200
    Design=1 Sample=0+1 Illness=0 Regimen=0 Measure=2+1 Definition=1
76. Burnip R, Erickson R, Barr GD, Shinefield H, Schoen EJ: Well-child care by
    pediatric nurse practitioners in a large group practice. *Am J Dis Child*
    130:51-55, 1976
    Controlled study of compliance with attendance for well child visits in
    patients allocated to nurse practitioner compared with those allocated
    to pediatrician.
    N=1,152
    Design=4 Sample=0+1 Illness=NA Regimen=0+1 Measure=2+1 Definition=1
77. Burns BH: Chronic chest disease, personality, and success in stopping
    cigarette smoking. *Br J Prev Soc Med* 23:23-27, 1969
    Report of variables related to success in giving up smoking among patients
    with chronic chest disease.
    N=94
    Design=2 Sample=0 Illness=1 Regimen=1 Measure=1 Definition=1
78. Burnum JF: Outlook for treating patients with self-destructive habits.
    Ann Intern Med 81:387-393, 1974
    Before-after study of effects of counseling upon compliance with stopping
    smoking, abstinence from alcohol or drugs, or losing weight.
    N=219
    Design=3 Sample=0+1 Illness=2+1 Regimen=1+1 Measure=1 Definition=1
79. Burt A, Thornley P, Illingworth D, White P, Shaw T, Turner R: Stopping
    smoking after myocardial infarction. *Lancet* 1:304-306, 1974
    Two methods of inducing heart attack victims to quit smoking were com-
    pared.
    N=223
    Design=3 Sample=0+1 Illness=1 Regimen=1 Measure=1 Definition=2
80. Bye C, Fowle AS, Letley E, Wilkinson S: Lack of effect of *Avena sativa* on
    cigarette smoking. *Nature* 252:580-581, 1974
    Controlled trial of extract of immature oats as an agent for reducing
    cigarette consumption by reducing craving.
    N=43
    Design=3 Sample=0+1 Illness=1 Regimen=1 Measure=1 Definition=2

81. Caine TM, Wijesinghe B: Personality, expectancies and group psycho-
    therapy. *Br J Psychiatry* 129:384-387, 1976
    A report on the use of personality and pretreatment expectancy tests for
    effective allocation of patients to group psychotherapy.
    N=182
    Design=1 Sample=0+1 Illness=0 Regimen=1 Measure=3+1 Definition=1
82. Caldwell JR, Cobb S, Dowling MD, De Jongh D: The dropout problem in
    antihypertensive therapy. *J Chronic Dis* 22:579-592, 1970
    Retrospective comparison of patients presenting to an emergency
    department in hypertensive crisis with unmatched hypertension clinic
    attenders.
    N=42 study, 24 control
    Design=2 Sample=1 Illness=2 Regimen=0 Measure=1 Definition=1
83. Campbell AH: Relapse in patients with tuberculosis. *Bull Int Union Tuberc*
    49:219-222, 1974
    An examination of the association of nonadherence to drug therapy and
    relapse rates in TB patients in Australia.
    N=3,280
    Design=1 Sample=2 Illness=1 Regimen=1 Measure=4+2 Definition=1
84. Campbell HG, Clarkson QD, Sinsabaugh LL: MMPI identification of non-
    rehabilitants among disabled veterans. *J Pers Assess* 41:266-269, 1977
    An assessment of some personality factors related to dropout rates in a
    rehabilitation program for disabled veterans.
    N=61
    Design=1 Sample=0+1 Illness=0 Regimen=1 Measure=2+1 Definition=1
85. Cann A, Sherman S, Elkes R: Effects of initial request size and timing of a
    second request on compliance: The foot in the door and the door in the
    face. *J Pers Soc Psychol* 32:774-782, 1975
    Report on the effect of magnitude of an initial verbal committment on
    compliance with a subsequent request.
    N=148
    Design=3 Sample=2 Illness=NA Regimen=0 Measure=3+1 Definiton=2
86. Caplan RD, Robinson E, French J, Caldwell J, Shinn M: Adhering to medi-
    cal regimens—pilot experiments in patient education and social support.
    Institute for Social Research, University of Michigan, Ann Arbor, 1976
    Psychosocial predictors and indicators of adherence with preliminary tests
    of parts of a model using educational and social support strategies.
    N=variable
    Design=3 Sample=2+1 Illness=2 Regimen=0 Measure=1+1 Definition=2
87. Carey R, Reid R, Ayers C, Lynch S, McLain W, Vaughan E: The Charlottes-
    ville blood-pressure survey: Value of repeated blood pressure measure-
    ments. *JAMA* 236: 847-851, 1976
    Results of repeated screening on hypertension prevalence with limited data
    on compliance with screening.
    N=533
    Design=1 Sample=2+1 Illness=2 Regimen=1 Measure=2 Definition=1

88. Carnahan J, Nugent C: The effects of self-monitoring by patients on the
    control of hypertension. *Am J Med Sci* 269:69-73, 1975
    Patients were taught to take their own blood pressures at home; the effect
    of this on response to treatment was assessed over six months.
    N=100
    Design=4 Sample=0+1 Illness=2 Regimen=1 Measure=2 Definition=1
89. Caron HS, Roth HP: Objective assessment of cooperation with an ulcer diet:
    Relation to antacid intake and to assigned physician. *Am J Med Sci*
    261:61-66, 1971
    Compliance with special diets was observed directly among hospitalized
    peptic ulcer patients who were given the opportunity to stray from
    their diet at a communal meal center.
    N=206
    Design=1 Sample=1+1 Illness=2 Regimen=1 Measure=3+1 Definition=2
90. ____: Patients' cooperation with a medical regimen. *JAMA* 203:922-926,
    1968
    Hopitalized peptic ulcer patients were rated for compliance with bedside
    antacids by ward residents and by objective measures, and the results
    compared.
    N=525
    Design=1 Sample=0 Illness=1 Regimen=1 Measure=2+1 Definition=2
91. Carpenter JO, Davis LJ: Medical recommendations—followed or ignored?
    Factors influencing compliance in arthritis. *Arch Phys Med Rehabil*
    57: 241-246, 1976
    A number of factors are examined in order to assess elements related to
    patient compliance with an exercise regimen for arthritis.
    N=54
    Design=1+1 Sample=1+1 Illness=2+1 Regimen=1 Measure=1 Definition=2
92. Carr JE, Whittenbaugh JA; Volunteer and nonvolunteer characteristics in
    an outpatient population. *J Abnorm Psychol* 73: 16-17, 1968
    Cohort analytic study of characteristics of psychiatric outpatients com-
    paring those who cooperate with those who did not cooperate with a
    telephone request to participate in a "psychotherapy outcome study"
    taking 1.5 hours of their time at a regularly scheduled clinic visit.
    N=78
    Design=2 Sample=0 Illness=1 Regimen=0 Measure=2 Definition=1
93. Carruthers S, Kelly J, McDevitt D: Plasma digoxin concentrations in pa-
    tients on admission to hospital. *Br Heart J* 30:707-712, 1974
    Patients who were receiving maintenance digoxin therapy before admission
    in emergency to a general hospital were studied for plasma digoxin con-
    centrations.
    N=101
    Design=1 Sample=0+1 Illness=0 Regimen=1 Measure=3+1 Definition=2
94. Chafetz ME, Blane HT, Abram HS, Golner J, Lacy E, McCourt WF, Clark E,
    Myers W: Establishing treatment relations with alcoholics. *J Nerv Ment
    Dis* 134(5): 395-409, 1962

Evaluation of the provision of immediate special counseling services for alcoholic patients referred from a casualty department.
N=200
Design=3 Sample=0+1 Illness=1 Regimen=1 Measure=2 Definition=2

95. Charney E, Bynum R, Eldredge D, Frank D, MacWhinney JB, McNabb N, Scheiner A, Sumpter E, Iker H: How well do patients take oral penicillin? A collaborative study in private practice. *Pediatrics* 40:188-195, 1967

Children presenting with acute streptococcal pharyngitis or otitis media at one of three private pediatric practices, and who were prescribed oral penicillin, were followed for compliance at five and nine days and the characteristics of compliers and noncompliers were compared.
N=459
Design=2 Sample=2 Illness=1 Regimen=2 Measure=3+1 Definition=2

96. Choi-Lao ATH: A preliminary study designed to explore the difference in effectiveness of group and individual teaching in self-medication. *Nurs Papers* 8:22-29, 1976

Report on a pilot experiment comparing the effects of group or individual teaching on adherence to self-medication.
N=9
Design=3 Sample=0+1 Illness=0 Regimen=1 Measure=2+1 Definition=2

97. Chubb JM, Winship HW: The pharmacist's role in preventing medication errors made by cardiac and hyperlipoproteinemic outpatients. *Drug Intell Clin Pharm* 8: 430-436, 1974

Controlled trial of the effect of pharmacist's instructions on medication compliance in two outpatient samples.
N=34
Design=4 Sample=0+1 Illness=1 Regimen=1 Measure=2 Definition=2

98. Cialdini R, Ascani K: Test of a concession procedure for inducing verbal, behavioral, and further compliance with a request to give blood. *J Appl Psychol* 61:295-300, 1976

Three compliance requests were compared to test their effectiveness in obtaining donors for a blood clinic.
N=189
Design=3 Sample=0 Illness=NA Regimen=2 Measure=3 Definition=2

99. Clark CM, Bayley EW: Evaluation of the use of programmed instruction for patients maintained on Warfarin therapy. *Am J Public Health* 62: 1135-1139, 1972

Controlled trial of ability of two methods of instruction (versus no instruction control group) to increase knowledge of patients with Warfarin therapy. Compliance was not assessed.
N=45
Design=4 Sample=0 Illness=0 Regimen=1 Measure=0 Definition=0

100. Clausen J, Seidenfeld M, Deasy L: Parent attitudes toward participation of their children in polio vaccine trials. *Am J Public Health* 44:1526-1536, 1954

Analysis of the differences in attitude and general orientation of mothers who gave or withheld their consent for their grade two children to participate in polio vaccine trials.
N=175
Design=1 Sample=2 Illness=NA Regimen=1 Measure=2 Definition=2

101. Clinite J, Kabat H: Improving patient compliance. *J Am Pharm Assoc* 16:74-76, 85, 1976
Evaluation of pharmacy interventions to improve compliance, including usual labeling, pharmacist's verbal instructions, printed instructions, and combinations of these.
N=62
Design=3 Sample=0+1 Illness=1 Regimen=1 Measure=2 Definition=2

102. Clinite JC, Kabat HF: Prescribed drugs, errors during self-administration. *J Am Pharm Assoc* NS9:450-452, 1969
Medication compliance of patients one week following hosptial discharge was assessed by interview and pill count.
N=30
Design=1 Sample=0 Illness=0 Regimen=1 Measure=2 Definition=1

103. Closson R, Kikugawa C: Noncompliance varies with drug class. *Hospitals* 49:89-93, 1975
Investigation of the relationship between patient compliance and the type of drug prescribed in a Veterans Administration population.
N=101
Design=1 Sample=0+1 Illness=0 Regimen=1 Measure=1 Definition=2

104. Cobb B, Clark R, McGuire C, Howe C: Patient-responsible delay of treatment in cancer: A social psychological study. *Cancer* 7:920-926, 1954
A comparison of two groups of cancer patients who delayed or were prompt in seeking assistance.
N=100
Design=2 Sample=1+1 Illness=1 Regimen=0 Measure=1+1 Definition=2

105. Cody J, Robinson A: The effect of low-cost maintenance medication on the rehospitalization of schizophrenic outpatients. *Am J Psychiatr* 134:73-76, 1977
A study of the relationship of cost of medications to treatment outcome among ambulatory schizophrenics.
N=90
Design=4 Sample=2+1 Illness=1 Regimen=1 Measure=NA Definition=2

106. Colcher IS, Bass JW: Penicillin treatment of streptococcal pharyngitis: A comparison of schedules and the role of specific counselling. *JAMA* 222:657-659, 1972
Pediatric outpatients with proven streptococcal pharyngitis were randomly assigned to three treatment groups: (1) I.M. penicillin; (2) oral penicillin, no instruction, (3) oral penicillin, specific counseling plus written instructions. Compliance in groups two and three was assessed by urine testing nine days after start of therapy.
N=300
Design=4 Sample=0 Illness=3 Regimen=2 Measure=3 Definition=1

107. Cole P, Emmanuel: Drug consultation: Its significance to the discharged hospital patient and its relevance as a role for the pharmacist. *Am J Hosp Pharm* 28:954-960, 1971

Hospitalized patients were assigned to one of three groups: (1) pharmacist consultation at time of discharge; (2) no consultation; (3) pharmacist consultation with self-administration of drugs two days prior to discharge. Compliance was assessed by telephone interview two weeks after discharge inquiring about pill taking and having patients count their own pills.

N=75

Design=3 Sample=0+1 Illness=0 Regimen=0 Measure=2+1 Definition=1

108. Collette J, Ludwig EG: Patient compliance with medical advice. *J Natl Med Assoc* 61:408-411, 1969

Compliance with various types of medical advice given social security disability applicants was compared with sociodemographic factors and antimedical attitudes as determined on an initial interview.

N=486

Design=2 Sample=1 Illness=0 Regimen=1 Measure=1 Definition=1

109. Cook D, Morch J, Noble E: Improving attendance at follow-up clinics. *Dimens Health Serv* 53:46-49, 1976

Before-after study evaluating letter reminders to improve appointment keeping.

N=514

Design=3 Sample=0+1 Illness=1 Regimen=0 Measure=2 Definition=2

110. Cooper B, Patterson R: The corticosteroid dose graph. *J Allergy Clin Immunol* 58:635-646, 1976

Evaluation of a medication-clinical event chart to monitor care for steroid-dependent asthmatics.

N=63

Design=1 Sample=0+1 Illness=3 Regimen=1 Measure=1 Definition=2

111. Copemann CD, Shaw, PL: Readiness for rehabilitation. *Int J Addict* 11:439-445, 1976

Some differences are described between successful and inactive residents in a drug rehabilitation center.

N=37

Design=2 Sample=0+1 Illness=0 Regimen=0 Measure=3 Definition=1

112. Coplin S, Hine J, Gormican A: Out-patient dietary management in the Prader-Willi syndrome. *J Am Diet Assoc* 68:330-334, 1976

Adherence to a low calorie diet by eight children with the Prader-Willi syndrome is reported.

N=8

Design=1 Sample=0 Illness=1 Regimen=2 Measure=4+1 Definition=0

113. Craig TJ, Huffine CL: Correlates of patient attendance in an inner-city mental health clinic. *Am J Psychiatr* 133:61-65, 1976

A report on the association of continuing treatment with the demographic and diagnostic attributes of low socioeconomic patients.

N=140

Design=1 Sample=1+1 Illness=1 Regimen=1 Measure=2 Definition=1

114. Crocco JA, Rooney JJ, Lyons HA: Outpatient treatment of tuberculosis in unreliable alcoholic patients. *NY State J Med* 76:58-61, 1976

Diagnosed alcoholics with tuberculosis were supervised closely and urged to maintain treatment through an outpatient clinic; they were followed for at least four years.

N=54

Design=3 Sample=0+1 Illness=3 Regimen=1+1 Measure=4 Definition=1

115. Cummings RE: A study of characteristics of patients who fail to complete a VA alcoholic treatment program. *Rehabil Lit* 36:139-141, 1975

Report of a comparative study of alcoholics who drop out and those who complete treatment in a VA hospital.

N=49

Design=2 Sample=0 Illness=1 Regimen=1 Measure=3+1 Definition=1

116. Currey H, Malcolm R, Riddle E, Schachte M: Behavioral treatment of obesity-limitations and results with the chronically obese. *JAMA* 237:2829-2831, 1977

Baseline and follow-up data are presented from a population of chronically obese female patients.

N=144

Design=1+1 Sample=0+1 Illness=1 Regimen=1 Measure=4 Definition=1

117. Curry FJ: Neighborhood clinics for more effective outpatient treatment of tuberculosis. *N Engl J Med* 279:1262-1267, 1968

Study of attendance rates by various groups of poorly attending tuberculous outpatients at a central chest clinic before and after decentralizing the clinic to form three neighborhood clinics and implementing home visiting.

N=variable (dystemporal samples)

Design=3 Sample=2 Illness=1 Regimen=1 Measure=2 Definition=1

118. _____: Study of irregular discharge TB patients at San Francisco General Hospital. *Pub Health Rep* 79:277-285, 1964

Incidence of irregular discharges of tuberculous patients from San Francisco General Hospital was reviewed before and after implementation of various enforcement procedures and social services.

N=variable

Design=3 Sample=0 Illness=1 Regimen=0 Measure=2 Definition=1

119. Curtis BD, Simpson D, Steven GC: Rapid puffing as a treatment component of a community smoking program. *J Community Psychiatr* 4:186-193, 1976

A three-week program of rapid puffing plus group discussion was compared to group discussion alone at follow-up periods of one week, two months, and five months.

N=26

Design=3 Sample=0+1 Illness=NA Regimen=2 Measure=1 Definition=2

120. Curtis EB: Medication errors made by patients. *Nurs Outlook* 9:290-291, 1961

Medication errors made at home by elderly patients were studied in a
special home care program.
N=26
Design=1 Sample=0 Illness=0 Regimen=0+1 Measure=1 Definition=1

121. Cuskey WR, Chambers CD, Wieland WF: Predicting attrition during the
outpatient detoxification of narcotic addicts. *Med Care* 9:108-116,
1971
This cohort analytic study of new patients to an addiction outpatient center followed subjects for attrition to establish intake features correlated
with this event.
N=86
Design=2 Sample=1+1 Illness=1 Regimen=2 Measure=3 Definition=2

122. Czaczkes JW, Kaplan DA: Selection of patients for regular haemodialysis,
pp 167-172, in Cameron JS (ed): *Dialysis and Renal Transplantation*,
Proceedings of the Ninth Conference. Florence, Italy, 1972
Analysis of psychiatric and psychological factors predictive of noncom-
pliance among chronic dialysis patients.
N=50
Design=1 Sample=3 Illness=1 Regimen=1 Measure=1 Definition=1

123. Dahl JC: Rational management of hypertension. *Minn Med* 60:311-314,
1977
Assessment of a program of physician and patient education on systemic
hypertension.
N=257
Design=1 Sample=0 Illness=2 Regimen=1 Measure=3 Definition=1

124. Daschner F, Marget W: Treatment of recurrent urinary tract infection in
children ii) Compliance of parents and children with antibiotic therapy
regimen. *Acta Paediatr Scand* 64:105-108, 1975
Documentation of the extent and role of noncompliance in the management of pediatric urinary infections.
N=105
Design=1 Sample=0 Illness=3 Regimen=1 Measure=3+1 Definition=2

125. Davidson N, Hudson B, Parry EHO: Defaulters from follow-up after peri-
partum cardiac failure. *Trop Geogr Med* 27:109-114, 1975
Problems of a subsistence agricultural economy as reasons for default
from follow-up of chronic diseases in rural Africa.
N=224
Design=2 Sample=1+1 Illness=2 Regimen=1 Measure=2+1 Definition=1

126. Davis KL, Estess FM, Simonton SC, Gonda TA: Effects of payment mode
on clinic attendance and rehospitalization. *Am J Psychiatry* 134:576-
578, 1977
An attempt to isolate factors distinguishing psychiatric patients who are
likely to remain in treatment from those who have a high risk of
dropping out.
N=115
Design=1 Sample=0+1 Illness=1 Regimen=1 Measure=3 Definition=2

127. Davis M, Eichhorn RL: Compliance with medical regimens: A panel study. *J Health Hum Behav* 4:240-249, 1963
     Interview population-based study of farm workers' health, attitudes, compliance with medical regimens, and their changes over a four-year period.
     N=variable
     Design=2 Sample=1 Illness=1 Regimen=1+1 Measure=1 Definition=1

128. Davis MS: Physiologic, psychological and demographic factors in patient compliance with doctors' orders. *Med Care* VI: 115-122, 1968
     New patients to a general medical clinic of a teaching hospital were interviewed at various stages throughout the course of their illness; initial attitudes and demographic features were analyzed with respect to compliance with therapy.
     N=154
     Design=1 Sample=1 Illness=1 Regimen=0 Measure=1+2 Definition=1

129. _____: Predicting non-compliant behavior. *J Health Soc Behav* 8:265-271, 1967
     Interviews with cardiac patients among a stratified sample of farmers were analyzed to derive "compliance indexes" that would predict adherence to medical recommendations. The various composite indexes were then applied prospectively to test their predictive value.
     N=not stated
     Design=2 Sample=2+1 Illness=1 Regimen=1+1 Measure=1 Definiton=1

130. _____: Variations in patients' compliance with doctors' orders: Analysis of congruence between survey responses and results of empirical investigations. *J Med Educ* 41:1037-1048, 1966
     Physicians' and medical students' perceptions of the magnitude and determinants of noncompliance were compared with results gleaned from a literature survey.
     N=132 physicians, 86 students
     Design=1 Sample=1 Illness=NA Regimen=NA Measure=1 Defintion=1

131. _____: Variations in patients' compliance with doctors' advice: An empirical analysis of patterns of communication. *Am J Public Health* 58:274-288, 1968
     Patterns of doctor-patient communication, assessed through analysis of tape recordings during clinical visits of new patients to a general medical OPD, were studied in relation to subsequent patient compliance with medical advice.
     N=variable
     Design=1 Sample=0 Illness=0 Regimen=0 Measure=1+2 Definition=1

132. _____: Variations in patients' compliance with doctors' orders: Medical practice and doctor-patient interaction. *Psychiatry In Med* 2:31-54, 1971
     Patient-physician interactions were assessed through tape recordings for new patients to a general medical clinic; the results of the interactional analysis over two or three visits, plus demographic characteristics of the patients, were compared with subsequent compliance.

N=154

Design=1 Sample=1 Illness=NA Regimen=0 Measure=1+2 Definition=2

133. De-Nour AK, Czaczkes JW: The influence of patient's personality on adjustment to chronic dialysis: A predictive study. *J Nerv Ment Dis* 162:323-333, 1976

An analysis of the influence of certain personality factors on compliance to a treatment program for chronic hemodialysis patients.

N=136

Design=1+1 Sample=3+1 Illness=2 Regimen=1 Measure=4+2 Definition=2

134. Deykin E, Weissman M, Tanner J, Prusoff B: A study of attendance patterns in depressed outpatients. *J Nerv Ment Dis* 160:42-48, 1975

The attendance patterns of lower class depressed women receiving outpatient psychotherapy were studied to determine the actual amount and frequency of therapy received in an 8-month period.

N=36

Design=2 Sample=1+1 Illness=1 Regimen=2 Measure=3+1 Definition=2

135. Diamond MD, Weiss AJ, Grynbaum B: The unmotivated patient. *Arch Phys Med Rehabil* 49:281-284, 1968

Patients undergoing rehabilitation for a variety of incapacitations were given an attitude-interview questionnaire. Results were compared to therapists' ratings of the patients' cooperation during treatments.

N=35

Design=1 Sample=1+1 Illness=1 Regimen=0 Measure=3 Definition=2

136. Dickey FF, Mattar ME, Chudzik GM: Pharmacist counseling increases drug regimen compliance. *Hospitals* 49:85-88, 1975

Description of two studies of pediatric compliance with ten-day courses of medication for otitis media. The first study documents the rate of noncompliance, and the second the effect of pharmacy counseling on improving compliance.

A. N=100

Design=1 Sample=0 Illness=1 Regimen=1+1 Measure=2 Definition=2

B. N=234

Design=3 Sample=0 Illness=1 Regimen=1+1 Measure=2 Definition=2

137. Dixon WM, Stradling P, Wootton ID: Outpatient PAS therapy. *Lancet* 2:871-872, 1957

Compliance was assessed among tuberculous outpatients for whom PAS had been prescribed.

N=151

Design=1 Sample=0+1 Illness=1 Regimen=1 Measure=3+1 Definition=2

138. Donabedian A, Rosenfeld LS: Follow-up study of chronically ill patients discharged from hospital. *J Chron Dis* 17:847-862, 1964

Compliance with medical recommendations was assessed at home interviews of chronically ill patients some three months after discharge from acute care hospitals.

N=82

Design=1 Sample=3+1 Illness=2+1 Regimen=1 Measure=1 Definition=1

139. Donovan JW: Randomized controlled trial of anti-smoking advice in pregnancy. *Br J Prev Soc Med* 31:6-12, 1977

Compliance was one outcome measured in an investigation of the effects of anti-smoking advice in pregnancy.

N=280 test, 308 control

Design=4 Sample=2+1 Illness=1 Regimen=1 Measure=1 Definition=1

140. Downie WW, Leatham PA, Rhind VM, Wright V: Steroid cards: Patient compliance. *Br Med J* 1:428, 1977

Descriptive study of extent of patient compliance in carrying notification of steroid drug use in patients with rheumatoid arthritis.

N=100

Design=1 Sample=0 Illness=1 Regimen=1 Measure =2 Definition=1

141. Drolet GJ, Porter DE: Why do patients in tuberculosis hospitals leave against medical advice? *NY TBC Health Assoc* 1-64, 1949

An analysis was done of several factors relating to leaving hospitals without medical consent for patients from four New York TB hospitals.

N=1828

Design=1 Sample=3+1 Illness=1 Regimen=1 Measure=3 Definition=2

142. Drury V, Wade O, Woolf E: Following advice in general practice. *J R Coll Gen Pract* 26:712-718, 1976

A random sample of patients in a single clinic was studied for compliance to tablet or capsule prescriptions.

N=521

Design=1 Sample=0+1 Illness=0 Regimen=0 Measure=2+2 Definition=2

143. Elinson J, Henshaw SK, Cohen SD: Response by a low income population to a multiphasic screening program: A sociological analysis. *Prev Med* 5:414-424, 1976

Results of household interviews to determine sociological factors affecting attendance or nonattendance at a free community screening centre.

N=1,351

Design=2+1 Sample=0 Illness=NA Regimen=NA Measure=2 Definition=2

144. Elling R, Whittemore R, Green M: Patient participation in a pediatric program. *J Health Hum Behav* 1:183-189, 1960

Study to discover relationships between family characteristics, the mother's conception of herself, and the child's participation in a clinic program for patients on rheumatic fever prophylaxis.

N=80

Design=1 Sample=0+1 Illness=1 Regimen=1 Measure=1+1 Definition=2

145. Eney RD, Goldstein EO: Compliance of chronic asthmatics with oral administration of theophylline as measured by serum and salivary levels. *Pediatrics* 57:513-517, 1976

Serum and salivary theophylline levels were assessed by gas chromatography and used to improve compliance among asthmatic children by selective increases in supervision.

N=47 study, 43 controls

Design=3 Sample=0+1 Illness=1 Regimen=1 Measure=3 Definition=2

146. Errera P, Davenport P, Decker L: Pre-intake dropout in a psychiatric
    clinic. *Ment Hygiene*. 49:558-563, 1965
    Discussion of factors preventing first time appointment makers from
    keeping their appointment.
    N=124
    Design=1+1 Sample=0+1 Illness=0 Regimen=0 Measure=2 Definition=2

147. Eshelman FN, Fitzloff J: Effect of packaging on patient compliance with
    an antihypertensive medication. *Curr Ther Res* 20:215-219, 1976
    Comparison of traditional prescription vials with special dispensers in
    compliance with chlorthalidone.
    N=100
    Design=4 Sample=0+1 Illness=1 Regimen=1 Measure=3+1 Definition=1

148. Etzwiler DD, Robb JR: Evaluation of programmed education among
    juvenile diabetics and their families. *Diabetes* 21:967-971, 1972
    The effectiveness of a programmed-instruction package in improving
    knowledge and clinical outcomes was assessed among juvenile diabetics
    and their parents.
    N=105 diabetics, 163 parents
    Design=3 Sample=0 Illness=1 Regimen=0 Measure=3+1 Definition=1

149. Evans RI, Rozelle RM, Lasater TM, Dembroski TM, Allen BP: Fear
    arousal, persuasion, and actual versus implied behavioral change. *J
    Pers Soc Psychol* 16:220-227, 1970
    Controlled trial of the ability of health messages containing varying
    amounts of information, fear arousal, and persuasions, to induce
    compliance with dental prophylaxis among junior high school children.
    N=139
    Design=4 Sample=2 Illness=NA Regimen=2 Measure=3+1 Definition=2

150. Evans RI, Rozelle RM, Mittlemark MB, Hansen WB, Bane AL, Havis J:
    Deterring the onset of smoking in children: Knowledge of immediate
    physiological effects and coping with peer pressure, media pressure,
    and parent modeling. *J Appl Psychol* 62:521-523, 1977
    Seventh grade students were randomly assigned to one of three experi-
    mental groups or to a control group in a study of methods designed
    to deter the onset of smoking.
    N=750
    Design=4 Sample=2 Illness=NA Regimen=0 Measure=1+1 Definition=2

151. Evenson RC, Altman H, Sletten IW, Cho DW: Accuracy of actuarial and
    clinical predictions for length of stay and unauthorized absence. *Dis
    Nerv Syst* 36:250-252, 1975
    Computer predictions using demographic and mental status data are
    compared with clinical predictions of patients' length of stay and
    unauthorized absence from five mental health institutions.
    N=210
    Design=2 Sample=2 Illness=0 Regimen=0 Measure=2 Definition=2

152. Ewalt P, Cohen M, Harmatz J: Prediction of treatment acceptance by
    child guidance clinic applicants. *Am J Orthopsychiatr* 42:857-864, 1972

Study of applicants to a child guidance center to determine factors pre-
dictive of postdiagnostic treatment.
N=253
Design=2+1 Sample=3+1 Illness=1 Regimen=1 Measure=3 Definition=2

153. Farberow N, Darbonne A, Stein K, Hirsch S: Self-destructive behavior of
uncooperative diabetics. *Psychol Rep* 27:935-946, 1970
Description of some demographic and psychological characteristics of
twelve uncooperative diabetic patients.
N=12
Design=1 Sample=0+1 Illness=1 Regimen=0 Measure=1 Definition=1

154. Farberow N, Stein K, Darbonne A, Hirsh S: Indirect self-destructive
behavior in diabetic patients. *Hosp Med* 6:123-135, 1970
An analysis of some psychosocial variables with respect to indirect self-
destructive behavior in an experimental group and a control group
of diabetic patients.
N=48
Design=3 Sample=0+1 Illness=1 Regimen=1 Measure=1 Definition=1

155. Farley OW, Peterson KD, Spanos G: Self-termination from a child
guidance centre. *Community Ment Health* J 11:325-334, 1975
Families of children undergoing psychotherapy were interviewed to find
reasons for termination of therapy.
N=52
Design=4 Sample=0 Illness=0 Regimen=0 Measure=2 Definition=2

156. Farquhar JW, Maccoby N, Wood PD, Alexander J.,Breitrose H, Brown B
Jr, Haskell W, McAlister A, Meyer A, Nash J, Stern M: Community
education for cardiovascular health. *Lancet* 1:1192-1195, 1977
A trial to determine whether preventive education can reduce the risk of
cardiovascular disease effectively.
N=2,151
Design=3 Sample=3 Illness=NA Regimen=1 Measure=3 Definition=1

157. Feinstein AR, Levitt M: The role of tonsils in predisposing to streptococcal infections and recurrences of rheumatic fever. *N Engl J Med* 282:
285-291, 1970
Children on penicillin prophylaxis were studied for the effect of tonsil
size on the recurrence of strep throat and rheumatic fever, comparing
compliers and noncompliers on different regimens.
N=532
Design=1 Sample=0 Illness=3 Regimen=1 Measure=1 Definition=1

158. Feinstein AR, Spagnuolo M, Jonas S, Levitt M, Tursky E: Discontinuation
of antistreptococcal prophylaxis. *JAMA* 197:949-952, 1966
Magnitude of noncompliance was assessed as a peripheral issue among
patients randomly assigned to a placebo group or oral penicillin group
to establish the safety of discontinuing antistreptococcal prophylaxis
among rheumatic fever victims with no residual cardiac damage.
N=161
Design=3 Sample=0 Illness=3 Regimen=2 Measure=1 Definition=2

159. Feinstein AR, Spagnuolo M, Jonas S, Kloth H, Tursky E, Levitt M: Prophylaxis of recurrent rheumatic fever. *JAMA* 206:565-568, 1968
   Children on penicillin prophylaxis for rheumatic fever prevention were studied for compliance. "Good" compliers were used to assess the relative efficacy of I.M. and oral preparations.
   N=1,046
   Design=4 Sample=0 Illness=1 Regimen=2 Measure=2+1 Definition=2

160. Feinstein AR, Wood HF, Epstein JA, Taranta A, Simpson R, Tursky E: A controlled study of three methods of prophylaxis against streptococcal infection in a population of rheumatic children, ii) Results of the first three years of the study, including methods for evaluating the maintenance of oral prophylaxis. *N Engl J Med* 260:697-702, 1959
   "Fidelity" to antibiotic prophylaxis for rheumatic fever was incorporated into interpretation of the results for two oral and one intramuscular regimen among children attending a special treatment clinic.
   N=391
   Design=3 Sample=0 Illness=2 Regimen=2 Measure=2+1 Definition=2

161. Feldman RG, Pippenger CE: The relation of anticonvulsant drug levels to complete seizure control. *J Clin Pharmacol* 3:51-59, 1976
   Noncompliance to drug therapy is mentioned as a possible cause of aberrant serum levels of DPH and PB in epileptic patients.
   N=25
   Design=2 Sample=0 Illness=3 Regimen=1 Measure=3 Definition=1

162. Fields WS, Lemak N, Frankowski R, Hardy R: Controlled trial of aspirin in cerebral ischemia. *Stroke* 8:301-314, 1977
   Compliance to medication is not central in this study of aspirin in the treatment of cerebral ischemia.
   N=88 aspirin, 90 placebo
   Design=4+1 Sample=2 Illness=3 Regimen=2 Measure=4+4 Definition=1

163. Fiester AR, Mährer AR, Giambra LM, Ormiston DW: Shaping a clinic population: The dropout problem reconsidered. *Community Ment Health J* 10:173-179, 1974
   A comparison of dropout and nondropout community outpatients on a pool of demographic variables.
   N=1,131
   Design=1 Sample=1+1 Illness=0 Regimen=1 Measure=2 Definition=1

164. Fiester AR, Rudestam KE: A multivariate analysis of the early dropout process. *J Consult Clin Psychol* 43:528-535, 1975
   Principal component factor analyses were performed on patient input, therapist input, and patient perspective therapy process variables that significantly differentiate early dropout from nonreport patients at two community mental health centers.
   N=181
   Design=1 Sample=0 Illness=0 Regimen=1 Measure=2 Definition=1

165. Fink D, Malloy MJ, Cohen M, Greycloud MA, Martin F: Effective patient care in the pediatric ambulatory setting: A study of the acute care

clinic. *Pediatrics* 43:927-935, 1969

Controlled trial of the ability of public health nurses, working through an acute care pediatric clinic, to improve care in terms of patient and parent knowledge of and compliance with medications, procedures, and appointments.

N=132 study, 142 controls

Design=4 Sample=0+1 Illness=0 Regimen=1 Measure=2+1 Defintion=2

166. Fink D, Martin F, Cohen M, Greycloud M, Malloy M: The management specialist in effective pediatric ambulatory care. *Am J Public Health* 59:527-533, 1969

Comprehensive planning by a nurse and/or a physician was compared with routine clinic care for pediatric patients presenting with acute respiratory infections.

N=85

Design=3 Sample=0 Illness=1 Regimen=0 Measure=2+2 Definition=1

167. Fink R: Delay behavior in breast cancer screening, pp 23-33, in Cullen JW, Fox BH, Isom RN (eds): *Cancer: The Behavioral Dimensions.* New York, Raven Press, 1976

A comparison of participation in a mass screening program for early breast cancer detection at centralized and decentralized clinics in New York City.

N=7,825

Design=2 Sample=2+1 Illness=1 Regimen=1 Measure=2 Definition=1

168. Finnerty FA, Mattie EC, Finnerty FA: Hypertension in the inner city i) Analysis of clinic dropouts. *Circulation* 47:73-75, 1973

The high dropout rate at a hypertension clinic was studied through finding and interviewing dropouts to determine their characteristics and stated reasons.

N=60 dropouts, 23 controls

Design=1 Sample=2 Illness=1 Regimen=0 Measure=2 Definition=2

169. Finnerty FA, Shaw LW, Himmelsbach CK: Hypertension in the inner city ii) Detection and follow-up. *Circulation* 47:76-78, 1973

Difficulties and results of a community hypertension screening program are discussed and a solution to the high referral no-show rate described, along with the success of specialized forms of treatment in maintaining attendance.

N=953

Design=4 Sample=0+1 Illness=3 Regimen=1 Measure=2 Definition=0

170. Fisher L, Johnson TS, Porter D, Bleich H, Slack W: Collection of a clear voided urine specimen: A comparison among spoken, written and computer-based instructions. *Am J Public Health* 67:640-644, 1977

The effectiveness of computerized instructions was compared with verbal and written forms.

N=99

Design=3 Sample=0+1 Illness=NA Regimen=1 Measure=3 Definition=1

171. Fleischman AI, Hayton T, Bierenbaum ML: Objective biochemical determination of dietary adherence in the young coronary male. *Am J Clin*

Nutr 20:333-337, 1967

Biochemical determinations of serum-free fatty acid fractions were used to assess adherence to prescribed diet among young male coronary patients. Nutritional interview histories were compared with the bio-chemical results.

N=33

Design=3 Sample=0 Illness=2 Regimen=1 Measure=3+1 Definition=2

172. Fletcher S, Appel F, Bourgois M: Management of hypertension: Effect of improving patient compliance for follow-up care. *JAMA* 233:242-244, 1975

Study of the effect of using a clerk to assist patients to return for follow-up care when found hypertensive at emergency room visits.

N=144

Design=4 Sample=1+1 Illness=2 Regimen=0 Measure=2+1 Definition=2

173. Fletcher SW, Appel FA, Bourgois M: Improving emergency-room patient follow-up in a metropolitan teaching hospital. *N Engl J Med* 291: 385-388, 1974

Controlled trial to assess whether addition of a follow-up clerk to the emergency room staff would improve compliance among emergency room patients requiring follow-up observation for nonurgent conditions.

N=291

Design=4 Sample=2+1 Illness=1 Regimen=0 Measure=2 Definition=1

174. Francis V, Korsch BM, Morris MJ: Gaps in doctor-patient communication. *N Engl J Med* 280:535-540, 1969

Doctor-patient interactions were taped and patients and their parents interviewed to assess the effects of doctor-patient communication on patient/parent satisfaction, reassurance, and compliance for pediatric patients.

N=587

Design=1 Sample=0 Illness=0 Regimen=0 Measure=2+1 Definition=1

175. Freedman JL, Fraser SC: Compliance without pressure: The foot-in-the-door technique. *J Pers Soc Psychol* 4:195-202, 1966

Two experimental studies of compliance with non-health-related requests.

A. N=156

Design=4 Sample=2 Illness=NA Regimen=2 Measure=1 Definition=2

B. N=112

Design=3 Sample=0 Illness=NA Regimen=2 Measure=1 Definition=2

176. Freemon B, Negrete V, Davis M, Korsch B: Gaps in doctor-patient com-munication: Doctor-patient interaction analysis. *Pediatr Res* 5:298-311, 1971

Taped recordings of doctor-patient interactions in a walk-in pediatric clinic were studied using the Bales Interaction Process Analysis. The depen-dent variables were patient satisfaction and compliance.

N=285

Design=3 Sample=0+1 Illness=0 Regimen=0 Measure=1 Definition=1

177. Freer CB, Ogunmuyiwa TA: Pre-school development screening in a
     health centre—the problem of non-attendance. *J R Coll Gen Prac* 27:
     428-430, 1977
     A study of attendance rates at a health center preschool child screening
     clinic.
     N=191
     Design=1+1 Sample=0+1 Illness=NA Regimen=0 Measure=1 Definition=1
178. Frisk PA, Cooper JW, Campbell NA: Community-hospital pharmacist
     detection of drug-related problems upon patient admission to small
     hospitals. *Am J Hosp Pharm* 34:738-742, 1977
     A study of drug-related problems, including noncompliance, that can be
     detected by pharmacy records and patient interviews.
     N=442
     Design=3 Sample=0+1 Illness=0 Regimen=0 Measure=1+1 Definition=2
179. Gabriel M, Gagnon J, Bryan C: Improved patient compliance through use
     of a daily drug reminder chart. *Am J Public Health* 67:968-969, 1977
     A controlled study was undertaken to examine the use of a daily drug
     reminder chart among geriatric hypertension patients in a community
     ambulatory care clinic.
     N=79
     Design=4 Sample=0+1 Illness=1 Regimen=1 Measure=2+1 Definition=2
180. Gabrielson IW, Levin LS, Ellison MD: Factors affecting school health
     follow-up. *Am J Public Health* 57:48-59, 1967
     A study to determine factors that influence parent behavior toward
     defects discovered in their children at school, in particular the parents'
     compliance with instructions to attend the appropriate health profes-
     sional.
     N=241
     Design=1 Sample=3+1 Illness=NA Regimen=0 Measure=2 Definition=1
181. Galasko C, Edwards D: The use of seat belts by motor car occupants in-
     volved in road traffic accidents. *Injury* 6:320-324, 1975
     A report on the effects of seat belt use on the reduction of mortality and
     severity of injury in automobile accidents.
     N=244
     Design=1 Sample=0+1 Illness=0 Regimen=0 Measure=3 Definition=0
182. Garb JR, Stunkard AJ: Effectiveness of a self-help group in obesity
     control: a further assessment. *Arch Intern Med* 134:716-720, 1974
     Twenty-one TOPS groups were studied in 1968 and 1970 to relate length
     of membership with weight loss.
     N=21 chapters of TOPS
     Design=1 Sample=2 Illness=NA Regimen=0 Measure=2 Definition=1
183. Garbus SB, Garbus SB: Analysis of mass hypertension screening. *Prev
     Med* 5:48-59, 1976
     Documentation of follow-up by questionnaire of screenees referred from
     mass hypertension screening to their physician for treatment.
     N=(30,329 screened) 8,875 hypertensives followed
     Design=2 Sample=2+1 Illness=2 Regimen=0 Measure=1 Definition=1

184. Gates SJ, Colborn DK: Lowering appointment failures in a neighborhood
     health center. *Med Care* 14:263-267, 1976
     Study of the effects of reminder letters and reminder calls on appointment
     keeping with an evaluation of the determinants of missing
     appointments.
     N=332
     Design=4 Sample=0+1 Illness=0 Regimen=1 Measure=2 Definition=2
185. Gatley MS:To be taken as directed. *J R Coll Gen Pract* 16:39-44, 1968
     Acutely ill patients who would admit to no errors in self-medication were
     studied by their general practitioner for compliance rates on the basis
     of pill count.
     N=86
     Design=1 Sample=0 Illness=0 Regimen=1 Measure=2 Definition=2
186. Geersten HR, Gray RM, Ward JR: Patient noncompliance within the
     context of seeking medical care for arthritis. *J Chron Dis* 26:689-698,
     1973
     Study of features of the therapeutic source, patient-therapist interaction,
     and patient characteristics and their relationship to compliance with
     rheumatoid arthritis regimens.
     N=123
     Design=1 Sample=0 Illness=3 Regimen=1 Measure=3+2 Definition=1
187. Geisler A, Andersen A, Vedso S: The co-operation of depressive patients
     in drug treatment. *Ugeskr Laeger* 130:1803-1806, 1968
     Psychiatric patients were treated for depression with either amitriptylin
     or a placebo with quinine added to all tablets as a tracer in order to
     assess the extent of adherence to the drug treatment.
     N=102
     Design=1 Sample=0 Illness=1 Regimen=0 Measure=3 Definition=2
188. Geisler A, Thomsen K: Failure to adhere to prescribed drug treatment.
     An investigation with labelled tablets. *Ugeskr Laeger* 135:1929-1932,
     1973
     Nonadherence to drug treatment was investigated in psychiatric patients
     who received amitriptylin, chlorprothixen, flupenthixol, or a placebo.
     N=272
     Design=1 Sample=0 Illness=1 Regimen=1 Measure=3 Definition=2
189. Gibberd FB, Dunne JF, Handley AJ, Hazleman BL: Supervision of
     epileptic patients taking phenytoin. *Br Med J* 1:147-149, 1970
     Epileptics on phenytoin were studied for serum levels of the drug,
     comparing inpatients and outpatients cross-sectionally and then follow-
     ing a group of outpatients prospectively for eight months, introducing
     several measures designed to improve compliance.
     N=14, 15, 12, respectively
     Design=3 Sample=0 Illness=1 Regimen=1 Measure=4+2 Definition=1
190. Gibson II, O'Hare MM: Prescription of drugs for old people at home.
     Gerontol Clin 10:271-280, 1968
     Home visits were made to determine number of drugs in the home and
     how they were being taken.

N=273
Design=1 Sample=0 Illness=0 Regimen=0 Measure=1 Definition=0

191. Glennon J A: Weight reduction—an enigma. *Arch Intern Med* 118:1-2, 1966

One year postdischarge patients who had been hospitalized for the treatment of obesity were assessed for weight reduction.
N=215
Design=2 Sample=0 Illness=1 Regimen=1 Measure=2 Definition=2

192. Glick BS: Dropout in an outpatient, double-blind drug study. *Psychosomatics* 6:44-48, 1965

Stated or implied reasons for dropouts were analyzed in a double-blind, placebo controlled drug study among depressed outpatients.
N=35
Design=3 Sample=0 Illness=1 Regimen=1+1 Measure=2 Definition=1

193. Glogow E: Effects of health education methods on appointment breaking. *Public Health Rep* 85:441-450, 1970

Glaucoma screenees were assigned randomly to a control group or to one of four informational modalities with attendance at a follow-up appointment as the dependent variable.
N=186
Design=4 Sample=2 Illness=3 Regimen=2 Measure=2 Definition=1

194. Glogow PH: Noncompliance—a dilemma. *Sight Sav Rev* :29-34, Spring 1973

Comparison of sociodemographic features of attenders and nonattenders in a glaucoma detection program.
N=186
Design=2 Sample=3+1 Illness=3 Regimen=1 Measure=3 Definition=2

195. Gold MA: Causes of patients' delay in diseases of the breast. *Cancer* 17:564-577, 1964

Description of reasons given by women with lesions of the breast for delay in seeking evaluation.
N=150
Design=1 Sample=1+1 Illness=2 Regimen=0 Measure=2 Definition=2

196. Goldstein M, Stein G, Smolen D, Perlini W: Bio-behavioral monitoring: A method for remote health measurement. *Arch Phys Med Rehabil* 57:253-258, 1976

Evaluation of a unique project in self-monitoring for cirrhotic patients.
N=26
Design=1 Sample=0+1 Illness=3 Regimen=1 Measure=4+2 Definition=2

197. Gopal PK: Study of defaulters in the treatment of leprosy. *Leprosy in India* 48:848-850, 1976

A descriptive analysis of the effect of a number of demographic variables on defaulting in a leprosy outpatient clinic.
N=282 males, 68 females
Design=1 Sample=1+1 Illness=1 Regimen=1 Measure=1 Definition=2

198. Gordis L, Markowitz M, Lilienfeld AM: Studies in the epidemiology and preventability of rheumatic fever iv) A quantitative determination of

compliance in children on oral penicillin prophylaxis. *Pediatrics* 43: 173-182, 1969
Children on penicillin prophylaxis for rheumatic disease were studied for compliance through determinations on urine samples collected both at regular clinic visits and on a randomized schedule at school.
N=136
Design=2 Sample=2 Illness=1 Regimen=1 Measure=4+2 Definition=2

199. _____: The inaccuracy in using interviews to estimate patient reliability in taking medications at home. *Med Care* 7:49-54, 1969
Comparison of objective and subjective patient compliance among children on oral penicillin prophylaxis with additional analysis of demographic, social, cognitive, and attitudinal factors among compliers and non-compliers.
N=103
Design=1 Sample=0 Illness=1 Regimen=1 Measure=4+3 Definition=2

200. _____: Why patients don't follow medical advice: A study of children on long-term antistreptococcal prophylaxis. *J Pediatr* 75:957-968, 1969
Black children on penicillin prophylaxis for rheumatic fever were studied for compliance by objective measures; results were compared with sociodemographic and clinical features.
N=111
Design=1 Sample=3+1 Illness=1 Regimen=1 Measure=4+1 Definition=2

201. Gordis L, Markowitz M: Evaluation of the effectiveness of comprehensive and continuous pediatric care. *Pediatrics* 48:766-776, 1971
Randomized trial of comprehensive pediatric care versus regular pediatric care for infants of primiparous adolescents. This is not a compliance study in the usual sense, though one can look at utilization rates for such factors as well-baby services, immunizations, etc.
N=120 study, 117 controls
Design=4 Sample=1 Illness=NA Regimen=1 Measure=1+1 Definition=1

202. _____: Evaluation of the effectiveness of comprehensive and continuous pediatric care. *Pediatrics* 48:766-776, 1971
Black children on rheumatic fever prophylaxis were stratified by compliance rates and then randomized to "continuous care" or the usual specialty clinic. Compliance with prophylaxis was monitored over the next fifteen months.
N=39 study, 38 controls
Design=4 Sample=1 Illness=1 Regimen=2 Measure=4 Definition=2

203. Gordon CGI: A method of controlled home treatment of pulmonary tuberculosis in Tanganyika. *Tubercle* 42:148-158, 1961
A descriptive report of a home treatment program for tuberculosis via patient and community education with emphasis on ensuring that patients would not be lost to treatment.
N=100
Design=1+1 Sample=0+1 Illness=1 Regimen=2 Measure=4+1 Definition=1

204. Gottlieb S, Kramer H: Compliance with recommendations following executive health examinations. *J Occup Med* 4:709-717, 1962

An evaluation of compliance with recommendations following executive
health examinations and identification of some of the factors operative
with respect to compliance/noncompliance.
N=574
Design=1 Sample=0+1 Illness=0 Regimen=0 Measure=2+1 Definition=2

205. Gotto A, Debakey M, Foreyt J, Scott L, Thornby J: Dietary treatment
of type IV hyperlipoproteinemia. *JAMA* 237:1212-1215, 1977
A two-year study of the effectiveness of special dietary counseling on
endogenous hypertriglyceridemia as measured by weight loss, plasma
lipid levels, and patient-reported diet.
N=278
Design=3+1 Sample=0+1 Illness=2 Regimen=2 Measure=4+2 Definition=1

206. Gottschalk LA, Mayerson P, Gottlieb AA: Prediction and evaluation of
outcome in an emergency brief psychotherapy clinic. *J Nerv Ment Dis*
144:77-96, 1967
Study of treatment success and dropout rates in a crisis-resolution short-
course psychotherapy outpatient clinic set up for urgent referrals.
N=53
Design=1 Sample=1+1 Illness=1 Regimen=1 Measure=3 Definition=2

207. Gould RL, Paulson I, Daniels-Epps L: Patients who flirt with treatment:
The silent population. *Am J Psychiatr* 127:166-171, 1970
Two studies of reasons for primary "no-shows" at a psychiatric OPD.
N=152, 233
Design=1 Sample=0+1 Illness=0 Regimen=0 Measure=2+1 Definition=2

208. Gray RM, Kesler JP, Moody PM: Effects of social class and friends'
expectations on oral polio vaccination participation. *Am J Public
Health* 56:2028-2032, 1966
A probability sample of mothers with children under five years of age
was studied to establish the effect of social class and of their
friends' (perceived) expectations of them on obtaining polio immunizations for their children.
N=846
Design=1 Sample=2 Illness=NA Regimen=2 Measure=1 Definition=0

209. Green J, Ray S, Charney E: Recurrence rate of streptococcal pharyngitis
related to oral penicillin. *J Pediatr* 75:292-294, 1969
Study of adherence rates to oral penicillin for streptococcal infections in a
private group practice.
N=222
Design=1 Sample=0+1 Illness=2 Regimen=1 Measure=3+1 Definition=2

210. Greiner GE: The pharmacist's role in patient discharge planning. *Am J
Hosp Pharm* 29:72-76, 1972
Report on a pilot study that provided input from the hospital pharmacist
in an attempt to increase compliance with drug therapies and to de-
crease readmittance rates of discharged patients.
N=156
Design=1 Sample=0+1 Illness=NA Regimen=0 Measure=0 Definition=0

211. Gross W, Nerviano V: The prediction of dropouts from an inpatient alcoholism program by objective personality inventories. *Q J Stud Alcohol* 34:514-515, 1973

Three personality inventories were assessed for ability to distinguish between completers and dropouts in an alcoholism treatment program. N=814

Design=2 Sample=0 Illness=1 Regimen=0 Measure=2 Definition=1

212. Grover P, Dean D, Livingston C, Snyder M, Miller D: Evaluating the effect of personalized risk factor education on patient compliance: Some research findings and methodologic issues. Presented at IXth International Health Education Conference, Ottawa, Ontario, August 1976

Report of experience with "canscreen," a low-cost, multisite cancer screening program based on the risk factor education approach. N=230

Design=3 Sample=0 Illness=NA Regimen=1 Measure=1 Definition=1

213. Gundert-Remy U, Remy C, Weber E: Serum digoxin levels in patients of a general practice in Germany. *Eur J Clin Pharmacol* 10:97-100. 1976

Evaluation of the effect of monitoring serum drug levels and feeding these back to patients on compliance with digoxin in a country general practice setting. N=33

Design=3 Sample=0 Illness=1 Regimen=1+1 Measure=4 Definition=2

214. Hadden DR, Montgomery DA, Skelly RJ, Trimble ER, Weaver JA, Wilson EA, Buchanan KD: Maturity onset diabetes mellitus: Response to intensive dietary management. *Br Med J* 3:276-278, 1975

Dietary management of maturity onset diabetes and the relationship of adherence to outcome are described. N=57

Design=3+1 Sample=0+1 Illness=2 Regimen=1+1 Measure=1 Definition=1

215. Haefner DP, Kirscht JP: Motivational and behavioral effects of modifying health beliefs. *Public Health Rep* 85:478-484, 1970

Volunteers from a university nonacademic staff were assessed for their health beliefs before and after viewing films on tuberculosis, cancer, and heart disease; they were then checked eight months later for beliefs and for compliance with a recommended health check. N=170

Design=4 Sample=0 Illness=NA Regimen=1 Measure=1 Definition=1

216. Hagan R, Foreyt J, Durham T: The dropout problem: Reducing attrition in obesity research. *Behav Ther* 7:463-471, 1976

Assessment of the effects of refundable monetary deposits upon attrition in obesity studies. N=42

Design=4 Sample=0+1 Illness=2 Regimen=1 Measure=4 Definition=2

217. Hammel RW, Williams PO: Do patients receive prescribed medication? *Am Pharm Assoc J* 4:331-334, 1964

Actual filling of prescriptions given out by private practitioners in four communities was studied and reasons for failure to fill the prescriptions within ten days were analyzed.
N=2,019
Design=1 Sample=2 Illness=0 Regimen=0 Measure=2 Definition=1

218. Hammond E, Percy C: Ex-smokers. *NY State J Med* 58:2956-2959, 1958
Mail survey of reasons ex-smokers give for quitting.
N=333
Design=1 Sample=0+1 Illness=1 Regimen=1 Measure=1 Definition=2

219. Handel S: Change in smoking habits in a general practice. *J R Coll Gen Pract* 23:149-150, 1973
Report of a G.P.'s attempt to reduce smoking among her patients.
N=100
Design=3 Sample=0 Illness=1 Regimen=1 Measure=1 Definition=2

220. Hansen A: Broken appointments in a child health conference. *Nurs Outlook* 1:417-419, 1953
Report on attendance at a pediatric clinic in a teaching hospital.
N=98
Design=1 Sample=0+1 Illness=0 Regimen=0 Measure=2 Definition=2

221. Hardy M: Parent resistance to need for remedial and preventive services. *J Pediatr* 48:104-114, 1956
Report of follow-through on recommendations made in a school screening program for hearing and vision.
N=6,731
Design=1 Sample=2+1 Illness=1 Regimen=1 Measure=1+1 Definition=1

222. Hardy MC: Follow-up of medical recommendations. *JAMA* 136:20-27, 1948
Families on welfare who brought their children for a free medical check-up were followed to assess compliance with medical and dental referrals that had been arranged for them.
N=1,068 children in 446 families
Design=2 Sample=3 Illness=NA Regimen=0 Measure=1 Definition=2

223. Hare EH, Willcox DR: Do psychiatric in-patients take their pills? *Br J Psychiatr* 113:1435-1439, 1967
Description of two biochemical methods for detecting phenothiazines and tricyclic antidepressants in urine with results for groups of psychiatric inpatients, day patients, and outpatients.
N=120, 27, 125 respectively
Design=1 Sample=0 Illness=0 Regimen=1 Measure=3+1 Definition=2

224. Harfouche J, Abi-yaghi M, Melidossian A, Azouri L: Factors associated with broken appointments in an experimental family health center. *Trop Doct* 3:128-133, 1973
Interview study of determinants of missing appointments at a new family health center in a previously underserviced area.
N=1,113
Design=1 Sample=1+1 Illness=1 Regmen=0 Measure=2 Definition=2

225. Harris MB, Bruner CG: A comparison of a self-control and a contract pro-

cedure for weight control. *Behav Res Ther* 9:347-354, 1971

A patient contract program proved superior to a self-control behavior modification program and to an attention placebo group after the three-month experimental period, but no differences remained seven months later.
  A. N=26 females, 6 males
     Design=4 Sample=0+1 Illness=3 Regimen=1 Measure=4+1 Definition=2
  B. N=18 females
     Design=4 Sample=0+1 Illness=3 Regimen=1 Measure=4+1 Definition=2

226. Hay DR, Turbott S: Changes in smoking habits in men under 65 years after myocardial infarction and coronary insufficiency. *Br Heart J* 32:738-740, 1970

Interview study up to two years after hospitalization for ischemic heart disease to determine smoking habit change.
N=340

Design=2 Sample=0 Illness=2 Regimen=1 Measure=1 Definition=1

227. Hayes P, Hickey K, Lovell S, Dugdale A: The storage of drugs in homes. *Med J Aust* 1:235-236, 1976

Household survey of stores of unused drugs in homes of children recently discharged from hospital.
N=84

Design=1 Sample=0+1 Illness=1 Regimen=0 Measure=2 Definiton=2

228. Haynes RB, Sackett DL, Gibson ES, Taylor DW, Hackett BC, Roberts, RS, Johnson AL: Improvement of medication compliance in uncontrolled hypertension. *Lancet* 1:1265-1268, 1976

A behavior modification program comprising increased supervision, home blood pressure, and tailoring was evaluated among noncompliant hypertensive patients.
N=38

Design=4+1 Sample=2+1 Illness=3 Regimen=1+1 Measure=2+1 Definition=2

229. Hecht AB: Improving medication compliance by teaching outpatients. *Nurs Forum* 13:112-129, 1974

Study of the effect of planned, individual instruction by nurses on medication errors of tuberculosis outpatients.
N=47

Design=3+1 Sample=1+1 Illness=3+1 Regimen=1 Measure=3+3 Definition=2

230. Hedstrand H, Aberg H: Treatment of hypertension in middle-aged men. *Acta Med Scand* 199:281-288, 1976

Results of a community hypertension survey and intervention program.
N=2,322

Design=1 Sample=2+1 Illness=3 Regimen=1 Measure=2 Definition=2

231. Heilbrun A: Improved detection of the early defecting counseling client. *J Consult Clin Psychol* 42:633-638, 1974

Report of an attempt to improve a "counseling readiness scale" in predicting dropouts from psychotherapy.
N=429

Design=2 Sample=0+1 Illness=1 Regimen=1 Measure=2 Definition=2

232. Heine RW, Trosman H: Initial expectations of the doctor-patient interaction as a factor in continuance in psychotherapy. *Psychiatry*
23:275-278, 1960
Cohort study of new referrals to a psychiatric outpatient department,
comparing initial assessments for those who continued to attend for
six weeks with assessments for those who did not.
N=46
Design=2 Sample=0+1 Illness=0 Regimen=1 Measure=3 Definition=2
233. Heinemann E, Moore B, Gurel M: Completion or termination of alcoholism treatment: Toward the development of a predictive index.
Psychol Rep 38:1340-1342, 1976
Self-concept, social support system, socioeconomic status, and physical
well-being were examined as possible predictors of completion of
alcoholism programs.
N=184
Design=2 Sample=2 Illness=1 Regimen=0 Measure=2 Definition=1
234. Heinzelmann F, Bagley RW: Response to physical activity programs and
their effects on health behavior. *Public Health Rep* 85:905-911, 1970
Middle-aged males believed to be at risk of coronary heart disease were
invited to participate in a fitness program. Attitudes, beliefs, and health
behaviors were assessed before entry into the program and every three-
four months thereafter in order to assess the reasons for entry and for
continuance (compared to a control group).
N=239 study, 142 controls
Design=1 Sample=2 Illness=NA Regimen=1 Measure=1 Definition=1
235. Heinzelmann F: Factors in prophylaxis behavior in treating rheumatic
fever: An exploratory study. *J Health Hum Behav* 3:73-81, 1962
College students with a history of rheumatic fever and/or rheumatic
heart disease were interviewed; the characteristics of those who were
and were not taking antibiotic prophylaxis were compared.
N=284
Design=1 Sample=3 Illness=1 Regimen=0 Measure=1 Definition=0
236. Hemminki E, Heikkila J: Elderly people's compliance with prescriptions, and quality of medication. *Scand J Soc Med* 3:87-92, 1975
Examination of how the quality of medication influences compliance
in homes for the aged.
N=217
Design=1 Sample=3+1 Illness=0 Regimen=1 Measure=1 Definition=2
237. Henderson M, Wood R: Compulsory wearing of seat belts in New South
Wales, Australia: An evaluation of its effect on vehicle occupant
deaths in the first year. *Med J Aust* 2:797-801, 1973
Temporal analysis of the effect of legislating compulsory seat belt use.
N=variable
Design=3 Sample=2+1 Illness=NA Regimen=2 Measure=2+1 Definition=0
238. Henke C, Yelin E, Ingbar M, Epstein W: The university rheumatic
disease clinic: Provider and patient perceptions of cost. *Arthritis
Rheum*, 20:751-758, 1977

A description of clinic and patient costs and the effect of costs on
   patients' attendance at appointments.
N=47
Design=1 Sample=1+1 Illness=1 Regimen=1 Measure=1 Definition=1

239. Hermann F: The outpatient prescription label as a source of medica-
   tion errors. *Am J Hosp Pharm* 30:155-159, 1973
   Analysis of outpatients' literal interpretations of prescription labels
   at the time of dispensing. Actual compliance not measured.
   N=uncertain
   Design=1 Sample=0 Illness=0 Regimen=1 Measure=1 Definition=1

240. Hertroijs A: A study of some factors affecting the attendance of
   patients in a leprosy control scheme. *Int J Lepr* 42:419-427, 1974
   Entry data on 8,655 patients who enrolled in a regional leprosy
   program were examined for differences between attenders and nonattenders.
   N=variable
   Design=2 Sample=3+1 Illness=2 Regimen=0 Measure=2 Definition=2

241. Hildebrandt DE, Davis JM: Home visits: A method of reducing the pre-
   intake dropout rate. *J Psychiatr Nurs* 13:43-44, 1975
   Study of the effect of home visits on reducing no-show rate for new
   referrals to an adolescent psychiatric clinic.
   N=91
   Design=4 Sample=2+1 Illness=0 Regimen=1 Measure=2 Definition=2

242. Hoehn-Saric R, Frank J, Imber S, Nash E, Stone A, Battle C: Systematic
   preparation of patients for psychotherapy—1) Effects on therapy
   behavior and outcome. *J Psychiatr Res* 2:267-281, 1964
   Evaluation of an intake interview (to give patients appropriate expectations) in order to improve patient cooperation with psychotherapy.
   N=40
   Design=4+1 Sample=1+1 Illness=2 Regimen=1 Measure=4+2 Definition=2

243. Hoenig F, Ragg N: The non-attending psychiatric outpatient: An administrative problem. *Med Care* 4:96-100, 1966
   Patients referred by general practitioners to a psychiatric OPD, but who
   failed to attend their first appointment, were compared with a
   random sample of attenders at the same clinic and with nonattenders
   at a neurology clinic.
   N=150 study, 150 attending + 95 nonattending controls.
   Design=1 Sample=0+1 Illness=1 Regimen=1 Measure=1 Definition=1

244. Hoffmann H, Noem A: Adjustment of Chippewa Indian alcoholics to
   a predominantly white treatment program. *Psychol Rep* 37:1284-
   1286, 1975
   Indians admitted to a state hospital treatment program were compared
   with white patients for sociodemographic and psychosocial features
   and for success in the program.
   N=51 Indians, 1,474 whites
   Design=2 Sample=1 Illness=1 Regimen=1 Measure=3 Definition=1

245. Hogarty G, Ulrich R, Goldberg S, Schooler N: Sociotherapy and the prevention of relapse among schizophrenic patients: An artifact of drug? *Proc Am Psychopathol Assoc* 64:285-293, 1976
Reanalysis of trial results to determine if "sociotherapy" improved medication compliance.
N=374
Design=4 Sample=2+1 Illness=3 Regimen=2 Measure=1 Definition=1

246. Hogarty GE, Goldberg SC, and the Collaborative Study Group: Drug and sociotherapy in the aftercare of the schizophrenic patients; one-year relapse rates. *Arch Gen Psychiatr* 28:54-64, 1973
Study of relapse rates and compliance among schizophrenic outpatients randomized to (1) chlorpromazine; (2) placebo; (3) placebo plus "major role therapy"; or (4) chlorpromazine plus "major role therapy" over two years.
N=374
Design=4 Sample=3+1 Illness=3 Regimen=1 Measure=1 Definition=1

247. Hogue C: Compliance in infant immunization. Paper presented at American Public Health Association Meeting, Florida, 20 October 1976
Test of a conceptual model of "health action" in an immunization program for infants.
N=66
Design=1 Sample=3+1 Illness=NA Regimen=1 Measure=3 Definition=2

248. Holder L: Effects of source, message, audience characteristics on health behavior compliance. *Health Serv Res* 87:343-350, 1972
Controlled trial of the effect on postnatal care compliance of two types of health messages delivered by two nurses and two mothers of different racial origin to new mothers of different racial backgrounds.
N=122
Design=3 Sample=0 Illness=NA Regimen=2 Measure=2+3 Definition=1

249. Horan V: Patient performance in the self-administration of dispensed medicines. *J Hosp Pharm*: 135-140, June 1973
Patients in a minimal care hospital ward were observed for compliance with self-administered medications.
N=31
Design=1 Sample=0+1 Illness=0 Regimen=1 Measure=2+1 Definition=2

250. Horenstein D, Houston B: The expectation-reality discrepancy and premature termination from psychotherapy. *J Clin Psychol* 32:373-378, 1976
Attempt to determine the relationship of dropping out to the disparity between a patient's initial expectations and subsequent experiences in psychotherapy.
N=154
Design=2 Sample=0+1 Illness=0 Regimen=1 Measure=2 Definition=2

251. Horenstein D: Correlates of initial client disturbance: Expectations for therapy, dropout, resistance, and demographic description. *J Clin Psychol* 31:709-715, 1975

Report of dropout rates from a university campus counseling service; no information on determinants despite article's title.
N=154
Design=1 Sample=0+1 Illness=0 Regimen=0 Measure=2 Definition=2

252. Howard K, Rickels K, Mock JE, Lipman RS, Covi L, Baumm NC: Theraputic style and attrition rate from psychiatric drug treatment. *J Nerv Ment Dis* 150:102-110, 1970

Droput rates were observed among neurotic outpatients in a placebo-controlled randomized drug trial, comparing therapeutic style used among dropouts to that among continuers and also comparing the therapeutic styles of "drug enthusiastic" physicians with those of "drug unenthusiastic" physicians.
N=variable
Design=2 Sample=1 Illness=3 Regimen=1 Measure=3 Definition=1

253. Howie VM, Ploussard JH: Compliance dose-response relationships in streptococcal pharyngitis. *Am J Dis Child* 123: 18-25, 1972

Study of the relative efficacy of three types of erythromycin and two types of penicillin, all in liquid suspensions, among pediatric patients with suspected streptococcal pharyngitis, taking into account compliance through measuring consumption of medication.
N=306
Design=4 Sample=0 Illness=3 Regimen=2 Measure=2 Definition=1

254. Huber N, Danahy S: Use of the MMPI in predicting completion and evaluating changes in a long-term alcoholism treatment program. *J Stud Alcohol* 36:1230-1237, 1975

Report of an attempt to predict cooperation with a ninety-day Veterans Administration hospital alcoholism program.
N=102
Design=2 Sample=1+1 Illness=1 Regimen=2 Measure=3 Definition=2

255. Hudson LD, Sbarboro JA: Twice weekly tuberculosis chemotherapy. *JAMA* 223:139-143, 1973

Results are presented of an outpatient treatment program for "unreliable" tuberculous patients, employing twice-weekly administration of high dose isoniazid and streptomycin by a nurse at a place of convenience to the patient.
N=101
Design=2 Sample=0 Illness=3 Regimen=2 Measure=4+1 Definition=1

256. Hulka B, Cassel J, Kupper L, Burdette J: Communication, compliance, and concordance between physicians and patients with prescribed medications. *Am J Public Health* 66:847-853, 1976

Further analysis of data relating to the relationship between compliance and doctor-patient communication.
N=357
Design=2 Sample=3+1 Illness=1 Regimen=1+1 Measure=1 Definition=2

257. Hulka B, Kupper L, Cassel J, Mayo F: Doctor-patient communication and outcomes among diabetic patients. *J Community Health* 1:15-27, 1975

Communication from physician to patient was studied to assess the effect of communication on subsequent patient compliance and outcomes.
N=242
Design=1 Sample=2+1 Illness=2 Regimen=1 Measure=2+1 Definition=1

258. Hulka B, Kupper L, Cassel J, Efird R, Burdette J: Medication use and misuse: Physician-patient discrepancies. *J Chron Dis* 28: 7-21, 1975
Study of the types of discrepancy between medication prescription and consumption.
N=357
Design=2 Sample=3+1 Illness=1 Regimen=1+1 Measure=1 Definition=2

259. Hulka BS: Motivation techniques in a cancer detection program. *Public Health Rep* 81:1009-1014, 1966
Evaluation of the effectiveness of various motivational techniques, namely telephone and mailed contacts and home vists, in eliciting participation in a cervical cancer detection program.
N=23,000
Design=1 Sample=2+1 Illness=NA Regimen=2 Measure=3 Definition=1

260. Hurtado A, Greenlick M, Columbo T: Determinants of medical care utilization: Failure to keep appointments. *Med Care* 11:189-198, 1973
Study of patient and physician characteristics related to appointment breaking in a prepaid multispecialty group practice.
N=10,466
Design=2 Sample=3+1 Illness=0 Regimen=0 Measure=2 Definition=2

261. Hyman MD: Social psychological determinants of patients' performance in stroke rehabilitation. *Arch Phys Med Rehabil* 53:217-226, 1972
Study of psychosociological factors associated with motivation and with the functional improvement of stroke patients in an inpatient rehabilitation program.
N=101
Design=2 Sample=0+1 Illness=2 Regimen=0 Measure=1+1 Definition=0

262. Hypertension Detection and Follow-up Program Cooperative Group: Mild hypertensives in the Hypertension Detection and Follow-up Program. *Ann NY Acad Sci* 304:254-266, 1978
First year experience in a multicentered, population-based screening and treatment program for mild to moderate hypertension.
N=variable
Design=4 Sample=2+1 Illness=3 Regimen=3 Measure=2+1 Definition=2

263. Intagliata J: A telephone follow-up procedure for increasing the effectiveness of a treatment program for alcoholics. *J Stud Alcohol* 37:1330-1335, 1976
A group of alcoholics was given either supportive follow-up telephone calls or no calls to test the effect on utilization of outpatient services and on general rehabilitation.
N=40
Design=4+1 Sample=0+1 Illness=1 Regimen=1 Measure=1+1 Definition=1

264. Inui T, Yourtee E, Williamson J: Improved outcomes in hypertension after physician tutorials. *Ann Intern Med* 84:646-651, 1976
Report of the effect of tutorials for physicians on the compliance of their hypertensive patients.
N=116, 102
Design=3 Sample=0+1 Illness=2 Regimen=1 Measure=2+2 Definition=2

265. Ireland HD: Outpatient chemotherapy for tuberculosis. *Am Rev Resp Dis* 82:378-383, 1960
Two-year follow-up of medication compliance among tuberculosis patients consecutively discharged from hospital, comparing rates for INH, PAS, and intramuscular streptomycin over time.
N=264
Design=2 Sample=0 Illness=1 Regimen=1 Measure=2 Definition=2

266. Irwin DS, Weitzell WD, Morgan DW: Phenothiazine intake and staff attitudes. *Am J Psychiatr* 127:1631-1635, 1971
Psychiatric patients on closed wards or open wards and as outpatients were studied for compliance using the Forrest rapid urine color tests; the results were compared with therapists' attitudes toward the efficacy of phenothiazines.
N=67, 19, 40
Design=1 Sample=2 Illness=1 Regimen=1 Measure=4 Definition=2

267. Isacsson SO, Janzon L: Results of a quit-smoking research project in a randomly selected population. *Scand J Soc Med* 4:25-29, 1976
Results of an intensive antismoking program aimed at a probability sample of heavy smokers.
N=58
Design=3+1 Sample=2+1 Illness=3 Regimen=2 Measure=3+1 Definition=2

268. Jackson H, Cooper J, Mellinger W, Olsen A: Streptococcal pharyngitis in rural practice. *JAMA* 197:105-108, 1966
Results of a dedicated effort in a general practice setting to provide high quality care for streptococcal pharyngitis.
N=1,052
Design=1 Sample=0+1 Illness=2 Regimen=1 Measure=2+1 Definition=1

269. Jacobs M: The addictive personality: Prediction of success in a smoking withdrawal program. *Psychosom Med* 34:30-38, 1972
A battery of psychological tests was given to smokers entering a treatment program, in order to determine correlates of success.
N=104
Design=2 Sample=1+1 Illness=2 Regimen=1 Measure=2+1 Definition=2

270. Jankowski CB, Drum DE: Diagnostic correlates of discharge against medical advice. *Arch Gen Psychiatr* 34:153-155, 1977
The medical histories of patients discharged against medical advice from a general hospital were studied to determine diagnostic correlates of this behavior.
N=73 test, 175 control
Design=2 Sample=0+1 Illness=0 Regimen=0 Measure=2+1 Definition=1

271. Jenkins BW: Are patients true to TID and QID doses? *GP* 9:66-69, 1954
     Patients of a private general practitioner who were prescribed medications
     on a TID or QID schedule were monitored for compliance.
     N=30
     Design=1 Sample=0 Illness=0 Regimen=1 Measure=2 Definition=2
272. Johannsen WJ, Hellmuth GA, Sorauf T: On accepting medical recom-
     mendations. *Arch Environ Health* 12:63-69, 1966
     Study of compliance and factors affecting compliance with recommenda-
     tions made for patients assessed at a cardiac work classification unit.
     N=127
     Design=2 Sample=1+1 Illness=1 Regimen=0 Measure=1 Definition=1
273. Johnson D, Freeman H: Long-acting tranquillizers. *Practitioner* 208:395-
     400, 1972
     Outpatient schizophrenics originally on oral phenothiazines were switched
     to intramuscular fluphenazine after a relapse and were compared for
     attendance and relapses for equal periods before and after initiation
     of the injections.
     N=179
     Design=3 Sample=0 Illness=1 Regimen=1 Measure=1 Definition=1
274. Johnson D: Treatment of depression in general practice. *Br Med J* 2:18-20,
     1973
     A descriptive study of physician and patient factors (including noncompli-
     ance by either) in the primary care of depression.
     N=73
     Design=1 Sample=0+1 Illness=2 Regimen=1 Measure=2+1 Definition=1
275. Jonas S: Appointment-breaking in a general medical clinic. *Med Care*
     9:82-88, 1971
     Appointment keepers were compared with breakers of scheduled appoint-
     ments at a general medical outpatient clinic.
     N=292 keepers, 273 breakers
     Design=1 Sample=1 Illness=0 Regimen=0 Measure=2 Definition=2
276. _____: Influence of the weather on appointment-breaking in a general
     medical clinic. *Med Care* 11:72-74, 1973
     Brief report of a study of the correlation between weather conditions and
     appointment breaking during two winter weeks.
     N=20 clinic appointments
     Design=1 Sample=0+1 Illness=NA Regimen=2 Measure=2 Definition=2
277. Joyce CR: Patient cooperation and the sensitivity of clinical trials. *J Chron
     Dis* 15:1025-1036, 1962
     The results of a double-blind crossover placebo-controlled trial of medica-
     tions for active rheumatoid arthritis were analyzed with and without
     compliance being taken into account, resulting in a difference in inter-
     pretation.
     N=78
     Design=3 Sample=1 Illness=1 Regimen=2 Measure=3+1 Definition=1
278. Kaback M, Becker M, Ruth M: Sociologic studies in human genetics: I.
     Compliance factors in a voluntary heterozygote screening program.

Birth Defects 10:145-163, 1974

An analysis of attitudinal and demographic differences between participants and nonparticipants in a Tay-Sachs screening program in the
Jewish communities in Baltimore and Washington.

N=500 compliers, 412 noncompliers

Design=2 Sample=3+1 Illness=NA Regimen=1 Measure=3 Definition=2

279. Kalb M: Social class, length of treatment contacts and the outpatient
treatment of alcoholism. *Br J Addict* 70:253-262, 1975

Attempt to separate the unique effects of social class and length of contact
on the type of treatment received by outpatient alcoholics.

N=80

Design=2 Sample=1+1 Illness=1 Regimen=2 Measure=2 Definition=2

280. Kanzler M, Jaffe J, Zeidenberg P: Long and short term effectiveness of a
large-scale proprietary smoking cessation program—a four year follow-
up of Smokenders participants. *J Clin Psychol* 32:661-669, 1976

One of the few long-term follow-ups of an antismoking program.

N=553

Design=3 Sample=0+1 Illness=1 Regimen=1 Measure=1+1 Definition=2

281. Kaplan DA, Czaczkes JW: Personality factors in chronic hemodialysis
patients causing noncompliance with medical regimen. *Psychosom Med*
34:333-344, 1972

Psychiatric assessments of patients on chronic hemodialysis were performed in order to study the relationship of personality factors to
compliance with diet as assessed by both objective and subjective
measures.

N=43

Design=2 Sample=3 Illness=0 Regimen=1 Measure=3+2 Definition=1

282. _____: The influence of patient's personality on adjustment to chronic
dialysis: A predictive study. *J Nerv Ment Dis* 162(5):323-333, 1976

A study of psychiatric personality assessment on compliance with diet,
rehabilitation, and psychological condition of chronic dialysis patients.

N=100 at six-month follow-up.

Design=2+1 Sample=2 Illness=1 Regimen=1 Measure=4+1 Definition=2

283. Karoly P, Doyle W: Effects of outcome expectancy and timing of self-
monitoring on cigarette smoking. *J Clin Psychol* 31:351-355, 1975

The effects of induced outcome expectancy and self-monitoring on smoking behavior were studied in college students.

N=56

Design=4 Sample=0+1 Illness=NA Regimen=2 Measure=3 Definition=1

284. Katholi R, Kiraly J, Hook E: The management of gonorrhea in an emergency room. *Intern Med* Feb: 101-104, 1977

Attendance at a follow-up session was part of the data collected in a study
of gonorrhea treatment in an emergency room situation.

N=81

Design=1+1 Sample=0+1 Illness=1 Regimen=1 Measure=3 Definition=1

285. Katz S, Vignos P, Moskowitz R, Thompson H, Svec K: Comprehensive
outpatient care in rheumatoid arthritis. *JAMA* 206:1249-1254, 1968

Patients with classical rheumatoid arthritis were assigned randomly to treatment and control groups in a study of effectiveness of multi-disciplinary clinic and home care.

N=40

Design=4 Sample=1+1 Illness=3 Regimen=1 Measure=4+1 Definition=1

286. Kearny T, Bonime HC: Problems of drug evaluation in outpatients. *Dis Nerv Syst* 27:604-606, 1966

Description of the problems created by patient dropout and lack of cooperation in a double-blind placebo-controlled drug trial among neurotic outpatients.

N=28

Design=4 Sample=0 Illness=1 Regimen=2 Measure=2 Definition=0

287. Kegeles SS: Why people seek dental care: A test of a conceptual formulation. *J Health Hum Behav* 4:166-173, 1963

Study of the utility of the "health belief model" in predicting, in both retrospective and prospective fashions, the use of prophylactic or symptomatic dental services among a random sample of factory workers.

N=426

Design=2 Sample=0 Illness=NA Regimen=0 Measure=1 Definition=1

288. Kellaway G, MaCrae E: Non-compliance and errors of drug administration in patients discharged from acute medical wards. *NZ Med J* 81:508-512, 1975

A report on the causes for drug defaulting in a group of outpatients from acute general wards in Auckland.

N=315

Design=1 Sample=0+1 Illness=1 Regimen=1 Measure=1 Definition=1

289. Kennell J, Soroker E, Thomas P, Wasman M: What parents of rheumatic fever patients don't understand about the disease and its prophylactic management. *Pediatrics* 43:160-167, 1969

Parents of rheumatic fever patients were interviewed to determine factors affecting the parents' understanding of prophylactic treatment (bicillin injections).

N=63 patients, 60 parents

Design=1 Sample=0 Illness=1 Regimen=1 Measure=3+1 Definition=0

290. Kidd AH, Euphrat JL: Why prospective outpatients fail to make or keep appointments. *J Clin Psychol* 27:394-395, 1971

Patients newly referred to a community mental health clinic but who failed to make or to keep a first appointment were interviewed by telephone to determine reasons for failure to come.

N=407

Design=3 Sample=0+1 Illness=0 Regimen=0 Measure=2 Definition=1

291. Kincey J, Bradshaw P, Ley P: Patients' satisfaction and reported acceptance of advice in general practice. *J R Coll Gen Pract* 25:558-566, 1975

Evaluation of patients' satisfaction with medical information, their views about compliance with medical advice, and the relationship between satisfaction and compliance.

N=61

Design=2+1 Sample=0+1 Illness=0 Regimen=0 Measure=1 Definition=2

292. Kingsley RG, Shapiro J: A comparison of three behavioral programs for the control of obesity in children. *Behav Ther* 8:30-36, 1977

A behaviorally oriented weight reduction program was taught to either mother and child, mothers alone, or children alone and weight loss was assessed at the end of the eight-week program, then six and twenty weeks later.

N=24 girls, 16 boys

Design=3 Sample=1+1 Illness=3+1 Regimen=1+1 Measure=4 Definition=2

293. Kirscht J, Haefner D: Effects of repeated threatening health communications. *Int J Health Educ* 16:268-277, 1973

Low and high fear messages urging health action for heart disease prevention were compared; varying the number of times of presentation was also tested.

N=120

Design=4+1 Sample=0+1 Illness=NA Regimen=0 Measure=1 Definition=1

294. Kirscht JP, Haefner DP, Eveland JD: Public responses to various written appeals to participate in health screening. *Public Health Rep* 90:539-543, 1975

Evaluation of response to mailed messages in neutral form, "threat" form, and "positive" form, recommending participation in a multiphasic screening program.

N=13

Design=3+1 Sample=0+1 Illness=NA Regimen=NA Measure=2 Defintion=1

295. Korsch BM, Negrete VF: Doctor-patient communication. *Sci Am* 227:66-74, 1972

Taped interviews and questionnaires were utilized to assess features of the doctor-parent-patient interaction and family characteristics of new visitors to a pediatric outpatient department; the results were compared with subsequent compliance.

N=800

Design=1 Sample=0 Illness=0 Regimen=0 Measure=1+1 Definition=0

296. Krasnoff A: Failure of MMPI scales to predict treatment completion. *J Stud Alcohol* 38:1440-1442, 1977

Completers and dropouts from a hospital treatment program for alcoholics were compared on four MMPI measures.

N=31 completers, 30 dropouts

Design=2 Sample=0+1 Illness=0 Regimen=0 Measure=3 Definition=1

297. Kutt H, Haynes J, McDowell F: Some causes of ineffectiveness of diphenylhydantoin. *Arch Neurol* 14:489-492, 1966

Uncontrolled epileptics with low serum diphenylhydantoin levels despite prescription of high doses were admitted to a metabolic ward for assessment.

N=16

Design=1 Sample=0 Illness=1 Regimen=1 Measure=3 Definition=1

298. Lando H: A comparison of excessive and rapid smoking in the modification of chronic smoking behavior. *J Consult Clin Psychol* 43:350-355, 1975
Report on a controlled study that compared two methods of aversive therapy designed to reduce smoking.
N=45
Design=4 Sample=0 Illness=NA Regimen=2 Measure=3+1 Definition=2

299. _____: Aversive conditioning and contingency management in the treatment of smoking. *J Consult Clin Psychol* 44:312, 1976
Brief report of short- and long-term results of various behavioral anti-smoking procedures.
N=49
Design=3 Sample=0 Illness=1 Regimen=1 Measure=1 Definition=1

300. Lane MF, Barbarite RV, Bergner L, Harris D: Child-resistant medicine containers: Experience in the home. *Am J Public Health* 61:1861-1868, 1971
Controlled study of the effect of safety lock pill containers on compliance among outpatients.
N=273
Design=3 Sample=0 Illness=0 Regimen=1 Measure=2+1 Definition=2

301. Langfeld SB: Hypertension: Deficient care of the medically served. *Ann Intern Med* 78:19-23, 1973
Blood pressures were measured on patients awaiting surgery and the treatment status of those found hypertensive was determined.
N=185
Design=1 Sample=2+1 Illness=2 Regimen=0 Measure=1 Definition=1

302. Latiolais CJ, Berry CC: Misuse of prescription medications by outpatients. *Drug Intell Clin Pharm* 3:270-277, 1969
Outpatients from six OPD clinics were interviewed at the time that they received prescriptions and were reinterviewed at home seven-ten days later to determine medication compliance.
N=180
Design=1 Sample=0+1 Illness=0 Regimen=0 Measure=2+1 Definition=2

303. Lawton MP: Group methods in smoking withdrawal. *Arch Environ Health* 14:258-265, 1967
Four different group methods: education, group discussion, education and discussion combined, and five-day discussion, were compared with waiting list controls.
N=73
Design=3 Sample=0 Illness=NA Regimen=2 Measure=1+1 Definition=2

304. Leistyna JA, Macaulay JC: Therapy of streptococcal infections; do pediatric patients receive prescribed oral medication? *Am J Dis Child* 111:22-26, 1966
Study of pediatric compliance with oral penicillin for streptococcal pharyngitis in a private practice setting.
N=162
Design=1 Sample=1+1 Illness=3 Regimen=2 Measure=3+3 Definition=2

305. Lester D, Narkunski A, Burkman J, Gandica A: An exploratory study of correlates of success in a vocational training program for ex-addicts. *Psychol Rep* 37:1212-1214,1975
   Results from six standard psychological tests were assessed for their ability to differentiate between ex-addicts who completed a vocational training program and those who failed to complete the program.
   N=51
   Design=1 Sample=0 Illness=0 Regimen=1 Measure=0 Definition=1

306. Levav I, Arnon A: Non-respondents in a psychiatric survey. *Am J Public Health* 66:989-991, 1976
   A comparison of demographic features and psychiatric ratings between respondents and nonrespondents in a psychiatric survey in six Israeli villages.
   N=unknown
   Design=1 Sample=0+1 Illness=2 Regimen=1 Measure=1 Definition=2

307. Levitz L, Stunkard A: A therapeutic coalition for obesity: Behavior modification and patient self-help. *Am J Psychiatr* 131:423-427, 1974
   Comparison of behavior modification and nutrition education programs in addition to usual procedures at sixteen TOPS chapters for weight reduction.
   N=234
   Design=3 Sample=2 Illness=3 Regimen=1 Measure=4+1 Definition=1

308. Levy R, Claravall V: Differential effects of a phone reminder on appointment keeping for patients with long and short between-visit intervals. *Med Care* 15:435-438, 1977
   Telephone reminders were used to improve attendance at a pediatric clinic.
   N=98
   Design=4 Sample=0+1 Illness=0 Regimen=0 Measure=2 Definition=2

309. Levy RL: Relationship of an overt commitment to task compliance in behavior therapy. *J Behav Ther Exper Psychiat* 8:25-29, 1977
   Investigation of the effect of verbal and written commitments on compliance with an assigned task (telephone call).
   N=44
   Design=4 Sample=0+1 Illness=NA Regimen=1 Measure=2 Definition=2

310. Ley P, Jain VK, Skilbeck CE: A method for decreasing patients' medication errors. *Psychol Med* 6:599-601, 1976
   Three versions of an information leaflet varying in readability were compared to a no-leaflet control group revealing a reduction in medication errors over one prescription period among psychiatric outpatients.
   N=80 anxious and 80 depressed patients
   Design=4 Sample=0 Illness=0 Regimen=0+1 Measure=2 Definition=2

311. Ley P, Whitworth M, Skilbeck C, Woodward R, Pinsent R, Pike L, Clarkson M, Clark P: Improving doctor-patient communication in general practice. *J R Coll Gen Pract* 26:720-724, 1976
   Test of the capability of simplified doctor-patient communications to increase patient recall of advice and compliance with therapy.
   N=258
   Design=3+1 Sample=0+1 Illness=0 Regimen=0 Measure=1 Definition=2

312. Lima J, Nazarian L, Charney E, Lahti C: Compliance with short term
     antimicrobial therapy: Some techniques that help. *Pediatrics* 57:383-
     386, 1976
     Compliance was improved by both a clock printed on the prescription
     label and a refrigerator sticker that indicated dosing times.
     N=53 controls, 45 test 1, 60 test 2
     Design=3 Sample=0 Illness=1 Regimen=1 Measure=2 Definition=2
313. Lindstrom CJ: No shows: A problem in health care. *Nurs Outlook* 23:
     755-759, 1975
     A comparison of regular and irregular users of a child health clinic as
     measured by appointment-keeping behavior in a small sample of Mexi-
     can-American mothers.
     N=30
     Design=2 Sample=1 Illness=NA Regimen=2 Measure=1 Definition=1
314. Linkewich JA, Catalano RB, Flack HL: The effect of packaging and
     instruction on outpatient compliance with medication regimens. *Drug
     Intell Clinic Pharm* 8:10-15, 1974
     Patients presenting to a hospital outpatient pharmacy with a prescription
     for oral penicillin tablets QID for ten days were assigned randomly
     to one of four groups receiving different modalities of instruction,
     packaging, and labeling, including a standard labeling control group.
     Compliance was assessed at a home interview between days seven and
     nine and the results were compared.
     N=120
     Design=4 Sample=0+1 Illness=0 Regimen=2 Measure=2+2 Definition=2
315. Lipman RS, Rickels K, Uhlenhuth EH, Park LC, Fisher, S: Neurotics who
     fail to take their drugs. *Br J Psychiatr* 3:1043-1049, 1965
     Anxious, tense neurotics were entered into a placebo-controlled, double-
     blind trial of meprobamate with compliance as one of the variables
     studied.
     N=254
     Design=3 Sample=3 Illness=2 Regimen=2+1 Measure=2+1 Definition=2
316. Low S, Pearson J: Do leprosy patients take dapsone regularly? *Lepr Rev*
     45:218-223, 1974
     Report on a study that compared urine dapsone/creatinine ratios of super-
     vised and outpatient lepers to determine the regularity of drug taking.
     N=104
     Design=2 Sample=0+1 Illness=1 Regimen=1 Measure=3 Definition=1
317. Lowe ML: Effectiveness of teaching as measured by compliance with
     medical recommendations. *Nurs Res* 19:59-63, 1970
     A prenatal education program had no effect on the expectant mother's
     compliance with recommended practices during pregnancy.
     N=56
     Design=4 Sample=0 Illness=NA Regimen=1 Measure=1 Definition=0
318. _____: Relationship between compliance with medical regimen and out-
     come of pregnancy. *Nurs Res* 22:157-160, 1973
     Study of compliance of black primigravidas with "usual instructions"

given to antenatal patients, and of the relationship between compliance and pregnancy outcome.
N=56
Design=2 Sample=0 Illness=2 Regimen=1 Measure=1+1 Definition=2

319. Lowenthal DT, Briggs WA, Mutterperl R, Adelman B, Creditor MA: Patient compliance for antihypertensive medication: The usefulness of urine assays. *Curr Ther Res* 19:405-409, 1976
Method for qualitative biochemical determination of thiazides and alphamethyldopa in urine with results in a hypertensive population.
N=207
Design=1 Sample=0+1 Illness=1 Regimen=1 Measure=3 Definition=2

320. Ludwig EG, Adams SD: Patient cooperation in a rehabilitation center: Assumption of the client role. *J Health Soc Behav* 9:328-336, 1968
Comparison of role characteristics and social positions of patients who completed rehabilitation services with those who did not.
N=406
Design=1 Sample=1 Illness=1 Regimen=0 Measure=1 Definition=1

321. Ludwig EG, Gibson G: Self perception of sickness and the seeking of medical care. *J Health Soc Behav* 10:125-133, 1969
Social security disability benefits applicants who perceived themselves as poor in health were categorized by recency of utilization of medical services; recent utilizers were compared to those who had not sought care for at least six months.
N=227
Design=1 Sample=0 Illness=1 Regimen=0 Measure=2 Definition=0

322. Ludy J, Gagnon J, Caiola S: The patient-pharmacist interaction in two ambulatory settings—its relationship to patient satisfaction and drug misuse. *Drug Intell Clin Pharm* 11:81-89, 1977
Clinic patients were assigned randomly to a satellite pharmacy with a private consultation room or to a traditional pharmacy with an open-window setting. Drug-taking behavior of the two groups was measured by questionnaires.
N=75
Design=4 Sample=1+1 Illness=NA Regimen=1 Measure=2+1 Defintion=2

323. Lue H, Chen C, Wei H: Some problems in long-term prevention of streptococcal infection among children with rheumatic heart disease in Taiwan. *Jpn Heart J* 17:550-559, 1976
An appraisal of factors leading to noncompliance in a long-term medication prophylaxis program.
N=130
Design=1+1 Sample=0+1 Illness=1 Regimen=2 Measure=3+1 Definition=2

324. Lund M, Jorgenson RS, Kuhl V: Serum diphenylhydantoin (phenytoin) in ambulant patients with epilepsy. *Epilepsia* 5:51-58, 1964
Controlled study of the effect on compliance of feeding back compliance-monitoring results to patients on diphenylhydantoin.
N=36 study, 40 control
Design=4 Sample=0+1 Illness=1 Regimen=1 Measure=3 Definition=2

325. MacCuish A, Munro J, Duncan L: Follow-up study of refractory obesity
     treated by fasting. *Br Med J* 1:91-92, 1968
     People who had been unable to lose weight in an ambulatory setting were
     fasted in hospital and then followed for several months after discharge.
     N=25
     Design=3 Sample=0+1 Illness=2 Regimen=2 Measure=4 Definition=2

326. MacDonald ET, MacDonald JB, Phoenix M: Improving drug compliance
     after hospital discharge. *Br Med J* 2:618-621, 1977
     The effects of pharmacist's counseling and three types of memory aids on
     medication errors were assessed in elderly outpatients.
     N=165
     Design=3 Sample=0+1 Illness=NA Regimen=1 Measure=2+2 Definition=2

327. Macdonald ME, Hagberg KL, Grossman BJ: Social factors in relation to
     participation in follow-up care of rheumatic fever. *J Pediatr* 62:503-
     513, 1963
     Pediatric patients on a rheumatic fever follow-up program were assessed
     for attendance and compliance with medical advice, comparing the re-
     sults with medical and social characteristics of the patients.
     N=123
     Design=2 Sample=1+1 Illness=3 Regimen=1 Measure=1 Definition=1

328. MacElveen PM: Cooperative triad in home dialysis care and patient out-
     comes. *Communicating Nurs Res* 5:134-147, 1972
     Cooperation among the patient, the assistant partner, and a significant
     staff member was studied for its effects on the outcome of home
     dialysis treatment.
     N=21
     Design=1 Sample=0+1 Illness=1 Regimen=1 Measure=4+4 Definition=1

329. Madden E: Evaluation of outpatient pharmacy patient counseling. *J Am
     Pharm Assoc* 13:437-443, 1973
     Military personnel were assigned randomly to a control group or an experi-
     mental group to determine the effects of pharmacist-patient consulta-
     tion on medical compliance.
     N=240
     Design=3 Sample=0+1 Illness=NA Regimen=1 Measure=2 Definition=2

330. Maddock RK: Patient cooperation in taking medicines; a study involving
     isoniazid and aminosalicylic acid. *JAMA* 199:137-140, 1967
     Compliance was studied among tuberculous outpatients, comparing re-
     sults from different methods and sites of monitoring and comparing
     results for different regimens.
     N=50
     Design=1 Sample=1 Illness=2 Regimen=1 Measure=4+1 Definition=2

331. Malahy B: The effect of instruction and labeling on the number of medi-
     cation errors made by patients at home. *Am J Hosp Pharm* 23:283-
     292, 1966
     Controlled study of the effect on the number of errors in self-administered
     medication of labeling prescriptions and of planned instruction.
     N=10 study, 10 control

Design=3 Sample=0 Illness=0 Regimen=0 Measure=1 Definition=2
332. Malik S, Singh VP, Goel BF: Follow-up results of occlusion and pleoptic
     treatment. *Acta Ophthalmol* 53:620-626, 1975
     Study of long-term results for various methods of treating amblyopia,
       showing correlation between compliance and achievement of the thera-
       peutic goal.
     N=not given
Design=1 Sample=0+1 Illness=1 Regimen=1 Measure=0 Definition=0
333. Malone JI, Hellrung JM, Malphus EW, Rosenbloom AL, Grgic A, Weber
     FT: Good diabetic control—a study in mass delusion. *J Pediatr* 88:943-
     947, 1976
     Evaluation of diabetic control and reliability of self-measurement of
       control among children at a diabetic camp.
     N=220
Design=1 Sample=0+1 Illness=3 Regimen=1 Measure=3+1 Definition=2
334. Mann L, Janis IL: A follow-up on the long-term effects of emotional
     role-playing. *J Pers Soc Psychol* 8:339-342, 1968
     Heavy-smoking female university student volunteers participated in a
       study to assess the effects on smoking of emotional role-playing versus
       passive listening in an anticancer demonstration.
     N=26
Design=4 Sample=0 Illlness=NA Regimen=0 Measure=1 Definition=2
335. Marsh WW, Perlman LV: Understanding congestive heart failure and self-
     administration of digoxin. *Geriatrics* 27:65-70, 1972
     Study to determine if an understanding of congestive heart failure was
       related to the reliability of self-administration of digoxin among out-
       patients.
     N=60
Design=1 Sample=1+1 Illness=1 Regimen=1 Measure=1 Definition=2
336. Marshall A, Barritt DW: Drug compliance in hypertensive patients. *Br Med
     J* 1:1278-1279, 1977
     A letter describing a double-blind comparison of atenolol with placebo
       given either twice or once daily in the treatment of asymtomatic hyper-
       tension.
     N=24
Design=3 Sample=0 Illness=1 Regimen=1 Measure=2 Definition=2
337. Martens LV, Frazier PJ, Hirt KJ, Meskin LH, Proshek J: Developing
       brushing performance in second graders through behavior modifica-
       tion. *Health Serv Res* 88:818-823, 1973
     Behavior modification techniques, discovery learning, and individual inter-
       action were utilized to improve dental hygiene among second grade
       schoolers.
     N=95 study, 102 control
Design=3 Sample=3 Illness=NA Regimen=1 Measure=4 Definition=2
338. Mason AS, Forrest IS, Forrest FM, Butler H: Adherence to maintenance
       therapy and rehospitalization. *Dis Nerv Syst* 24:103-104, 1963
     Compliance with prescribed phenothiazines was assessed among chronic

ambulatory schizophrenics on their return to the hospital in relapse.
N=48
Design=1 Sample=0 Illness=0 Regimen=1 Measure=3 Definition=1

339. Mason RM, Barnardo DE, Fox WR, Weatherall M: Assessment of drugs in outpatients with rheumatoid arthritis. *Ann Rheum Dis* 26:373-388, 1967
Two studies of the efficacy of four drugs for the treatment of established rheumatoid arthritis among separate groups of outpatients with compliance monitoring as a feature of the design.
N=36, 36
Design=4 Sample=0+1 Illness=2 Regimen=1+1 Measure=3+2 Definition=1

340. Mattar ME, Markello J, Yaffe SJ: Inadequacies in the pharmacologic management of abulatory children. *J Pediatr* 87:137-141, 1975
Thorough evaluation of various aspects of noncompliance among pediatric patients with otitis media.
N=674
Design=2+1 Sample0+1 Illness=1 Regimen=1+1 Measure=2 Definition=2

341. _____: Pharmaceutic factors affecting pediatric compliance. *Pediatrics* 55:101-108, 1975
Study of the effect of verbal and written instructions from hospital pharmacy personnel on poor compliance among pediatric patients with otitis media.
A. N=100
Design=2+1 Sample=0+1 Illness=1 Regimen=1+1 Measure=2 Definition=2
B. N=233
Design=3+1 Sample=0 Illness=1 Regimen=1 Measure=2 Definition=2

342. Mausner J, Mausner B, Rial WY: The influence of a physician on the smoking of his patients. *Am J Public Health* 58:46-53, 1968
Report on the effect of a general practitioner's advice plus special pamphlet on smoking cessation.
N=125
Design=3 Sample=0+1 Illness=1 Regimen=1 Measure=1 Definition=2

343. Mausner JS: Cigarette smoking among patients with respiratory disease. *Am Rev Resp Dis* 102:704-713, 1970
Report of smoking cessation among patients of chest physicians.
N=111
Design=2 Sample=2+1 Illness=1 Regimen=1 Measure=1 Definition=1

344. McClellan TA, Cowan G: Use of antipsychotic and antidepressant drugs by chronically ill patients. *Am J Psychiatr* 126:113-115, 1970
Study of compliance among outpatients on antipsychotic and antidepressant medications using objective and subjective measures.
N=286
Design=1 Sample=0+1 Illness=0 Regimen=1+1 Measure=3+2 Definition=0

345. McInnis JK: Do patients take antituberculosis drugs? *Am J Nurs* 70:2152-2153, 1970
Verbal reports were compared with an objective measure of compliance among tuberculous outpatients at five county health clinics.

N=144
Design=1 Sample=0 Illness=1 Regimen=1 Measure=3+1 Definition=1
346. McIntire M, Angle C, Sathees K, Lee P: Safety packaging—what does the public think? *Am J Public Health* 67:169-171, 1977
A telephone survey was used to collect data on attitudes toward and use of prescription safety packaging.
N=636
Design=1 Sample=3 Illness=NA Regimen=0 Measure=1 Definition=2
347. McKenney JM, Harrison WL: Drug-related hospital admissions. *Am J Hosp Pharm* 33:792-795, 1976
The association between hospital admissions and drug-related problems including noncompliance was studied in a large teaching hospital.
N=216
Design=1 Sample=0+1 Illness=1 Regimen=1 Measure=1+1 Definition=2
348. McKenney JM, Slining JM, Henderson HR, Devins D, Barr M: The effect of clinical pharmacy services on patients with essential hypertension. *Circulation* 48:1104-1111, 1973
Hypertensive outpatients of a comprehensive health care clinic were assigned alternately to control or study groups, the latter receiving the special attention of a community pharmacist who "educated" the patients, monitored blood pressure control, and assisted in the management of questions and problems that arose. Compliance and blood pressure levels were compared in the two groups.
N=25 study, 25 control
Design=3 Sample=0 Illness=2 Regimen=0 Measure=2 Definition=1
349. McKercher PL, Rucker TD: Patient knowledge and compliance with medication instructions. *J Am Pharm Assoc* 17:282-291, 1977
The relationship between compliance and patient knowledge was examined in a random sample of elderly outpatients from a general medicine and an internal medicine clinic.
N=60
Design=1 Sample=1+1 Illness=0 Regimen=1 Measure=2+1 Definition=1
350. Mealey SA, Kane RL: Factors that influence Navajo patients to keep appointments. *Nurse Pract* 2:18-22, 1977
A study of some factors affecting appointment keeping in Navajo community clinic.
N=351 follow-up appointments
Design=2 Sample=0+1 Illness=1 Regimen=1 Measure=2 Definition=2
351. Mealey SA: Navajos can and do keep appointments. *Nurse Pract* 1:13-15, 1975
A brief description of appointment-keeping behavior by Navajos at a family health clinic.
N=375 appointments
Design=1 Sample=0+1 Illness=NA Regimen=1 Measure=2 Definition=1
352. Meller W, Anderson A: Medical compliance, the effect of appointment reminders on keeping appointments in a core city pediatric outpatient department. *Minn Med* 59:625-626, 1976

Mailed appointment reminders decreased broken appointments compared
to a concurrent, but nonrandom control group.
N=566 experimental, controls not stated
Design=3 Sample=0 Illness=0 Regimen=0 Measure=2 Definition=1

353. Meyer AJ, Henderson JB: Multiple risk factor reduction in the prevention
of cardiovascular disease. *Prev Med* 3:225-236, 1974
Business firm employees at "high risk" for cardiac disease were assigned
randomly to control, counseling, or a behavior modification program
with exercise, weight reduction, and smoking reduction as the behavioral endpoints.
N=36
Design=4 Sample=0+1 Illness=NA Regimen=1 Measure=4+1 Definition=2

354. Meyers A, Dolan TF, Mueller D: Compliance and self-medication in cystic
fibrosis. *Am J Dis Child* 129:1011-1013, 1975
Patients with cystic fibrosis were studied to determine the relationship
between compliance with antibiotics and the serverity of the disease.
N=61
Design=1 Sample=0 Illness=1 Regimen=1+1 Measure=4 Definition=2

355. Michaux WW: Side-effects, resistance and dosage deviations in psychiatric
outpatients treated with tranquilizers. *J Nerv Ment Dis* 133:203-212,
1961
Report of compliance and side effect aspects of a double-blind randomized
trial of three medications or placebo among psychiatric outpatients at
22 mental hygiene clinics.
N=180
Design=4 Sample=2+1 Illness=0 Regimen=2 Measure=1 Definition=1

356. Miettinen M, Turpeinen O, Karvonen MJ, Elosuo R, Paavilainen E: Effect
of cholesterol-lowing diet on mortality from coronary heart-disease and
other causes. *Lancet* 2:835-838, 1972
Study of the efficacy of a low saturated fat diet on coronary heart disease
mortality and morbidity at two mental hospitals. Individual compliance
records were not kept but "compliance" was monitored through yearly
biopsies of adipose tissue.
N=29,217 "person years"
Design=3 Sample=0+1 Illness=0 Regimen=1 Measure=4 Definition=1

357. Miller JR, Pless IB: Child automobile restraints: Evaluation of health
education. *Pediatrics* 59:907-911, 1977
Three methods of instructions (pamphlet alone; pamphlet plus verbal
instructions by the pediatrician; and pamphlet, verbal instructions,
plus a tape slide show) were compared to a control group.
N=654
Design=4 Sample=0+1 Illness=NA Regimen=2 Measure=1 Definition=2

358. Miller W: Drug usage: Compliance of patients with instructions on medi-
cation. *J Am Osteopath Assoc* 75:401-404, 1975
Questionnaire survey of patients with chronic diseases to assess compli-
ance.
N=57
Design=1 Sample=0 Illness=1 Regimen=0 Measure=1 Definition=2

359. Mitchell R, Robson H: Patients' compliance with follow-up after treatment of gonococcal urethritis. *Can Med Assoc J* 116:48-50, 1977
A comparison of some variables in two groups of men treated for gonococcal urethritis who returned for follow-up study on their own initiative or required telephone tracing before follow-up.
N=302
Design=1 Sample=0+1 Illness=1 Regimen=2 Measure=3+1 Definition=2
360. Mohler DN, Wallin DG, Dreyfus EG, Bakst HF: Studies in the home treatment of streptococcal disease. *N Engl J Med* 254:45-50, 1956
The effectiveness of oral and intramuscular penicillin for treatment of proven b-hemolytic streptococcal pharyngitis was compared among two dystemporal samples of pediatric outpatients, with the greater efficacy of the intramuscular preparation being allowed for.
N=127, 196
Design=3 Sample=0+1 Illness=0 Regimen=2 Measure=1+1 Definition=1
361. Mojonnier L, Hall Y: The national diet-heart study—assessment of dietary adherence. *J Am Diet Assoc* 52:288-292, 1968
Description of methods of dietary adherence in the national diet-heart study.
N=variable
Design=2 Sample=0 Illness=0 Regimen=0 Measure=4+2 Definition=0
362. Moon MH, Moon BA, Black WA: Compliancy in splint-wearing behaviour of patients with rheumatoid arthritis. *NZ Med J* 83:360-365, 1976
Descriptive study of frequency of and reasons for noncompliance with wearing hand and wrist splints.
N=46
Design=1 Sample=0+1 Illness=1 Regimen=1 Measure=1+2 Defintion=1
363. Morrow G, Del Gaudio A, Carpenter P: The dropout and the terminator: A methodological note on definitions. *J Clin Psychol* 33:867-869, 1977
A study indicating the difference between the definitions for dropouts and for terminators in a sample of psychotherapy outpatients.
N=221
Design=1+1 Sample=1+2 Illness=1 Regimen=0 Measure=3 Definition=2
364. Moulding T, Onstad GD, Sbarbaro JA: Supervision of outpatient drug therapy with the medication monitor. *Ann Intern Med* 73:559-564, 1970
Uncontrolled study of compliance of tuberculous outpatients with medication, utilizing a vertical-stack unit-dose medication dispenser-monitor.
N=122
Design=1 Sample=1 Illness=1 Regimen=1 Measure=2+1 Definition=2
365. Moulding T: Preliminary study of the pill calendar as a method of improving the self-administration of drugs. *Am Rev Resp Dis* 84:284-287, 1961
Pilot study of the use of a pill calendar to improve the compliance with antituberculous medication of Navajo Indians.
N=29
Design=2 Sample=0 Illness=0 Regimen=2 Measure=2+2 Definition=2

366. Moulding TS, Halper AR, Mkutu MP, Halper S: Self-administration of isoniazid and thiacetazone studied by the medication monitor. Unpublished paper
A medication monitor employing stack loading of unit doses of isoniazid and thiacetazone tablets with a spring-loaded uranium source and a photographic film strip to record package removal was used to study compliance among tuberculous outpatients at a district hospital in Malawi.
N=13
Design=2 Sample=0 Illness=1 Regimen=1 Measure=4+1 Definition=2
367. Murthy RS, Ghosh A, Anuradha D: Patients who refuse psychiatric help— a follow-up study. *Bull Pgi (India)* 10:22-26, 1976
Reasons for dropping out of psychiatric care after initial evaluations were studied.
N=21
Design=1 Sample=0+1 Illness=2 Regimen=0 Measure=2 Definition=1
368. Murthy RS, Ghosh A, Wig N: Drop-outs from psychiatric walk-in clinic. *Indian J Psychiatr* 19:11-17, 1977
Report of various demographic, social, and clinical variables affecting acceptance or nonacceptance of treatment at a walk-in psychiatric clinic.
N=110
Design=1 Sample=1+1 Illness=1 Regimen=1 Measure=3 Definition=2
369. Murthy RS, Ghosh A, Wig NN: Treatment acceptance patterns in a psychiatric out-patient clinic: Study of demographic and clinical variables. *Indian J Psychiatr* 16:323-329, 1974
A study of treatment acceptance patterns in a psychiatric outpatient clinic and some variables related to compliance.
N=135
Design=1 Sample=1+1 Illness=NA Regimen=1 Measure=2 Definition=2
370. Mushlin AI, Appel FA: Diagnosing patient noncompliance. *Arch Intern Med* 137: 318-321, 1977
Patient compliance with return appointments and medication taking was predicted by interns and residents at discharge from hospital and compared with subsequent compliance.
N=187 for appointments, 71 for pill counts
Design=2 Sample=0+1 Illness=0 Regimen=0+1 Measure=2+1 Definition=2
371. Mushlin AI: A study of physicians'ability to predict patient compliance. Master's thesis, Johns Hopkins University, Baltimore, May 1972
Interns' and residents' predictions of short-term compliance of their patients immediately following discharge from hospital were compared with objective determinations at the time of the first clinic visit.
N=191
Design=2 Sample=3+1 Illness=0 Regimen=1 Measure=2+1 Definition=1
372. Myers E, Calvert E: The effect of forewarning on the occurrence of side-effects and discontinuances of medication in patients on dothiepin. *J Intern Med Res* 4:237-240, 1976
Depressed patients were given either information about the possible side

effects of dothiepin or no information and after two weeks were questioned about their compliance.
N=89

Design=3+1 Sample=0+1 Illness=1 Regimen=2 Measure=1 Definition=2
373. Myers ED: Age, persistence and improvement in an open out-patient group. *Br J Psychiatr* 127: 157-159, 1975
Relationship between age and treatment continuance and outcome was assessed among psychiatric outpatients.
N=87

Design=2 Sample=0+1 Illness=0 Regimen=1 Measure=3+1 Definition=1
374. Nakielna EM, Cragg R, Grzybowski S: Lifelong follow-up of inactive tuberculosis: Its value and limitations. *Am Rev Resp Dis* 112:765-772, 1975
Report of experience in British Columbia with lifelong surveillance of patients with inactive tuberculosis.
N=300

Design=2 Sample=2+1 Illness=2 Regimen=2 Measure=2+1 Definition=2
375. Nazarian L, Mechaber J, Charney E, Coulter M: Effect of a mailed appointment reminder on appointment keeping. *Pediatrics* 53:349-352, 1974
Study of the effect of a simple postal card reminder on attendance at a pediatric clinic.
N=663

Design=3 Sample=0+1 Illness=1 Regimen=1 Measure=2 Definition=1
376. Neely E, Patrick ML: Problems of aged persons taking medications at home. *Nurs Res* 17:52-55, 1968
A random sample of patients over the age of sixty years, in a prepaid group practice was studied for medication errors at home.
N=59

Design=1 Sample=1+1 Illness=1 Regimen=0+1 Measure=1 Definition=2
377. Nelson A, Gold B, Hutchinson R, Benezra E: Drug default among schizophrenic patients. *Am J Hosp Pharm* 32:1237-1242, 1975
Study of the relationship to compliance of patients' attitudes and the treatment milieu among schizophrenic patients. An in-hospital self-medication program was also evaluated.
N=40

Design=4 Sample=0+1 Illness=1 Regimen=1 Measure=4 Definition=2
378. Neve HK: Demonstration of largactil (chlorpromazine hydrochloride) in the urine. *J Ment Sci* 104:488-490, 1958
Description of a qualitative biochemical method of detecting chlorpromazine in urine.
N=109

Design=1 Sample=0 Illness=1 Regimen=1 Measure=3+1 Definition=1
379. Nielsen HB, Bjerre P: How do discharged patients administer the prescribed medicine? An investigation by questionnaire sent to patients discharged from a medical department. *Ugeskr Laeger* 135:2171-2174, 1973
Study of post-hospital discharge compliance rates in Denmark.

N=150

Design=1 Sample=0+1 Illness=0 Regimen=0 Measure=0 Definition=0

380. Nikias MK: Social class and the use of dental care under prepayment. *Med Care* 6:381-393, 1968

Utilization of dental services by subscribers to a group prepaid dental plan was studied, comparing social characteristics of those who used the service for symptomatic or for prophylactic purposes.

N=5,980

Design=1 Sample=2+1 Illness=NA Regimen=0 Measure=1 Definition=0

381. Normand J, Legendre M, Kahn J, Bourdarias J, Mathivat A: Comparative efficacy of short-acting and long-acting quinidine for maintenance of sinus rhythm after electrical conversion of atrial fibrillation. *Br Heart J* 38:381-387, 1976

Sinus rhythm was measured by electrocardiogram in patients admitted for atrial fibrillation to compare BID and QID administration of quinidine.

N=40

Design=4+1 Sample=0+1 Illness=2 Regimen=1 Measure=4 Definition=1

382. Nugent CA, Ward J, Macdiarmid WD, McCall JC, Baukol J, Tyler FH: Glucocorticoid toxicity. Single contrasted with divided daily doses of prednisolone. *J Chron Dis* 18:323-332, 1965

Study of intermittent versus continuous prednisolone for rheumatoid arthritis patients (cross-over) with analysis of compliance with medication and of dropouts.

N=38

Design=4 Sample=0 Illness=2 Regimen=2 Measure=2 Definition=1

383. O'Leary MR, Rohsenow DJ, Donovan DM: Locus of control and patient attrition from an alcoholism treatment program. *J Consult Clin Psychol* 44:686-687, 1976

A brief report of the association between locus of control and drop-out rates in two groups of male alcoholics.

N=153 dropouts

Design=1+1 Sample=0+1 Illness=1 Regimen=1 Measure=2 Definition=2

384. Oakes TW, Ward JR, Gray RM, Klauber MR, Moody PM: Family expectations and arthritis patient compliance to a hand resting splint regimen. *J Chron Dis* 22:757-764, 1970

Married arthritic outpatients who were given splints to wear while sleeping were assessed for compliance and the results compared with ratings of the spouses' expectations that the patient should wear the splint.

N=66

Design=1 Sample=0+1 Illness=1 Regimen=1 Measure=1 Definition=2

385. Oh SB: A clinical and sociomedical study for defaulting tuberculosis treatment. *Int Union Tuberc Bull* 47:223-224, 1974

A brief account of a study examining the effects of some clinical and demographic factors on defaulting from tuberculosis treatment in Korea.

N=112 defaulters, 88 control

Design=2 Sample=0+1 Illness=1 Regimen=0 Measure=2 Definition=0

386. Oja P, Teraslinna P, Parjanen T, Karava R: Feasibility of an 18 months'
     physical training program for middle-aged men and its effect on physi-
     cal fitness. *Am J Public Health* 64:459-465, 1974
     Report on participation and results in a rigorous exercise program offered
     to middle-aged manager-executives.
     N=178
     Design=1 Sample=0+1 Illness=NA Regimen=2 Measure=2 Definition=1
387. Onstad GD, Sbarboro JA, Rotenberg L: Post hospital chemotherapy of the
     unreliable patient. *Am Rev Resp Dis* 101:258-263, 1970
     Study of several methods utilized to achieve compliance with antituber-
     culous medication among outpatients deemed particularly unreliable
     due to poor attendance, lack of cooperativeness, and positive sputum
     cultures.
     N=57
     Design=2 Sample=0 Illness=2 Regimen=2 Measure=3 Definition=2
388. Ottens AJ: The effect of transcendental meditation upon modifying the
     cigarette smoking habit. *J Sch Health* 45:577-583, 1975
     Report of a study that compared the effectiveness of transcendental
     meditation, self-control, and no treatment on reducing smoking.
     N=54
     Design=4 Sample=1 Illness=NA Regimen=2 Measure=1 Definition=1
389. Palmer A, Ayers WR, Abraham S, Wilbur M: Spirometry using motiva-
     tional techniques. *J Chron Dis* 24:643-650, 1971
     In order to achieve maximum patient effort in the measurement of lung
     function through spirometry, a simple motivational device was de-
     veloped.
     N=890
     Design=3 Sample=0 Illness=NA Regimen=2 Measure=3 Definition=2
390. Pam A, Bryskin L, Rachlin S, Rosenblatt: Community adjustment of self-
     discharged patients. *Psychiatr Q* 47:175-183, 1973
     Comparison of community adjustment between elopers and normal
     discharges from an open psychiatric hospital.
     N=42
     Design=2 Sample=0 Illness=0 Regimen=0 Measure=2 Definition=1
391. Panepinto W, Higgins M: Keeping alcoholics in treatment. *Q J Stud
     Alcohol* 30:414-419, 1969
     Study of the effect of process changes and letter reminders in improving
     attendance of alcoholics at an alcohol clinic.
     N=variable
     Design=3 Sample=0+1 Illness=1 Regimen=0 Measure=2 Definition=2
392. Park LC, Lipman RS: A comparison of patient dosage deviation reports
     with pill counts. *Psychopharmacologia* 6:299-302, 1964
     Verbal reports were compared to pill counts as measures of compliance
     among neurotically depressed outpatients as part of a controlled study
     of imipramine and placebo.
     N=42
     Design=2 Sample=0 Illness=1 Regimen=2 Measure=2+1 Definition=2

393. Parker LB, Bender LF: Problem of home treatment in arthritis. *Arch Phys Med Rehabil* 38:392-394, 1957
     A questionnaire was administered to patients returning to an arthritis clinic to assess compliance and reasons for noncompliance with physical therapy.
     N=56
     Design=1 Sample=1+1 Illness=1 Regimen=1 Measure=1 Definition=1

394. Parkes CM, Brown GW, Monck EM: The general practitioner and the schizophrenic patient. *Br Med J* 1:972-976, 1962
     One-year follow-up of schizophrenics discharged from hospital with attention focused on source of care, medications, compliance, and relapse rates.
     N=96
     Design=1 Sample=2 Illness=2 Regimen=0 Measure=1 Definition=0

395. Parkin DM, Henney CR, Quirk J, Crooks J: Deviation from prescribed drug treatment after discharge from hospital. *Br Med J* 2:686-688, 1976
     Patient compliance and medication knowledge were studied following discharge from general medical wards.
     N=130
     Design=1 Sample=0+1 Illness=1 Regimen=1+1 Measure=2+1 Definition=2

396. Pathmanathan I: The improvement of immunization status in children attending child health clinics. *J Trop Med Hyg* 76:294-296, 1973
     Before-after study of effect of changing schedule and increasing convenience for immunization in children.
     N=56,000
     Design=3 Sample=2 Illness=NA Regimen=1 Measure=3+1 Definition=0

397. Paulson P, Bauch R, Paulson M, Zilz D: Medication data sheets—an aid to patient education. *Drug Intell Clin Pharm* 10:448-453, 1976
     Knowledge of medication regimen rather than actual compliance was measured to determine the effectiveness of written and verbal instructions.
     N=1,500
     Design=4 Sample=0+1 Illness=0 Regimen=0 Measure=1 Definition=1

398. Penman HG, Wraith DG: Two simple tests to detect omission of prescribed para-aminosalicylic acid. *Lancet* 2:552-553, 1956
     Details of laboratory techniques given, as well as description of results of tests, in patients with tuberculosis who were taking or not taking PAS.
     N=22
     Design=1 Sample=0 Illness=1 Regimen=1 Measure=3 Definition=1

399. Pentecost R, Zwerenz B, Manuel J: Intrafamily identity and home dialysis success. *Nephron* 17:88-103, 1976
     Evaluation of the predictive value of a measure of family cohesiveness and personal identity with respect to success in home dialysis.
     N=40
     Design=2+1 Sample=0+1 Illness=1 Regimen=1 Measure=4 Definition=2

400. Perry C, Mullen G: The effects of hypnotic susceptibility on reducing smoking behavior treated by an hypnotic technique. *J Clin Psychol* 31:498-505, 1975
Smokers were tested for their susceptibility to hypnotism; this measure was compared to smoking behavior after hypnotic therapy.
N=38
Design=1+1 Sample=0+1 Illness=2 Regimen=1 Measure=1 Definition=2
401. Piper G, Jones J, Matthews V: The Saskatoon Smoking Study: Results of the second year. *Can J Public Health* 65:127-129, 1974
Assessment of the effects of a student-directed program in smoking education among junior high school students.
N=uncertain
Design=3 Sample=2 Illness=1 Regimen=0 Measure=1 Definition=1
402. Pitman ER, Benzier EE, Katz M: Clinic experience with a urine PAS test. *Dis Chest* 36:1-2, 1959
Clinical validation of a urinary test for PAS among "suitable" tuberculous outpatients.
N=61
Design=1 Sample=0 Illness=1 Regimen=1 Measure=3+1 Definition=2
403. Podell RN, Kent D, Keller K: Patient psychological defenses and physician response in the long-term treatment of hypertension. *J Fam Pract* 3:145-149, 1976
Descriptive study of patient and physician factors contributing to dropping out and pill noncompliance in a private family practice.
N=53
Design=1 Sample=0+1 Illness=3 Regimen=0 Measure=2+2 Definition=2
404. Porter AM, McCullough DM: Counselling against cigarette smoking. *Practitioner* 209:686-689, 1972
Controlled trial of the effect on patients' smoking habits of counseling by a private general practitioner.
N=191
Design=4 Sample=1 Illness=NA Regimen=2 Measure=1 Definition=2
405. Porter AM: Drug defaulting in a general practice. *Br Med J* 1:218-222, 1969
Compliance rates were assessed in a general practice among groups of patients with depression, acute infections, various chronic diseases, and in pregnancy.
N=variable
Design=1 Sample=0 Illness=1 Regimen=1 Measure=3+1 Definition=2
406. Powell B, Othmer E, Sinkhorn C: Pharmacological aftercare for homogeneous groups of patients. *Hosp Community Psychiatr* 28:125-127, 1977
The effect of psychopharmacological support groups was studied for outpatients being treated with prolixin, lithium carbonate, or antidepressants.
N=85
Design=1+1 Sample=0+1 Illness=1 Regimen=1 Measure=3 Definition=1

407. Pozen M, Stechmiller J, Harris W, Smith S, Fried D, Voigt G: A nurse
     rehabilitator's impact on patients with myocardial infarcation. *Med
     Care* 15:830-837, 1977
     The effectiveness of a nurse rehabilitator in facilitating patients' recovery
     was assessed in high and low risk cardiac patients.
     N=102
     Design=4+1 Sample=1+1 Illness=3 Regimen=1 Measure=1+1 Definition=1
408. Pragoff H: Adjustment of tuberculosis patients one year after hospital
     discharge. *Pub Health Rep* 77:671-679, 1962
     Compliance of tuberculosis patients one year following hospital discharge
     was studied in relation to social and environmental factors.
     N=66
     Design=1 Sample=1+1 Illness=1 Regimen=1 Measure=1 Definition=1
409. Pratt T, Linn M, Carmichael J, Webb N: The alcoholic's perception of the
     ward as a predictor of aftercare attendance. *J Clin Psychol* 33:915-918,
     1977
     An analysis of background and attitudinal factors of attenders and non-
     attenders at outpatient services for discharged alcoholic patients.
     N=35
     Design=1+1 Sample=1+1 Illness=1 Regimen=1 Measure=3 Definition=2
410. Preston DF, Miller FL: The tuberculosis outpatient's defection from
     therapy. *Am J Med Sci* 247:21-25, 1964
     Tuberculosis outpatients' compliance statements and their physicians'
     estimates of compliance were compared with the results of urinary
     measures of INH and PAS.
     N=25
     Design=1 Sample=0+1 Illness=1 Regimen=1 Measure=3+1 Definition=2
411. Prickman LE, Koelsche GA, Berkman JM, Carryer HM, Peters GA, Hender-
     son LL: Does the executive health program meet its objective? *JAMA*
     167:1451-1455, 1958
     Compliance with medical advice was studied among executives who had
     had at least two complete periodic health assessments at the Mayo
     Clinic.
     N=231
     Design=1 Sample=0 Illness=1 Regimen=1 Measure=1 Definition=1
412. Quinn R, Federspiel C, Lefkowitz L, Christie A: Recurrences and sequelae
     of rheumatic fever in Nashville. *JAMA* 238:1512-1515, 1977
     Those who adhered to penicillin prophylaxis were compared to those who
     did not in a follow-up study of patients with rheumatic fever.
     N=269
     Design=1+1 Sample=0+1 Illness=1 Regimen=1 Measure=1 Definition=1
413. Radelfinger S: Some effects of fear-arousing communications on pre-
     ventive health behavior. *Health Educ Monogr* 19:2-15, 1965
     Study of the effect of high-fear, low-fear, and neutral messages about
     tetanus in inducing compliance with recommendations to obtain a
     tetanus shot among college students.
     N=194
     Design=4 Sample=0+1 Illness=NA Regimen=2 Measure=3+1 Definition=2

414. Rae JB: The influence of the wives on the treatment outcome of alco-
     holics: A follow-up study of two years. *Br J Psychiatr* 120:601-613,
     1972
     Study of the personality traits of wives of alcoholics in relation to treat-
     ment success for their husbands.
     N=62
     Design=2 Sample=2+1 Illness=1 Regimen=1 Measure=2 Definition=2

415. Raw M: Persuading people to stop smoking. *Behav Res Ther* 14:97-101,
     1976
     Report of an experiment studying the effect on smoking of a physician's
     advice to stop and of whether or not the interviewer wore a white
     coat.
     N=40
     Design=3+1 Sample=0+1 Illness=1 Regimen=1 Measure=1 Definition=1

416. Rayner JF: Socioeconomic status and factors influencing the dental health
     practices of mothers. *Am J Public Health* 60:1250-1259, 1970
     Descriptive study of demographic, attitudinal, perceptual, and dental
     health behavior responses to a questionnaire administrated to mothers
     of children aged eleven to fourteen years.
     N=524
     Design=1 Sample=2+1 Illness=NA Regimen=1 Measure=1 Definition=1

417. Raynes AE, Warren G: Some characteristics of "drop-outs" at first contact
     with a psychiatric clinic. *Community Ment Health J* 7:144-150, 1971
     Comparison of sex, source of referral, and waiting period between at-
     tenders and nonattenders.
     N=738
     Design=1 Sample=0+1 Illness=1 Regimen=0 Measure=2 Definition=1

418. Recruitment in large-scale clinical trials pp 47-49, in Weiss SM (ed): *Heart
     and Lung Institute Working Conference on Health Behavior*, Bethesda,
     NIH, 1975
     People were asked to participate in a blood donor clinic in one of three
     ways: an extreme request (donate every two months for three years)
     followed by the critical request (donate tomorrow); a minimal request
     (display a blood bank card) followed by the critical request; and the
     critical request only.
     N=189
     Design=3 Sample=0 Illness=NA Regimen=2 Measure=3 Definition=1

419. Rehder T, McCoy L, Blackwell B, Whitehead W, Robinson A: Improving
     compliance by counseling and pill container. *Am J Pharm* (In press)
     Factorial evaluation of medication counseling and special pill containers
     in improving compliance with antihypertensive medications.
     N=100
     Design=3 Sample=0 Illness=1 Regimen=2 Measure=2+2 Definition=2

420. Reibel EM: Study to determine the feasibility of a self-medication
     program for patients at a rehabilitation center. *Nurs Res* 18:65-68, 1969
     Patients on a hospital rehabilitation ward were issued their medications
     for self-administration and then interviewed periodically to assess the
     accuracy of their medication use.

N=27

Design=1 Sample=0 Illness=1 Regimen=1 Measure=1 Definition=2

421. Reid RA, Lantz KH: Physician profiles in training the graduate internist. *J Med Educ* 52:301-307, 1977

This study compared the return rate of patients of doctors who received feedback information about their practice and of doctors who received no feedback information.

N=13 control, 8 experimental

Design=4 Sample=0+1 Illness=1 Regimen=0 Measure=2 Definition=2

422. Reisin E, Abel R, Modan M, Silverberg D, Eliahou H, Modan B: Effect of weight loss without salt restriction on the reduction of blood pressure in hypertensive patients. *N Engl J Med* 298:1-5, 1978

Compliance to a dietary weight reduction program is described in a controlled study of the effect of weight loss on hypertension.

N=107

Design=1 Sample=0+1 Illness=2 Regimen=2 Measure=4 Definition=2

423. Richards AD: Attitude and drug acceptance. *Br J Psychiatr* 110:46-52, 1964

Attitudes of institutionalized psychiatric patients judged "extreme noncompliers" were analyzed.

N=30

Design=2 Sample=0 Illness=1 Regimen=1 Measure=3+1 Definition=1

424. Rickels K, Anderson J, Howard K: Dropout contact by mail: A useful research tool. *Dis Nerv Syst* 29:545-548, 1968

Comparison of medication intake and reasons for missed appointments between nonattenders and those who miss an appointment but attend a rescheduled appointment.

N=123

Design=1 Sample=1 Illness=0 Regimen=0 Measure=1 Definition=1

425. Rickels K, Boren R, Stuart HM: Controlled psychopharmacological research in general practice. *J New Drugs* 4:138-147, 1964

Analysis of dropouts, side effects, and dosage deviation among acute ambulatory neurotic patients in a double-blind randomized trial of placebo , meprobamate, or phenobarbitol in a general practice setting.

N=89

Design=4 Sample=1+1 Illness=1 Regimen=2 Measure=2 Definition=1

426. Rickels K, Briscoe E: Assessment of dosage deviation in outpatient drug research. *J Clin Pharmacol* 10:153-160, 1970

Report of compliance aspects of two controlled clinical trials of medications among neurotic outpatients, with a comparison of verbal reports and pill counts.

N=176, 301

Design=3 Sample=1+1 Illness=0 Regimen=1 Measure=2+1 Definition=1

427. Rickels K, Raab E, Gordon PE, Laquer KG, Desilverio RV, Hesbacher P: Differential effects of chlordiazepoxide and fluphenazine in two anxious patient populations. *Psychopharmacologia* 12:181-192, 1968

Neurotic ambulatory patients at a large city hospital and at four private

general practices were placed in a double-blind clinical trial of oral
fluphenazine and chlordiazepoxide. Medication consumption and continuance in the study were analyzed.
N=93
Design=1 Sample=3 Illness=1 Regimen=2+1 Measure=2+1 Definition=1

428. Ritson B: Involvement in treatment and its relation to outcome amongst
alcoholics. *Br J Addict* 64:23-29, 1969
Assessment of relationship of program cooperation and attitudes with
subsequent abstinence among alcoholics.
N=50
Design=2+1 Sample=1+1 Illness=1 Regimen=1 Measure=1+1 Definition=2

429. Robbins GF, Conte AJ, Leach JE, Macdonald M: Delay in diagnosis and
treatment of cancer. *JAMA* 143:346-348, 1950
Interview study of reasons given by cancer patients for delay in seeking
care. The study spans three years during which a massive anticancer
publicity campaign was launched.
N=1,839
Design=1 Sample=0+1 Illness=1 Regimen=0 Measure=1 Definition=2

430. Robertson L, Haddon W: The buzzer-light reminder system and safety
belt use. *Am J Public Health* 64:814-815, 1974
Brief report comparing seat belt use in cars with and without buzzer-light
reminder systems.
N=5,745
Design=2 Sample=2 Illness=NA Regimen=1 Measure=3 Definition=1

431. Robertson L, Kelley A, O'Neill B, Wixom C, Eiswirth R, Haddon W:
A controlled study of the effect of television messages on safety belt
use. *Am J Public Health* 64:1071-1080, 1974
Cleverly controlled study of the effect of prolonged exposure to tele-
vision car seat belt safety messages.
N=162,835
Design=3 Sample=2+1 Illness=NA Regimen=2 Measure=4 Definition=2

432. Robertson L, O'Neill B, Wixom C: Factors associated with observed safety
belt use. *J Health Soc Behav* 13:18-24, 1972
Drivers were observed for their use of seat belts, traced via license number,
and interviewed by phone.
N=548 interviews
Design=2 Sample=0+1 Illness=NA Regimen=1 Measure=3 Definition=2

433. Robertson LS: Safety belt use in automobiles with starter-interlock and
buzzer-light reminder systems. *Am J Public Health* 65:1319-1325, 1975
Data from visual observation of use or nonuse of safety belts by drivers
are used to compare the effectiveness of buzzer-light and starter-interlock systems in automobiles.
N=5,557
Design=1 Sample=2+1 Illness=NA Regimen=1 Measure=3+1 Definition=2

434. Rockart JF, Hofmann PB: Physician and patient behavior under different
scheduling systems in a hospital outpatient department. *Med Care*
7:463-470, 1969

Descriptive study of patient mean arrival time, waiting time, and no-show rate and of physician mean arrival time at several outpatient departments using different scheduling methods.
N=1,500
Design=1 Sample=2 Illness=0 Regimen=1 Measure=2 Definition=0

435. Rogers RW, Deckner CW: Effects of fear appeals and physiological arousal upon emotion, attitudes, and cigarette smoking. *J Pers Soc Psychol* 32:222-230, 1975
In two experiments physiological arousal, situational cues, and degree of reassurance were manipulated to study the effect on subsequent smoking behavior.
A. N=119
Design=4 Sample=0+1 Illness=1 Regimen=1 Measure=1 Definition=1
B. N=160
Design=4 Sample=0+1 Illness=1 Regimen=1 Measure=1 Definition=1

436. Romm FJ, Armstrong PS, Prior AP: A comparison of program and contraceptive use continuation rates in a family planning clinic. *Am J Public Health* 65:693-699, 1975
Report of patient participation in a rural Georgia family planning program.
N=168
Design=2+1 Sample=2+1 Illness=NA Regimen=1 Measure=2+2 Definition=2

437. Rosenberg CM, Liftik J: Use of coercion in the outpatient treatment of alcoholism. *J Stud Alcohol* 37:58-65, 1976
Comparison of attendance rates at an alcoholism clinic for voluntary patients and for those required by parole to attend.
N=155
Design=2+1 Sample=1+1 Illness=1 Regimen=1 Measure=2+1 Definition=2

438. Rosenberg SG: Patient education leads to better care for heart patients. *HSMHA Health Reports* 86:793-802, 1971
Various "patient education" techniques were applied to a group of outpatients with congestive heart failure to improve knowledge about the disease and its therapy and to reinforce the importance of adherence.
N=50
Design=3 Sample=2 Illness=2 Regimen=1 Measure=3+1 Definition=1

439. Rosenzweig SP, Folman R: Patient and therapist variables affecting premature termination in group psychotherapy. *Psychother Theory Res Pract* 11:76-79, 1974
A study of the relationship between therapists' attitudes toward patients and outcome of therapy.
N=26
Design=2+1 Sample=0+1 Illness=1 Regimen=1 Measure=3 Definition=2

440. Rosser WW, Flett DG: How patients follow hospital discharge instructions in an urban family practice. *Can Fam Physician* 57-59, 1971
Comparison of written versus verbal discharge instructions in affecting compliance.
N=33
Design=4 Sample=0+1 Illness=1 Regimen=1 Measure=1 Definition=1

441. Roth HP, Berger DG: Studies on patient cooperation in ulcer treatment
     i) Observation of actual as compared to prescribed antacid intake on a
     hospital ward. *Gastroenterology* 38:630-633, 1960
     Report of two studies in which compliance of hospitalized patients for
     whom antacid had been prescribed was assessed.
     N=86
     Design=2 Sample=0+1 Illness=2 Regimen=2 Measure=2+1 Definition=2
442. Roth HP, Caron HS, Hsi BP: Measuring intake of a prescribed medication:
     A bottle count and a tracer technique compared. *Clin Pharmacol Ther*
     II:228-237, 1970
     Antacid intake was assessed among peptic ulcer outpatients utilizing bottle
     count and tracer techniques.
     N=105
     Design=2 Sample=0 Illness=3 Regimen=2+1 Measure=3+2 Definition=2
443. _____: Estimating a patient's cooperation with his regimen. *Am J Med Sci*
     262:269-273, 1971
     Compliance among outpatients on atropine plus antacid was assessed by
     objective measures.
     N=160
     Design=2 Sample=3 Illness=3 Regimen=2 Measure=4+2 Definition=1
444. Rubenstein HS: Behavior in a medical clinic of patients with well con-
     trolled bronchial asthma. *Lancet* 1:1011-1012, 1976
     Brief report of two studies of appointment keeping by asthmatic patients
     and other patients at a university health service.
   A. N=82
     Design=2 Sample=0+1 Illness=0 Regimen=1 Measure=2 Definition=2
   B. N=40
     Design=3 Sample=0+1 Illness=1 Regimen=1 Measure=2 Definition=2
445. Rubinstein EA, Lorr M: A comparison of terminators and remainders in
     outpatient psychotherapy. *J Clin Psychol* 12:345-349, 1956
     Remainers and terminators in psychotherapy were compared on selected
     psychological and demographic variables.
     N=128
     Design=2+1 Sample=2+1 Illness=1 Regimen=1 Measure=3 Definition=2
446. Rud B, Kisling E: The influence of mental development on children's
     acceptance of dental treatment. *Scand J Dent Res* 81:343-352, 1973
     Descriptive study comparing mental and chronologic age with acceptance
     of dental treatment.
     N=108
     Design=1 Sample=2+1 Illness=1 Regimen=2 Measure=3 Definition=2
447. Russel M, Wilson C, Feyerabend C, Cole PV: Effect of nicotine chewing
     gum on smoking behavior and as an aid to cigarette withdrawal. *Br Med
     J* 2:391-393, 1976
     Placebo-controlled double-blind clinical evaluation of 2 mg nicotine chew-
     ing gum in smoking reduction and cessation.
     N=43
     Design=4 Sample=0 Illness=1 Regimen=2 Measure=4+2 Definition=2

448. Russell M, Armstrong E, Patel U: Temporal contiguity in electric aversion therapy for cigarette smoking. *Behav Res Ther* 14:103-123, 1976
   Four treatment groups and one control group were evaluated on their success or failure in stopping smoking.
   N=70
   Design=4+1 Sample=0+1 Illness=2 Regimen=1 Measure=1 Definition=1

449. Sackett DL, Haynes RB, Gibson ES, Hackett BC, Taylor DW, Roberts RS, Johnson AL: Randomized clinical trial of strategies for improving medication compliance in primary hypertension. *Lancet* 1:1205-1207, 1975
   Evaluation of the effect on compliance of treatment at the work site and of a special education program among new hypertensive patients.
   N=230
   Design=4 Sample=2+1 Illness=3 Regimen=1+1 Measure=2+1 Definition=2

450. Sansom CD, MacInerney J, Oliver V, Wakefield J: Differential response to recall in a cervical screening programme. *Br J Prev Soc Med* 29:40-47, 1975
   Analysis of characteristics of responders and nonresponders to a letter request to return for a repeat cervical screening program in patients with previous normal cervical smears.
   N=93
   Design=1 Sample=2 Illness=NA Regimen=1 Measure=2 Definition=1

451. Sarnat H, Peri J, Nitzan E, Perlberg A: Factors which influence cooperation between dentist and child. *J Dent Educ*: 9-15, December 1972
   Analysis of child's anxiety and parental permissiveness variables on child's cooperation in a dental situation.
   N=34
   Design=1 Sample=0 Illness=NA Regimen=1 Measure=3 Definition=2

452. Schmahl DP, Lichtenstein E, Harris DE: Successful treatment of habitual smokers with warm smoky air and rapid smoking. *J Consult Clin Psychol* 38:105-111, 1972
   Rapid smoking plus either warm smoky air or warm mentholated air and telephone follow-up checks at two or four week intervals were experimentally evaluated in a two by two factorial design.
   N=28
   Design=4 Sample=0 Illness=NA Regimen=2 Measure=1+1 Definition=2

453. Schroeder SA: Lowering broken appointment rates at a medical clinic. *Med Care* 11:75-78, 1973
   Comparison of three techniques designed to improve appointment-keeping rates among patients of low socioeconomic status.
   N=503 follow-up visits
   Design=3 Sample=0+1 Illness=0 Regimen=2 Measure=3 Definition=1

454. Schwab PJ, Smith BH: A supportive clinic: Who comes, how often, and for what? *Compr Psychiatr* 18:503-509, 1977
   Appointment-keeping rates were included in data reported for a sample of psychiatric outpatients at a supportive clinic over a three-year period.
   N=346
   Design=1 Sample=0+1 Illness=1 Regimen=1 Measure=1+1 Definition=1

455. Schwartz D, Wang M, Zeitz L, Goss ME; Medication errors made by elderly, chronically ill patients. *Am J Public Health* 52:2018-2029, 1962

Ambulatory patients over the age of sixty years were interviewed to determine the accuracy of their usage of medication with errors classified by type and error makers examined for characteristics.
N=178
Design=1 Sample=2+1 Illness=0 Regimen=0+1 Measure=1 Definition=1

456. Schwartz D: The elderly patient and his medications. *Geriatrics* 20:517-520, 1965

Study of medication errors made by elderly, chronically ill, ambulatory patients.
N=not given
Design=1 Sample=0+1 Illness=0 Regimen=0+1 Measure=1+1 Definition=1

457. Sear AM: Clinic discontinuation and contraceptive need. *Fam Plann Perspect* 5:80-88, 1973

Study of the relationships between some demographic and clinical factors and continuance in a family planning clinic.
N=362 interviews
Design=1 Sample=1+1 Illness=NA Regimen=1 Measure=2 Definition=1

458. Shafil M, Lavely R, Jaffe R: Meditation and the prevention of alcohol use. *Am J Psychiatr* 132:942-945, 1975

Comparison of reported alcohol consumption among practitioners of transcendental meditation and a matched control group.
N=216
Design=2 Sample=0+1 Illness=3 Regimen=NA Measure=1 Definition=2

459. Shapiro RJ: Therapist attitudes and premature termination in family and individual therapy. *J Nerv Ment Dis* 159:101-107, 1974

Dropouts from child psychotherapy analysis were studied in relation to therapists' affective response to patients, degree of psychopathology, and assessment of treatment program.
N=51
Design=3 Sample=0+1 Illness=1 Regimen=1 Measure=3 Definition=1

460. Sharpe TR, Mikeal RL: Patient compliance with antibiotic regimens. *Am J Hosp Pharm* 31:479-484, 1974

Study of the relationship between written drug therapy information provided by pharmacists and the degree of patient compliance with ten-day courses of antibiotics.
N=80
Design=3+1 Sample=1+1 Illness=0 Regimen=3 Measure=2+1 Defintion=2

461. Shepard DS, Moseley TA: Mailed versus telephoned appointment reminders to reduce broken appointments in a hospital outpatient department. *Med Care* 14:268-273, 1976

Report of an attempt to improve attendance at three children's outpatient clinics with a cost-effectiveness analysis of the strategies employed.
N=1,039
Design=4 Sample=0+1 Illness=0 Regimen=0 Measure=2 Definition=2

462. Sherwin AL, Robb JP, Lechter M: Improved control of epilepsy by monitoring plasma ethosuximide. *Arch Neurol* 28:178-181, 1973
Study of ethosuximide dose-response relationships in the treatment of petit mal epilepsy and the effect of blood level monitoring on improving compliance among patients.
N=70
Design=3 Sample=0 Illness=3 Regimen=1+1 Measure=4 Definition=2

463. Siegel E, Thomas D, Coulter E, Tuthill R, Chipman S: Continuation of contraception by low income women: A one year follow-up. *Am J Public Health* 61:1886-1898, 1971
Initiates to a lower class family planning clinic were followed up at one year to assess continuance of contraceptives.
N=682
Design=3 Sample=1 Illness=NA Regimen=1 Measure=1 Definition=2

464. Silverman S, Silverman SI, Silverman B, Garfinkel L: Self-image and its relation to denture acceptance. *J Prosthet Dent* 35:131-141, 1976
"Focused interviews," "embedded-figures tests," and "projective figure drawings" were used to assess self-image of geriatric acceptance of dentures.
N=40
Design=1 Sample=1 Illness=NA Regimen=0 Measure=1 Definition=1

465. Silverstone JT, Solomon T: The long-term management of obesity in general practice. *Br J Clin Pract* 19:395-398, 1965
A one-year study of weight loss incorporating a double-blind study of diethylpropion (an anorectic) and close supervision by appointments with the general practitioner.
N=32
Design=4 Sample=0+1 Illness=3+1 Regimen=3 Measure=4+1 Definition=1

466. Sivin I: Two years of experience with the copper T(TCU 200): A study in four developing countries, pp 249-282, in Hefnawi F, Segal SJ (eds): *Analysis of Intrauterine Contraception*, Proceedings of Third International Conference on Intrauterine Contraception. Amsterdam, North Holland, 1975
A lengthy report of IUD continuation and termination rates in four countries.
N=4,700 cooper T, 2,750 Lippe's loop
Design=2 Sample=3+1 Illness=NA Regimen=1 Measure=1+1 Definition=1

467. Slaikeu KA, Tulkin SR, Speer, DC: Process and outcome in the evaluation of telephone counseling referrals. *J Consult Clin Psychol* 43:700-707, 1975
Attempt to validate concreteness and motivation as predictors of appointment compliance on referral from a telephone suicide and crisis service.
N=89
Design=2+1 Sample=0+1 Illness=0 Regimen=1 Measure=2 Definition=2

468. Sloan CL, Tobias DL, Stapell CH, Ho MT, Beagle WS: A weight control program for students using diet and behavior therapy. *J Am Diet Assoc* 68:466-468, 1976

Overweight female students were enrolled in a program encompassing diet and behavioral therapy for eating habits.
N=15
Design=2 Sample=0 Illness=NA Regimen=1 Measure=4 Definition=2

469. Slocumb JC, Odoroff CL, Kunitz SJ: The use-effectiveness of two contraceptive methods in a Navejo population: The problem of program dropouts. *Am J Obstet Gynecol* 122:717-726, 1975
Study of contraception utilization rates for the pill and the IUD in a Navajo reservation population with description and comparison of several actuarial methods for handling dropouts.
N=834
Design=2+1 Sample=3+1 Illness=NA Regimen=1 Measure=2+2 Definition=2

470. Soutter B, Kennedy M: Patient compliance assessment in drug trials: Usage and methods. *Aust NZ J Med* 4:360-364, 1974 (see also comment, *Aust NZ J Med* 5:72, 1975)
Evaluation of the extent to which published drug trials report the use of methods of assessing or insuring compliance in the execution of efficacy studies. Also contains an excellent brief review of methods for measuring compliance.
N=324
Design=1 Sample=0+1 Illness=2 Regimen=2 Measure=1 Definition=2

471. Spaeth GL: Visual loss in a glaucoma clinic I. Sociological considerations. *Invest Ophthalmol* 9:73-82, 1970
Patients from a glaucoma clinic were interviewed in an attempt to study the relationships between the clinic patient and his disease including the factor of compliance with medication use.
N=69 attenders, 25 poor attenders
Design=2 Sample=1+1 Illness=1 Regimen=1 Measure=1 Definition=2

472. Stadt ZM, Blum H, Kent G, Fletcher E, Keyes G, Frost L: Direct mail dental motivation of parents of three year old children. *Am J Public Health* 53:572-57, 1963
Report of the effects of mailing dental health brithday cards from a county health department to families with preschool children.
N=2,662
Design=3 Sample=2+1 Illness=NA Regimen=0 Measure=1 Definition=0

473. Stamler R, Stamler J, Civinelli J, Pritchard D, Gosch F, Ticho S, Restivo B, Fine D: Adherence and blood-pressure response to hypertension treatment. *Lancet* 2:1227-1230, 1975
Descriptive study that includes figures on dropouts from first phase of the Hypertension Detection and Follow-up Program at one center.
N=116
Design=1 Sample=0+1 Illness=2 Regimen=2 Measure=2+1 Definition=1

474. Starfield B, Sharp E: Ambulatory pediatric care: The role of the nurse. *Med Care* 6:507-515, 1968
Randomized clinical trial of the role of the nurse in increasing compliance with an exercise regimen for enuretic children of families enrolled at a public hospital OPD.

N=231 children in 146 families
Design=4 Sample=1 Illness=3 Regimen=2 Measure=2+1 Definition=2
475. Starfield B, Sharp ES, Mellits ED: Effective care in the ambulatory setting:
       The nurse's contribution. *J Pediatr* 79:504-507, 1971
       Randomized clinical trial of the role of the nurse in inducing compliance
          of enuretic children with an exercise program compared with control
          families who received no special attention.
       N=70 study, 73 control families
       Design=4 Sample=0 Illness=1 Regimen=1 Measure=1 Definition=1
476. Starnbach HK, Kaplan A: Profile of an excellent orthodontic patient.
       Angle Orthod 45:141-145, 1975
       By evaluating retrospectively orthodontic patients as excellent, average,
          and poor and sending a questionnaire to the parents, the author identi-
          fies some demographic variables that could predict successful treat-
          ment.
       N=362
       Design=1 Sample=0 Illness=NA Regimen=0 Measure=1+1 Defintion=1
477. Steckel SB, Swain MA: Contracting with patients to improve compliance.
       J Am Hosp Assoc 51:81-84, 1977
       Hypertensive patients were assigned randomly to one of three groups to
          test the effect of patient education and written contracts on compli-
          ance.
       N=115
       Design=4 Sample=0+1 Illness=1 Regimen=1 Measure=3+1 Definition=1
478. Steger H, Chisholm S: Predicting adjustment of heart patients with the
       cardiac adjustment scale. *J Clin Psychol* 33:735-739, 1977
       The cardiac adjustment scale was evaluated as a means of predicting the
          outcome of a rehabilitation program.
       N=74
       Design=1+1 Sample=0+1 Illness=1 Regimen=1 Measure=3 Definition=2
479. Stern MP, Farquhar JW, Maccoby N, Russel S: Results of a two-year
       health education campaign on dietary behavior: The Stanford three
       community study. *Circulation* 54:826-833, 1976
       Controlled study of the effect of mass media communications and per-
          sonal counseling of high risk individuals on dietary habits and on serum
          lipids in three California communities.
       N=1,204
       Design=3+1 Sample=2 Illness=NA Regimen=1 Measure=1 Definition=2
480. Stine OC, Chuaqui C, Jimenez C, Oppel WC: Broken appointments at a
       comprehensive clinic for children. *Med Care* 6:332-339, 1968
       Characteristics of families of black patients enrolled in a comprehensive
          pediatric clinic were compared to appointment compliance.
       N=203
       Design=2 Sample=1 Illness=0 Regimen=1 Measure=2+1 Definition=2
481. Stone DB: A study of the incidence and causes of poor control in patients
       with diabetes mellitus. *Am J Med Sci* 241:436-442, 1961
       Most diabetic outpatients under poor control were judged noncompliant

due to ignorance; after a period of instruction, compliance and control were reassessed.
N=160
Design=1 Sample=0+1 Illness=2 Regimen=1 Measure=1 Definition=1

482. Stone WN, Green BL, Gleser GC, Whitman RM, Foster BB: Impact of psychosocial factors on the conduct of combined drug and psycho-therapy research. *Br J Psychiatr* 127:432-439, 1975
The effect of attitudes of therapists, patients, and researchers on the con-duct and outcome of combined drug and psychotherapy research was examined in a brief crisis-oriented psychotherapy clinic.
N=77
Design=3 Sample=1 Illness=0 Regimen=1 Measure=0 Definition=0

483. Stott H: Drug acceptability and chemoprophylaxis in under-developed countries. WHO-UNICEF assisted tuberculosis project Nairobi Kenya. *Bull U Int Tuberc* 29:285-292, 1959
Pill counts were made in the homes of tuberculosis suspects assigned randomly to isoniazid treatment.
N=98
Design=4 Sample=0 Illness=1 Regimen=1 Measure=2 Definition=1

484. Straker M, Davanloo H, Moll A: Psychiatric clinic dropouts. *Laval Medical* 38:71-77, 1967
Study of dropout rates in a "model" psychiatric outpatient clinic offering short-term psychotherapy
N=440
Design=3+1 Sample=0+1 Illness=1 Regimen=1 Measure=3 Definition=1

485. Stuart RB: Behavioral control of overeating. *Behav Res Ther* 5:357-365, 1967
A behavioral treatment for overeating, utilizing operant and respondent conditioning techniques.
N=8
Design=3 Sample=0 Illness=2 Regimen=2 Measure=4 Definition=2

486. Stunkard A, McLaren-Hume M: The results of treatment for obesity. *Arch Intern Med* 103:79-85, 1959
Review of the literature on the success of treatment for obesity and a report of a series in the authors' own work.
N=100
Design=2 Sample=0+1 Illness=1+1 Regimen=1+1 Measure=4 Definition=2

487. Suchman EA: Preventive health behavior: A model for research on com-munity health campaigns. *J Health Soc Behav* 8:197-209, 1967
An "epidemiological model" of acceptance of preventive health measures was proposed and tested among Puerto Rican sugar cane cutters who were subjected to a community health campaign designed to get them to use safety gloves.
N=115
Design=1 Sample=3 Illness=NA Regimen=1 Measure=2+1 Definition=2

488. Sudak HS, Sawyer JB, Spring GK, Coakwell CM: High referral success rates in a crisis center. *Hosp Community Psychiatr* 28:530-532, 1977

Report of data from a crisis clinic that used an active referral method
where a worker phoned to make appointment for clients and followed
up to check that the appointment was kept.
N=1,921
Design=1+1 Sample=0+1 Illness=0 Regimen=1 Measure=3 Definition=1

489. Sullivan J, Suyono H, Bahrawi W, Hartoadi A: Contraceptive use-effective-
ness in Mojokerto Regency, Indonesia: A comparison of regular pro-
gram and special drive acceptors. *Stud Fam Plann* 7:188-196, 1976
Study of recruiting methods in population-based family planning projects.
N=2,421
Design=3+1 Sample=3 Illness=NA Regimen=1 Measure=1+1 Definition=1

490. Svarstad BL: Physician-patient communication and patient conformity
with medical advice, pp 220-235, in Mechanic D (ed): *The Growth
of Bureaucratic Medicine*. New York, Wiley, 1974
A review of determinants of compliance and a study of physicians' influence in transmitting their expectations and motivating their patients.
N=131
Design=2 Sample=0 Illness=0 Regimen=0 Measure=2+1 Definition=0

491. Tagliacozzo DM, Ima K: Knowledge of illness as a predictor of patient
behavior. *J Chron Dis* 22:765-775, 1970
Chronically ill black patients attending an outpatient department were
assessed for their demographic characteristics, beliefs, clinical features,
and their knowledge of their disease and its complications; the results
were compared with attendance.
N=159
Design=1 Sample=1 Illness=1+1 Regimen=0 Measure=2 Definition=2

492. Tagliacozzo DM, Ima K, Lashof JC: Influencing the chronically ill: The
role of prescriptions in premature separations of outpatient care.
Med Care 11:21-29, 1973
Study of the effect of diet prescriptions and medication loads on con-
tinued attendance at a general medical outpatient department.
N=195
Design=1 Sample=1 Illness=1+1 Regimen=1 Measure=2 Definition=2

493. Tagliacozzo DM, Luskin DB, Lashof JC, Ima K: Nurse intervention and
patient behavior. *Am J Public Health* 64:596-603, 1974
Experimental evaluation of effect on compliance of an extensive instructional program in a lecture format delivered by nurses among patients
with chronic medical diseases.
N=192
Design=4+1 Sample=1+1 Illness=1+1 Regimen=0 Measure=2+2 Definition=0

494. Tapp JT, Slaikeu KA, Tulkin SR: Toward an evaluation of telephone
counseling; process and technical variables influencing "shows" and
"no shows" for a clinical referral. *Am J Community Psychol* 2:357-
364, 1975
Report of the interrelationships among process variables, technical
effectiveness, caller motivation, and shows and no-shows at referrals
made by telephone counselors at a suicide and crisis service.

N=20, 20

Design=2 Sample=0 Illness=0 Regimen=1 Measure=2 Definition=2

495. Tash RH, O'Shea RM, Cohen LK: Testing a preventive-symptomatic theory of dental health behavior. *Am J Public Health* 59:514-521, 1969

Results of a dental health behavior questionnaire administered to a population-based sample of adults were analyzed for correlates of "preventive" dental visits and "symptomatic" dental visits.

N=1,862

Design=1 Sample=2 Illness=NA Regimen=0 Measure=1 Definition=2

496. Taubman AH, King J, Weisbuch J, Little F, French D: Noncompliance in initial prescription filling. *Apothecary* 87:14-46, 1975

An improved record-keeping system and a closer pharmacist-patient relationship were promoted to enhance compliance to initial prescription filling.

N=1,251

Design=1+1 Sample=0 Illness=0 Regimen=0 Measure=2 Definition=2

497. Thawrani YP, Mukherji B, Taluja RK, Kaul KK: A study of patient compliance in urban out-patient pediatric practice. *Indian Pediatr* 12:679-683, 1975

Parents of 500 children were interviewed to find out whether the regimens were being followed, and reasons for deviance.

N=500

Design=1 Sample=0 Illness=0 Regimen=0 Measure=1 Definition=2

498. Treusch JV, Krusen FH: Physical therapy applied at home for arthritis: A followup study, with a supplementary summary of the sedimentation rate of erythrocytes in 229 cases of arthritis. *Arch Intern Med* 72:231-238, 1943

A questionnaire was mailed to determine whether physiotherapy was being continued one to two years after it was initiated; reasons for discontinuing are analyzed.

N=218

Design=1 Sample=2 Illness=1 Regimen=1 Measure=1 Definition=1

499. Tuomilehto J, Rajala A, Puska P: A study on the drop-outs of the hypertension register of the North Karelia project. *Community Health* 7:149-152, 1976

Cooperation rates in a WHO Community hypertension project designed to promote compliance.

N=229

Design=2 Sample=2 Illness=1 Regimen=2 Measure=2 Definition=2

500. Tyroler H, Johnson A, Fulton J: Patterns of preventive health behavior in populations. *J Health Hum Behav* 6:128-140, 1965

Report of two studies investigating (1) acceptance of oral poliomyelitis vaccine and (2) levels of carious tooth salvage within families.

A. N=333

Design=2 Sample=0+1 Illness=NA Regimen=1 Measure=3 Definition=1

B. N=128 families

Design=2 Sample=0+1 Illness=NA Regimen=1 Measure=3 Definition=1

418   REFERENCE MATERIALS

501. Uehling D, Hussey J, Weinstein A, Wank R, Bach F: Cessation of immuno-suppression after renal transplantation. *Surgery* 79:278-282, 1976
Case reports of evident and admitted noncompliance and its consequences among renal transplant recipients.
N=5
Design=1 Sample=0+1 Illness=1 Regimen=1 Measure=1 Definition=1
502. Uhlenhuth EH, Park LC, Lipman RS, Rickels K, Fisher S, Mock J: Dosage deviation and drug effects in drug trials. *J Nerv Ment Dis* 141:95-99, 1965
Analysis of changes in outcomes in two drug trials of anxiolytic agents among neurotic outpatients, comparing compliant patients with all patients entered into the trials.
N=164, 190
Design=4 Sample=0 Illness=1 Regimen=1 Measure=2+1 Definition=2
503. Vannecelli M, Pfav B, Ryback R: Data attrition in follow-up studies of alcoholics. *J Stud Alcohol* 37:1325-1330, 1976
Staff ratings of compliance were compared for responders and nonres-ponders to a follow-up questionnaire in an alcoholic treatment program.
N=60
Design=2 Sample=0+1 Illness=0 Regimen=1 Measure=1+1 Definition=1
504. Vertinsky PA, Yang Chung-Fang, Macleod PJM, Hardwick DF: A study of compliance factors in voluntary health behaviour. *Int J Health Educ* 19:3-15 1976
Factors determining attendance at a Tay-Sachs screening program are assessed by a mailed questionnaire.
N=392 (15% of mailed questionnaire)
Design=1 Sample=1 Illness=1 Regimen=NA Measure=2 Definition=2
505. Vincent P: Factors influencing patient noncompliance: A theoretical approach. *Nurs Res* 20:509-516, 1971
Glaucoma outpatients were questioned regarding attitudes, demographic factors, knowledge of glaucoma and its therapy, and the results were compared with reported compliance.
N=62
Design=1 Sample=1+1 Illness=1 Regimen=1 Measure=1 Definition=2
506. Walfish S, Tapp J, Tulkin S, Slaikeu K, Russel M: The prediction of "shows" and "no-shows" to a crisis center. *Am J Community Psychol* 3:367-370, 1975
Determinants affecting appointment keeping as a result of referrals received through telephone crisis intervention.
N=70
Design=2 Sample=0 Illness=NA Regimen=0 Measure=2 Definition=1
507. Wallace HM, Losty MA, Oliver-Smith F, Azzaretti L, Rich H: Study of follow-up of children recommended for rheumatic fever prophylaxis. *Am J Public Health* 46:1563-1570, 1956
Providers of initial care of children referred to rheumatic fever prophy-laxis are questioned to determine the current care status of the children.

N=664
Design=1 Sample=0+1 Illness=1 Regimen=1 Measure=1 Definition=1
508. Wallston BS, Wallston KA, Kaplan GD, Maides SA: Development and
validation of the health locus of control (HLC) scale. *J Consult Clin
Psychol* 44:580-583, 1976
Relationships were found between the HLC scale and health information
seeking in one study and between the HLC scale and satisfaction with
two weight loss programs differing in degree of self-direction in a
second study.
   A. N=44 female college students
Design=1 Sample=0 Illness=NA Regimen=1 Measure=3 Definition=2
   B. N=34 overweight women
Design=4 Sample=0 Illness=2 Regimen=0 Measure=4+1 Definition=2
509. Wandless I, Davie J: Can drug compliance in the elderly be improved?
Br Med J 1:359-361, 1977
Three instruction schemes for self-medication in older patients were com-
pared to see whether they improved drug compliance during self-ad-
ministration in hospital.
N=46
Design=4 Sample=0+1 Illness=0 Regimen=1 Measure=2 Definition=2
510. Waters WH, Gould NV, Lunn JE; Undispensed prescriptions in a mining
general practice. *Br Med J* 1:1062-1063, 1976
The type of illness, age, and sex of patient were all found to relate to the
proportion of prescriptions presented for filling.
N=1,611 prescriptions
Design=1 Sample=0+1 Illness=1 Regimen=0 Measure=3+1 Definition=2
511. Watkins JD, Williams TF, Martin DA, Hogan MD, Anderson E: A study of
diabetic patients at home. *Am J Public Health* 57:452-459, 1967
Study of level of control, knowledge of regimen, and compliance with
regimen at home among diabetic outpatients.
N=60
Design=1 Sample=2 Illness=1 Regimen=1 Measure=3+1 Definition=2
512. Watts TE: The regularity of attendance of male tuberculosis patients
diagnosed at Mulago hospital between January and July in 1968 and in
1970. *Tubercle* 53:174-181, 1972
Study of defaulting rates for males on outpatient tuberculosis therapy
before and after implementation of special recording procedures and
the use of two health assistants to trace and retrieve defaulters.
N=variable
Design=3 Sample=0+1 Illness=1 Regimen=1 Measure=3 Definition=1
513. Weintraub M, Au WY, Lasagna L: Compliance as a determinant of serum
digoxin concentration. *JAMA* 224:481-485, 1973
Outpatients for whom digoxin had been prescribed were questioned
about their compliance; the results were compared with serum levels
of digoxin and with social and clinical characteristics of the patients.
N=72
Design=1 Sample=2 Illness=1 Regimen=1 Measure=1 Definition=2

514. Werner W: "Technical failures" in lithium prophylaxis, pp 329-334, in Ban TA, Lehmann HE (eds): *Psychopharmacology, Sexual Disorders and Drug Abuse*. Amsterdam, North Holland, 1972

Manic depressives were interviewed concerning their consistent lithium taking and many factors were analyzed to find determinants of continuation with therapy.

N=120

Design=1 Sample=0+1 Illness=1 Regimen=1 Measure=1 Definition=1

515. Wescott WB, Starcke EN, Shannon IL: Chemical protection against post-irradiation dental caries. *Oral Surg Oral Medicine Oral Pathology* 40:709-719, 1975

Patients at high risk to dental caries were trained and encouraged to practice strict dental hygiene. Compliance dictated the success of the treatment.

N=24

Design=2 Sample=0+1 Illness=2 Regimen=2 Measure=1 Definition=0

516. West D, Graham S, Swanson M, Wilkinson G: Five year follow-up of a smoking withdrawal clinic population. *Am J Public Health* 67:536-544, 1977

Data from a five-year follow-up were examined to determine the relationship between smoking status and clinic protocols and among selected social and psychological factors.

N=559

Design=2 Sample=0+1 Illness=NA Regimen=1 Measure=1 Definition=1

517. White MK, Alpert JJ, Kosa J: Hard-to-reach families in a comprehensive care program. *JAMA* 201:123-128, 1967

Study of the provision of comprehensive pediatric care for groups of easy and hard to reach families with analysis of characteristics and response of the various groups.

N=variable

Design=2 Sample=1+1 Illness=NA Regimen=0 Measure=2 Definition=1

518. Whyte R: Psychiatric new-patient clinic non-attenders. *Br J Psychiatr* 127:160-162, 1975

Of 50 nonattenders, 22 were contacted and paired with 22 attenders to determine factors affecting compliance with referral.

N=22 nonattenders, 22 attenders

Design=2+1 Sample=2+1 Illness=1 Regimen=0 Measure=2 Definition=2

519. Wikler L, Stoycheff J: Parental compliance with post discharge recommendations for retarded children. *Hosp Community Psychiatr* 25:595-598, 1974

Parents were interviewed to determine the extent to which they followed recommendations for care of their retarded child after hospitalization.

N=80

Design=1 Sample=1+1 Illness=1 Regimen=1 Measure=1 Definition=1

520. Wilber JA, Barrow JG: Hypertension—a community problem. *Am J Med* 52:653-663, 1972

Community survey for hypertension giving the treatment status of discovered hypertension.

N=6,012

Design=2 Sample=3 Illness=NA Regimen=0 Measure=1+1 Definition=2

521. _____: Reducing elevated blood pressure: Experience found in a community. *Minn Med* 52:1303-1305, 1969

Selected individuals found hypertensive during a community hypertension screening program were asked to participate in a special home service program involving periodic home visits by a public health nurse. Compliance rates and blood pressures were compared after two and four years for those who did and did not accept the service.

N=220

Design=3 Sample=0 Illness=2 Regimen=1 Measure=3+1 Definition=2

522. Wilhelmsen L, Ljungberg S, Wedel H, Werko L: A comparison between participants and non-participants in a primary preventive trial. *J Chron Dis* 29:331-339, 1976

Participants and nonparticipants in a primary preventive trial against coronary heart disease were compared for mortality, autopsy findings, morbidity, and sobriety.

N=9,968

Design=2 Sample=2+1 Illness=3 Regimen=1 Measure=2 Definition=2

523. Willcox DR, Gillan R, Hare EH: Do psychiatric out-patients take their drugs? *Br Med J* 2:790-792, 1965

Psychiatric outpatients on imipramine and/or chlorpromazine were monitored for compliance; results were compared with demographic factors and clinical data.

N=125

Design=1 Sample=1 Illness=1 Regimen=1 Measure=3+1 Definition=2

524. Williams A, Duncan B: A commercial weight-reducing organization: A critical analysis. *Med J Aust* 1:781-785, 1976

"Outside" analysis of the records of Weight Watchers International in Australia.

N=5,558

Design=1 Sample=2 Illness=2 Regimen=1 Measure=4+1 Definition=2

525. Williams TF, Anderson E, Watkins JD, Coyle V: Dietary errors made at home by patients with diabetes. *J Am Diet Assoc* 51:19-25, 1967

Report of two studies of dietary adherence among adult diabetic outpatients assessed at home by (1) a twenty-four hour recall method and (2) a seven-day food record.

N=60, 17

Design=1 Sample=0+1 Illness=1 Regimen=1 Measure=1 Definition=2

526. Williams W, Lee J: Methadone maintenance: A comparison of methadone treatment subjects and methadone treatment dropouts. *Int J Addict* 10:599-608, 1975

Demographic and psychosocial variables were compared between treatment subjects and dropouts in a methadone maintenance program.

N=119

Design=2+1 Sample=1+1 Illness=2 Regimen=1 Measure=3 Definition=2

527. Willis FN, Dunsmore NM: Work orientation, health attitudes, and compliance with therapeutic advice. *Nurs Res* 16:22-25, 1967

Post-myocardial infarction patients were assessed for work orientation and observed for cooperation with hospital and postdischarge medical advice.

N=28

Design=2 Sample=0 Illness=1 Regimen=0+1 Measure=3+1 Definition=1

528. Wilson JD, Enoch MD: Estimation of drug rejection by schizophrenic in-patients, with analysis of clinical factors. *Br J Psychiatr* 113:209-211, 1967

Hospitalized schizophrenic patients on chlorpromazine tablets three times per day were assessed for compliance by single urinary FPN test and then switched to liquid chlorpromazine and rechecked in five to six days.

N=50

Design=3 Sample=0 Illness=1 Regimen=1+1 Measure=3+1 Definition=1

529. Winkelman NW: A clinical and socio-cultural study of 200 psychiatric patients started on chlorpromazine 10½ years ago. *Am J Psychiatr* 120:861-869, 1964

Compliance was found best among patients at higher socioeconomic levels where attitudes toward the illness and therapy were more positive.

N=200

Design=2+1 Sample=1+1 Illness=2 Regimen=1 Measure-0 Definition=1

530. Winokur MZ, Czaczkes JW, De-Nour AK: Intelligence and adjustment to chronic hemodialysis. *J Psychosom Res* 17:29-34, 1973

Psychological and intelligence assessments prior to the initiation of patients into chronic dialysis programs were compared with dietary adherence and work levels six months after the start of therapy.

N=38

Design=1 Sample=2 Illness=1 Regimen=1 Measure=4+1 Definition=1

531. Witters L, Herbert P, Shulman R, Krauss R, Levy R: Therapeutic failure in familial type II hyperlipoproteinemia. *Metabolism* 25:1017-1026, 1976

A study of reduction of plasma cholesterol comparing responders and nonresponders in the treatment program.

N=16

Design=2 Sample=0 Illness=2 Regimen=1 Measure=4+2 Definition=2

532. Wolf S, Carr A, Davis D, Davidson S, Dale E, Forsythe A, Goldenberg E, Hanson R, Lulejian G, Nelson M, Treitman P, Weinstein A: The value of phenobarbitol in the child who has had a single febrile seizure: A controlled prospective study. *Pediatrics* 59:378-385, 1977

Compliance is cited as a major problem in a continuous phenobarbitol regimen to prevent recurrences of febrile convulsions.

N=355

Design=3+1 Sample=0+1 Illness=3 Regimen=1 Measure=4 Definition=1

533. Woodwark GM, Gauthier MR: Hospital education program following myocardial infarction. *Can Med Assoc J* 106:665-667, 1972

Report of the use and utility of a patient education program among survivors of myocardial infarctions.

N=19 study, 19 controls
Design=3 Sample=0 Illness=1 Regimen=1 Measure=1 Definition=0

534. Woody G, O'Hare K, Mintz J, Obrien C: Rapid intake: A method for increasing retention rate of heroin addicts seeking methadone treatment. *Compr Psychiatr* 16:165-169, 1975
Quasi-experimental evaluation of the value of shortening the intake procedures to reduce dropout rates at an addiction treatment clinic.
N=42, 43
Design=3 Sample=1+1 Illness=1 Regimen=1 Measure=0 Definition=1

535. Wynn-Williams N, Arris M: On omitting PAS. *Tubercle* 39:138-142, 1958
Urine samples were tested for PAS and the importance of maintaining treatment was stressed to outpatient adults being treated for respiratory tuberculosis.
N=153
Design=2 Sample=0+1 Illness=1 Regimen=1 Measure=3+1 Definition=2

536. Zaki MH, Edelstein S, Josephson RA, Weisberg SR: Regularity of drug administration among hospitalized and ambulatory tuberculous patients. *Am Rev Resp Dis* 97:136-139, 1968
Matched pairs of tuberculous inpatients and outpatients were studied to evaluate compliance and patient characteristics.
N=132 pairs
Design=2 Sample=2 Illness=1 Regimen=1 Measure=3+1 Definition=2

537. Zielinski JJ: Epileptics not in treatment. *Epilepsia* 15:203-210, 1974
A study comparing treatment patterns for known epileptics and those diagnosed in a field survey.
N=410
Design=2 Sample=2+1 Illness=2 Regimen=1 Measure=1 Definition=1

SPECIAL ARTICLES ON MEASUREMENT METHODS

538. Belles QC, Littleman ML: A sensitive filter paper spot test for the detection of isoniazid (INH) metabolites in urine. *Med J Aust* 2:588-590, 1962
Description of a simple test for detection of INH in urine.

539. Biron P, Boyer L, Brouillet J, Boyer A, Senecal L, Moisan R: Dietary compliance in obesity: Ketonuria versus weight loss. *Soc Occup Med* 5:70, 1977
Empirical validation of the use of ketostix in monitoring adherence of obese patients to a low calorie, low carbohydrate diet.

540. Bradshaw P, Ley P, Kincey J, Bradshaw J: Recall of medical advice: Comprehensibility and specificity. *Br J Soc Clin Psychol* 14:55-62, 1975
Three experiments investigated the effect of readability of medical advice on subsequent recall.

541. Chaves AD: A simple paper strip urine test for para-aminosalicylic acid. *Am Rev Resp Dis* 80:585-586, 1959
An evaluation of the use of phenistix in detecting PAS in urine.

542. _____: Results of the PAS urine test (phenistix); study done in May and June, 1959. *Am Rev Resp Dis* 81:111-112, 1960
Comparison of urinary test and interview rating of adherence to PAS.

543. Curry SH, Davis JM, Janowsky DS, Marshal JH: Factors affecting chlorpromazine plasma levels in psychiatric patients. *Arch Gen Psychiatr* 22:209-215, 1970
Description of gas chromatography quantitative determination of chlorpromazine in plasma, urine, feces, applied to assess relationship between blood levels and various routes of administration.

544. Dawson KP, Jamieson A: Value of blood phenytoin estimation in management of childhood epilepsy. *Arch Dis Child* 46:386-388, 1971
Description of a modified Dill technique for measuring blood phenytoin levels.

545. Deuschle K, Jordahl C, Hobby G: Clinical usefulness of riboflavin-tagged isoniazid for self-medication in tuberculous patients. *Am Rev Resp Dis* 82:1-10, 1960
Inpatient-outpatient evaluation of riboflavin in compliance monitoring both separately and in combination with INH.

546. Eadie MJ: Plasma level monitoring of anticonvulsants. *Clin Pharmacokinet* 1:52-66, 1976
A discussion of the theory and practice of plasma level monitoring of several anticonvulsant drugs.

547. Evans R, Rozelle R, Lasater T, Dembroski T, Allen B: New measure of effects of persuasive communications: A chemical indicator of toothbrushing behavior. *Psychol Rep* 23:731-736, 1968
A preliminary study on the use of a disclosing agent (erythrosin) as an indicator of bacterial plaque on teeth.

548. Feldman RG, Pippenger CE: The relation of anticonvulsant drug levels to complete seizure control. *J Clin Pharmacol* 29:51-59, 1976
Descriptive study showing that serum levels of phenytoin are not closely related to seizure control.

549. Fitzloff J, Eshelman F: Quantitative urine analysis for measuring compliance. *Am J Hosp Pharm* 33:990-992, 1976
Comparison of results of UV spectrophotometry and gas chromatographic methods for detecting the primary metabolite of tolbutamide in urine.

550. Forrest FM, Forrest IS, Mason AS: Review of rapid urine tests for phenothiazine and related drugs. *Am J Psychiatr* 118:300-307, 1971
Review of urinary tests for phenothiazines and related substances.

551. Gold S, Griffiths PD, Huntsman RG: Phenothiazines in urine. *Br J Psychiatr* 108:88-94, 1962
Comparison of results given by several urinary tests for phenothiazines and imipramine among hospitalized psychiatric patients.

552. Goldstein A, Brown BW: Urine testing schedules in methadone maintenance treatment of heroin addiction. *JAMA* 214:311-315, 1970
Discussion proposing the use of randomized schedules for urine testing to ascertain abstinence among heroin addicts.

553. Haerer AF, Grace JB: Studies of anticonvulsant levels in epileptics. *Acta Neurol Scand* 45:18-31, 1969

Attempts to correlate various recognized side effects of diphenylhydantoin with actual serum levels. No direct information on compliance per se.

554. Hobby GL, Deuschle KW: The use of riboflavin as an indicator of isoniazid ingestion in self-medicated patients. *Am Rev Resp Dis* 80:415-423, 1959
Complete description of the method of use of riboflavin as a urinary marker for medication intake.

555. Jusko W, Levy G, Yaffe S: Effect of age on intestinal absorption of riboflavin in humans. *J Pharm Sci* 59:487-490, 1970
Useful article for those interested in using riboflavin as a compliance marker.

556. Khalil S, Salama R: A new colormetric method for the determination of methyldopa. *J Pharm Pharmac* 26:972-974, 1974
Biochemical details of a rapid method for quantitative measurement of methyldopa in vitro.

557. Krebs R: Using attendance as a means of evaluating community mental health programs. *Community Ment Health J* 7:72-77, 1971
Report on the efficacy of using attendance as a measure in evaluating success or failure of a community mental health program.

558. Lewis LA, Brown HB, Page IH: Ten years dietary treatment of primary hyperlipidemia. *Geriatrics* 25:64-81, 1970
As a noncentral issue, methods of compliance surveillance are discussed in relation to diet studies in this report of hyperlipidemia intervention attempts.

559. Likes K, Eshelman F: Pharmacokinetic calculations in determining compliance (letter). *Am J Hosp Pharm* 33:20-21, 1976
Description of use of pharmacokinetic theory to predict serum drug levels, which may be compared with actual blood levels in order to determine compliance.

560. Luchins D, Ananth J: Therapeutic implications of tricyclic antidepressant plasma levels. *J Nerv Ment Dis* 162:430-436, 1976
Though not on compliance, this article outlines the difficulty in correlating body fluid drug levels with achievement of the therapeutic goal.

561. Lund L, Alvan G: Phenytoin dosage nomogram. *Lancet* 2:1305-1306, 1975
Letter recommending serum phenytoin levels for monitoring epileptic therapy and showing that the drug kinetics need to be evaluated on an individual basis, while discouraging use of nomogram.

562. Madden P, Goodman S, Guthrie H: Validity of the 24-hr recall. *J Am Diet Assoc* 68:143-147, 1976
Unobtrusive direct observations were used to asses the validity of twenty-four hour food recall among elderly, noninstitutionalized individuals.

563. Mayer TC: Drug defaulting in general practice (letter). *Br Med J* 1:705, 1969
Prescribing in multiples of seven makes it easier to assess whether drugs have been taken in correct dosage.

564. Melchoic JC: The clinical use of serum determinations of phenytoin and phenobarbital in children. *Dev Med Child Neurol* 7:387-391, 1965
Description of the laboratory measurement of serum phenytoin and phenobarbital levels with dose-level correlations among epileptic children.

565. Middleton EJ, Davies JM, Morrison AB: Relationship between rate of dissolution, disintegration time, and physiological availability of riboflavin in sugar-coated tablets. *J Pharm Sci* 53:1378-1380, 1964
Description of test of and results for in vitro dissolution and distintegration of riboflavin compared to its bioavailability.

566. Mitchison DA, Allen BW, Miller AB: Detection of rifampicin in urine by a simple microbiological assay. *Tubercle* 51:300-304, 1970
A technique for the detection of rifampicin in urine by microbiological assay is described.

567. Moulding T, Knight SJ, Colson JB: Vertical pill-calendar dispenser and medication monitor for improving the self-aministration of drugs. *Tubercle* 48:32-37, 1967
Description of a pill calendar/medication monitor.

568. Moulding T: Proposal for a time-recording pill dispenser as a method for studying and supervising the self-administration of drugs. *Am Rev Resp Dis* 85:754-757, 1962
Description of a round variant of Moulding's vertical pill dispenser.

569. _____: The medication monitor for studying the self-administration of oral contraceptives. *Am J Obstet Gynecol* 110:1143-1144, 1971
Description of the methods applicable to the use of a special medication monitor in assessing compliance problems among women on oral contraceptives.

570. Oakes M, Human RP, Meers PD: Serum-levels of four antibiotics administered orally to patients in general practice. *Lancet* 1:222-224, 1973
Methods are described for the measurement of four antibiotics in serum as utilized among 50 outpatients with presumed bacterial infections. Implications for the monitoring of compliance are discussed.

571. Paulson SM, Krause S, Iber F: Development and evaluation of a compliance test for patients taking disulfiram. *Johns Hopkins Med J* 141:119-125, 1977
Development of a breath test to detect carbon disulfide, a metabolite of disulfiram that is used in the treatment of alcoholism.

572. Plaa GL, Hine CH: Hydantoin and barbiturate blood levels observed in epileptics. *Arch Int Pharmacodyn* 128:375-382, 1960
Description of the biochemical measurement of diphenylhydantoin, n-methylethylphenylhydantoin (mesantoin), and barbiturates in blood.

573. Pollack B: The validity of the Forrest reagent test for the detection of chlorpromazine or other phenothiazines in the urine. *Am J Psychiatr* 115:77-78, 1958
Study of the specificity and sensitivity of urine testing with Forrest's reagent for phenothiazines in the urine.

574. Roberts RW: Comparative study of urine tests for the detection of isoniazid. *Am Rev Resp Dis* 80:904-908, 1959

Two procedures for testing urine for presence of isoniazid were evaluated in ambulatory and hospitalized patients at different time intervals after ingestion.

575. Rosenberg A: Fall in carbon-monoxide blood levels after stopping smoking (letter). *Lancet* 1:593, 1972
Brief report of carboxyhemoglobin levels among smokers and of the time required to reach zero levels after quitting.

576. Ryan WL, Carver MJ, Haller J: Phenolsulfonphthalein as an index of drug ingestion. *Am J Pharm* 134:168-171, 1962
Description of the use of phenolsulfonphthalein (phenol red, PSP) as a urinary marker of drug ingestion.

577. Schork MA, Remington RD: The determination of sample size in treatment-control comparisons for chronic disease studies in which dropout or non-adherence is a problem. *J Chron Dis* 20:233-239, 1967
A description and rationale for a method of determining sample size in treatment-control studies.

578. Sheiner L, Rosenberg B, Marathe V, Peck C: Differences in serum digoxin concentrations between outpatients and inpatients: An effect of compliance? *Clin Pharmacol Ther* 15:239-246, 1974
Report of the quantification of outpatient digoxin compliance based on pharmacodynamic interpretation of serum digoxin levels.

579. Silberstein R, Blackman S: A method to evaluate whether patients take prescribed medication. *Clin Pediatr* 5:239-240, 1966
Very brief account of the use of riboflavin tablets to determine pill compliance.

580. Simpson J: Simple tests for the detection of urinary PAS. *Tubercle* 37:333-340, 1956
Two straightforward tests for detecting PAS in the urine are clearly described.

581. Stark JE, Ellard G, Gammon P, Fox W: The use of isoniazid as a marker to monitor the self-administration of medicaments. *Br J Clin Pharm* 2:355-358, 1975
The effectiveness of isoniazid as a compliance monitor was tested in a group of male student volunteers.

582. Stensrud PA, Palmer H: Serum phenytoin determinations in epileptics. *Epilepsia* 5:364-370, 1964
Laboratory and clinical correlation of serum phenytoin levels.

REVIEWS, COMMENTARIES, AND EDITORIALS

583. A position in support of a national health program. Position paper adopted by the board of trustees, Society for Public Health Education, 4 November 1973
Claims in favor of widespread implementation of health education programs with relevance for compliance implied.

584. Aberg H: Patient compliance. *Acta Med Scand* (Suppl) 606:25-31, 1977

A review of some of the literature concerning compliance with hypertension therapy plus suggestions to improve compliance.

585. Arthur H, Dawson D: The role of intake procedures and community education in reducing no-show rates. *Hosp Community Psychiatry* 28:511-512, 1977

A brief report on appointment-keeping rates at a community psychiatric service.

586. Atkinson A, Skegg J: Anti-smoking publicity and the demand for tobacco in the UK, *Manch Sch Soc Stud* 44:265-282, 1973

A reevaluation of data describing the effect of publicity and taxation on tobacco use in the UK.

587. Atkinson L, Gibson I, Andrews J: The difficulties of old people taking drugs. *Age Aging* 6:144-150, 1977

Review article outlining problems that lead to nonadherence to medication regimens in elderly patients.

588. Auger T, Wright E, Simpson R: Posters as smoking deterrents. *J Appl Psychol* 56:169-171, 1972

Brief review of two studies assessing the effect of "no smoking" posters on cigarette consumption in public areas.

589. Ayd FJ: Single daily dose of antidepressants (editorial). *JAMA* 230:263-264, 1974

Commentary on compliance aspects of reducing the frequency of pill taking for depressed patients and results of a letter survey of psychiatrists' prescribing habits.

590. Azarnoff DL, Abrams WB, Cuttner J, Hewitt WL, Hailman HF: Panel 3: Phase III investigations. *Clin Pharmacol Ther* 18:650-652, 1975

Expert panel recommendations on Phase III trials of new therapeutic agents including requirements to monitor and insure patient compliance.

591. Baekeland F, Lundwall L: Dropping out of treatment: A critical review. *Psychol Bull* 82:738-783, 1975

Extensive review of patient dropout from programs dealing with addiction, alcoholism, psychiatric ailments, and a few medical disorders.

592. Ball WL: Improving patient compliance with therapeutic regimens: Hamilton symposium examines the problems and solutions. *Can Med Assoc J* 111:268-282, 1974

General review article of determinants of compliance and proposed interventions.

593. Baretz RM, Stephenson GR: Unrealistic patient. *NY State J Med* 76:54-57, 1976

Reviews problem of psychiatric patients who refuse to comply with therapy due to denial and depression and suggests strategies for management.

594. Barmes D: Gaining acceptance of preventive measures. *NZ Soc Periodont Bull* 42:3-12, 1976

Commentary on the need to gain public cooperation with the various aspects of preventive dental measures.

595. Barnes ST, Jenkins CD: Changing personal and social behaviour: Experiences of health workers in a tribal society. *Soc Sci Med* 6:1-15, 1972
Review discussion of an epidemiologic analysis of resistance to an anti-malaria campaign in an underdeveloped country and solutions offered.
596. Barofsky I (ed): *Medication Compliance: A Behavioral Management Approach*. Thorofare, NJ, Slack, 1977
This book contains 19 articles concerned with compliance to medication regimens with emphasis on the treatment of hypertension.
597. Barofsky I: Behavioral therapeutics and the management of therapeutic regimens, pp 100-109, in Sackett DL, Haynes RB (eds): *Compliance with Therapeutic Regimens*, Baltimore, Johns Hopkins University Press, 1976
Discussion of the application of behavior modification techniques to the management of patient compliance with therapeutic regimens.
598. _____: *Compliance, Adherence and the Therapeutic Alliance*, Proceedings of the First International Congress on Patient Counselling. Amsterdam, Excerpta Medica Foundation 1976
A review of some of the patient-therapy interactions that affect compliance and the development of self-care.
599. _____: Introduction, pp xv-xvii, in Barofsky I (ed): *Medication Compliance: A Behavioral Management Approach*, Thorofare, NJ, Slack, 1977
Initial statement concerning scope and justification of the book.
600. _____: Sociological and psychological aspects of medication compliance, pp 29-44, in Barofsky I (ed): *Medication Compliance: A Behavioral Management Approach*. Thorofare, NJ, Slack, 1977
Review of some of the sociopsychological factors that affect compliance to medication regimens.
601. _____: Summary, pp 215-221, in Barofsky I (ed): *Medication Compliance: A Behavioral Management Approach*, Thorofare, NJ, Slack, 1977
Summary of Barofsky's volume on medication compliance.
602. Bebbington PE: The efficacy of Alcoholics Anonymous: The elusiveness of hard data. *Br J Psychiatr* 128:572-580, 1976
Review of studies of effectiveness of Alcoholics Anonymous upon compliance with abstinence from alcohol.
603. Becker M (ed): The health belief model and personal health behavior. *Health Educ Monogr* 2:324-473, 1974
A monograph that explores the origin and characteristics of the health belief model and its relation to preventive illness and sick role behavior.
604. Becker MH, Green LW: A family approach to compliance with medical treatment—a selective review of the literature. *Int J Health Educ* 18:1-11, 1975
This paper attempts to demonstrate the value of studying patient-family interactions to identify determinants of compliance and strategies for improving compliance.
605. Becker MH: Sociobehavioral determinants of compliance, pp 40-50, in

Sackett DL, Haynes RB (eds): *Compliance with Therapeutic Regimens,* Baltimore, Johns Hopkins University Press, 1976
Review of the sociobehavioral factors associated with patient compliance and an in-depth description of the health belief model.

606. Berkanovic E: Behavioral science and prevention. *Prev Med* 5:92-105, 1976
Examination of the health belief model plus social networks that influence individual behavior and through which behavior modifying techniques must function.

607. Birch D: Control: Cigarettes and calories. *Can Nurse* 71:33-35, 1975
Description of a strategy to avoid an increase in weight when stopping smoking.

608. Biron P, Carignan R: Chromoconfusion, a new type of pill-pill "interaction". *Can Med Assoc J* 110:1346-1347, 1974
Commentary on the confusion created by similarity of pill sizes, shapes, and color when patients are placed on regimens involving more than one pill type.

609. Biron P: Dosage, compliance and bioavailability in perspective. *Can Med Assoc J* 115:102-103, 1976
A thoughtful review of the relative importance of compliance, dose, and bioavailability as determinants of effective plasma concentrations of prescribed drugs.

610. Blackwell B: Chemical coping. Self-control and compliance in hypertension, pp 57-67, in Barofsky I (ed); *Medication Compliance: A Behavioral Management Approach.* Thorofare, NJ, Slack, 1977
Discussion of the relative merits of psychological and drug therapies in the management of hypertension.

611. _____: Drug deviation in psychiatric patients, pp 17-31, in Ayd FJ (ed): *The Future of Pharmacotherapy in New Drug Delivery Systems.* Baltimore, International Drug Therapy Newsletter, 1973
Review article on compliance among psychiatric patients with special focus on measurement and determinants; additional comments on magnitude and possible interventions.

612. _____: Patient compliance. *N Engl J Med* 289:249-253, 1973
General review article of determinants of compliance and proposed interventions.

613. _____: Treatment adherence. *Br J Psychiatr* 129:513-531, 1976
A general review of the magnitude, determinants, and strategies for improving compliance, with an emphasis on medical and psychiatric disorders.

614. _____: Treatment adherence in hypertension. *Am J Pharm* 148:75-85, 1976
Thorough review of and commentary on compliance and strategies to improve compliance in hypertension and other chronic diseases.

615. _____: The drug defaulter. *Clin Pharmacol Ther* 13:841-848, 1972
Review of methods of measurement, magnitude, and correlates of noncompliance.

616. Boyd J, Covington T, Stanaszek W, Coussons R: Drug defaulting part 1: Determinants of compliance. *Am J Hosp Pharm* 31:362-367, 1974
A review of factors influencing drug defaulters and some suggested strategies pharmacists could use to increase compliance.
617. Bryan CK: Patient information vs patient education. *Drug Intell Clin Pharm* 10:314-318, 1976
Commentary on the importance of educating the patient about the need to comply with medical advice rather than merely to present the information.
618. Buskirk ER: Obesity: A brief overview with emphasis on exercise. *Fed Proc* 33:1948-1951, 1974
Review of prevention and treatment of obesity.
619. Canada AT: The pharmacist and drug compliance, pp 129-134, in Sackett DL, Haynes RB (eds): *Compliance with Therapeutic Regimens*, Baltimore, Johns Hopkins University Press, 1976
A review of the pharmacist's involvement in measuring and promoting patient compliance with medication therapy.
620. Caplan R, Robinson E, French J, Caldwell J, Shinn M: *Adhering to Medical Regimens: Pilot Experiments in Patient Education and Social Support.* Ann Arbor, Institute for Social Research, 1976
Volume containing chapters discussing models, methods, and predictors of adherence to medical regimens.
621. Chambers DW: Behavior management techniques for pediatric dentists: An embarrassment of riches. *J Dent Child* 44:30-34, 1977
A review of behavior modification methods used by dentists in the management of children.
622. Charney E: Compliance and prescribance. *Am J Dis Child* 129:1009-1010, 1975
Excellent editorial viewing noncompliance from the perspective of poor drug efficacy and prescribing.
623. _____: Patient-doctor communication: Implications for the clinician. *Pediatr Clin North Am* 19:263-279, 1972
General review article.
624. Clark JR: Oral hygiene in the orthodontic practice: Motivation, responsibilities, and concepts. *Am J Orthod* 69:72-82, 1976
An article reviewing the importance of oral hygiene and some methods that can promote dental care habits.
625. Compliance, pp 41-46, in Weiss SM (ed): *Proceedings of the National Heart and Lung Institute Working Conference on Health Behavior.* Bethesda, NIH, 1975
Recommendations of research focusing on the health belief model.
626. Crawford JJ, Pell J: The Rand Report: A brief critique. *Addict Behav* 2:141-146, 1977
A critical review of a publication of the Rand Corporation about alcoholism and its treatment, including identification of several methodological problems one of which was the high subject loss to follow-up interviews.

627. Cristol AH: Techniques to reduce drop outs in a psychiatric clinic. *Penn Psychol Q* 3:32-35, 1963
     A brief comment on maintaining the traditional doctor-patient relationship in psychoanalysis with the aim of continuing therapy.

628. Crooks J, Shepherd A, Stevenson I: Drugs and the elderly, the nature of the problem. *Health Bull* 33:222-226, 1975
     A brief reference to poor drug compliance in the elderly and some suggested improvements.

629. Darrow WW: Approaches to the problem of venereal disease prevention. *Prev Med* 5:165-175, 1976
     A review of methods and successes in preventing venereal disease.

630. Davidoff F: Compliance with antihypertensive therapy: The last link in the chain. *Conn Med* 40:378-383, 1976
     Review of compliance-improving programs in hypertension and diabetes.

631. Davis MS: Documenting the need, pp 13-26, in *Proceedings of the Second Invitational Conference on Health Education in the Hospital*, Chicago, American Hospital Association, 1969
     Position paper promoting the use of patient education to improve compliance.

632. Davis P: Compliance structures and the delivery of health care: The case of dentistry. *Soc Sci Med* 10:329-337, 1976
     A theoretical discussion of issues concerning dental health and care in New Zealand. The conceptual orientation is within the framework of a compliance model.

633. Dembroski TM: Clarification of the relationship between the development and modification of life-style and chronic disease: Is it possible? pp 108-121, in Weiss SM (ed): *Proceedings of the National Heart and Lung Institute Working Conference on Health Behavior*. Bethesda, NIH, 1975
     Review of literature relating chronic disease prevention and control to lifestyle and health behaviors.

634. Demone H: Experiments in referral to alcoholism clinics. *Q J Stud Alcohol* 24:495-502, 1963
     Review of four studies of improving treatment links with problem alcoholics.

635. Dengler HJ, Lasagna L: Report of a workshop on fixed-ratio drug combinations. *Eur J Clin Pharmacol* 8(2):149-154, 1975
     Report on various pros and cons of fixed-ratio drug combinations including convenience, compliance, cost, efficacy, and safety.

636. Dollery CT: Pharmacological basis for combination therapy of hypertension. *Annu Rev Pharmacol Toxicol* 17:311-323, 1977
     A discussion of the use of drug combinations in the treatment of hypertension with an addendum about the compliance problems associated with multiple medications.

637. Dooley BJ: The effect of compulsory seat belt wearing on the mortality and pattern of injury to car occupants. Proceedings Reports, *J Bone Joint Surg* 57b:252, 1975

Abstract of report concerning the effectiveness of seat belt legislation in Victoria, Australia.

638. Dunbar JM, Stunkard AJ: Adherence to diet and drug regimen, pp 391-423 in Levy R, Rifkind B, Dennis B, Ernst N (eds): *Nutrition,Lipids, and Coronary Heart Disease*. New York, Raven Press, 1979.
Extensive and thorough review of the literature of compliance with a special focus on dietary problems.

639. Editorial: Keep on taking the tablets. . .*Lancet* 2:195-196, 1970
Commentary on the demerits of available biochemical methods of medication compliance monitoring.

640. Editorial: Cheek-pouches. *Lancet* 1:888, 1972
Commentary on methods of monitoring compliance.

641. Editorial: Acceptance of measles vaccine. *Lancet* 2:387-388, 1977
Brief comment on measles vaccination rates in the USA and the UK.

642. Editorial: Keep on taking the tablets. *Br Med J* 1:793, 1977
Brief comment on nonadherence to drug treatments.

643. Editorial: The need for patient education. *Am J Public Health* 61:1277-1279, 1971
Commentary on the recommendations of the Committee on Educational Tasks in Chronic Illness.

644. Editorial: Successes, failures and prospects of the anti-smoking programme. *Med J Aust* 2:815-816, 1975
Comments on the effectiveness of the antismoking program in Australia.

645. Edsall JR, Awe R, Bunyan S, Hackney R, Iseman N, Reagan W: Treatment of tuberculosis in alcohlic patients. *Am Rev Resp Dis* 116:559-561, 1977
Guidelines to assist in maintenance of treatment of tuberculosis in alcoholic patients.

646. Effects of treatment on morbidity in hypertension. III) Influence of age, diastolic pressure and prior cardiovascular disease; further analysis of side effects. Veterans Administration Cooperative Study Group on Antihypertensive Agents. *Circulation* 45:991-1004, 1972
Discussion of endpoints in the VA hypertension trials, including a description of side effects among study and control subjects and the changes in therapy necessitated by them.

647. Effects of treatment on morbidity in hypertension: Results in patients with diastolic blood presssure averaging 115 through 129 mm Hg. Veterans Administration Cooperative Study Group on Antihypertensive Agents. *JAMA* 202:1028-1034, 1967
Results of the VA studies on the efficacy of antihypertensive agents, with a description of prerandomization compliance screening maneuvers.

648. Emrick CD: A review of psychologically oriented treatment of alcoholism: I) The use and interrelationships of outcome criteria and drinking behavior following treatment. *Q J Stud Alcohol* 35:523-549, 1974
A summary of results of 271 studies that evaluated outcome following psychologically oriented treatment.

649. _____: A review of psychologically oriented treatment of alcoholism: II) The relative effectiveness of different treatment approaches and the effectiveness of treatment versus no treatment. *J Stud Alcohol* 36:88-108, 1975
Review of 384 studies. Degree of abstinence from alcohol used as end result to measure difference between treated and untreated patients.

650. Ensor PG, Rosenberg SG: Principles of learning, patient education and hypertension, pp 167-179, in Barofsky I (ed): *Medication Compliance: A Behavioral Management Approach*. Thorofare, NJ, Slack, 1977
Review of patient education as it relates to compliance with medication therapy for hypertension.

651. Epstein LH, McCoy JF: Issues in smoking control. *Addict Behav* 1:65-72, 1975
A review of the effectiveness of current intervention strategies related to reduction of smoking and the maintenance of effects.

652. Evans R, Kirk R, Walker P, Rosenbluth S, McDonald J: Medication maintenance of mentally ill patients by a pharmacist in a community setting. *Am J Hosp Pharm* 33:835-838, 1976
Study of the ability of a community pharmacy to assist in the care of mentally ill outpatients by monitoring compliance, side effects, drug interactions, and by making minor alterations in treatment according to the patient's mental status.

653. Evans RI: Smoking in children: Developing a social psychological strategy of deterrance. *Prev Med* 5:122-127, 1976
Description of technique under study to prevent children from starting to smoke.

654. Faigel HC: Getting patients to follow advice: The art of communication. *Clin Pediatr* 11:666-667, 1972
A brief review of three studies of doctor-patient communications and suggestions to improve cooperation.

655. Feinstein AR: Biostatistical problems in compliance bias. *Clin Pharmacol Ther* 16:846-857, 1974
Review of features of compliance that can affect biostatistical data and interpretations.

656. _____: "Compliance bias" and the interpretation of therapeutic trials, pp 152-166, in Sackett DL, Haynes RB (eds): *Compliance with Therapeutic Regimens*. Baltimore, Johns Hopkins University Press, 1976
Discussion of six features of compliance that can affect biostatistical data and interpretations.

657. Ferguson T: The non-compliant patient. *J Tenn Med Assoc* 70:248-251, 1977
A brief review of some factors affecting compliance with hypertension therapy plus a report of a case study of a noncompliant patient.

658. Fink DL: Tailoring the consensual regimen, pp 110-118, in Sackett DL, Haynes RB (eds): *Compliance with Therapeutic Regimens*. Baltimore, Johns Hopkins University Press, 1976

Prescribing the therapeutic regimen so that it is agreeable to provider and patients.

659. Fink JL: On pharmacist's role in patient behavior. *Am J Public Health* 67:269-270, 1977
A brief letter commenting on the pharmacist's influence on patient behavior.

660. Finnerty FA: The DC general hospital experience, pp 211-214, in Barofsky I (ed): *Medication Compliance: A Behavioral Management Approach*. Thorofare, NJ, Slack, 1977
Article advocating changes in the health care delivery system in order to improve patient adherence to therapy.

661. Fitzgerald JD: The influence of the medication on compliance with therapeutic regimens, pp 119-128, in Sackett DL, Haynes RB (eds): *Compliance with Therapeutic Regimens*. Baltimore, Johns Hopkins University Press, 1976
Examination of some aspects of the relationship between drug characteristics and compliance.

662. Foldvary LA, Lane JC: The effectiveness of compulsory wearing of seatbelts in casualty reduction. *Accid Anal Prev* 6:59-81, 1974
A descriptive report of the effectiveness of seat belt use in reducing traffic accident casualties before and after legislation for compulsory wearing in Victoria, Australia.

663. Fox EM: Drug compliance in the elderly. *Br Med J* 1:578, 1977
This short letter comments on the efficacy of using distinctive tablets and combined preparations to increase drug compliance in elderly patients.

664. Fox W: Self-administration of medicaments; a review of published work and a study of the problems. *Bull Union Against Tuber* 32:307-331, 1962
Review of measurement of compliance, some selected aspects of compliance problems, and some methods of improving compliance.

665. _____: The problem of self-administration of drugs: With particular reference to pulmonary tuberculosis. *Tubercle* 39:269-274, 1958
Review article plus anecdotal account of compliance monitoring and determinants at a tuberculosis control center.

666. Fredrickson D: Helping smokers quit: The physician's role (editorial interview). *Ca* 26:236-241, 1976
Advice on formal and informal methods physicians can use or prescribe for helping patients quit smoking.

667. Gagnon MA: Subjective phenomena in drug trials. *Int J Clin Pharmacol* 15:155-160, 1977
A discussion of the types of problems arising from subjective elements in pharmacological studies.

668. Garfield SL: A note on the confounding of personality and social class characteristics in research on premature termination. *J Consult Clin Psychol* 45:483-485, 1977

A brief critical evaluation of an earlier article in terms of its appraisal of research in the area of early termination in psychotherapy.

669. Gavrin JB, Tursky E, Albam B, Feinstein AR: Rheumatic fever in children and adolescents, II) Maintenance and preservation of the population. *Ann Intern Med* 60(5): 18:30, 1964
Résumé of procedures utilized to maintain compliance among children receiving prophylaxis for rheumatic fever at a special treatment center.

670. Gillum RF, Barsky AJ: Diagnosis and management of patient noncompliance. *JAMA* 228:1563-1567, 1974
A review of current understanding with recommendations to physicians for anticipating and minimizing noncompliance.

671. Gold S: Plaque-control motivation in orthodontic practice. *Am J Orthod* 68:8-14, 1975
Article describing use of patient contracts and psychotherapeutic techniques in orthodontics.

672. Goldsmith CH: The effect of differing compliance distributions on the planning and statistical analysis of therapeutic trials, pp 137-151, in Sackett DL, Haynes RB (eds): *Compliance with Therapeutic Regimens*. Baltimore, Johns Hopkins University Press, 1976
A proposal of a uniform compliance measure and a study of the effects of differing compliance distributions on the outcome of clinical trials.

673. Gordis L: Methodologic issues in the measurement of patient compliance, pp 51-66, in Sackett DL, Haynes RB (eds): *Compliance with Therapeutic Regimens*. Baltimore, Johns Hopkins University Press, 1976
Discussion of difficulties in and solutions to the measurement of noncompliant patient behavior.

674. Gordon J: Evaluation of communications media in two health projects in Baltimore. *Public Health Rep* 82:651-655, 1967
Description of the relative impact of various forms of mass media and personal messages in influencing people to use prenatal and diabetic screening facilities.

675. Gori G: Artificial tobacco substitutes. *JAMA* 234:489-490, 1975
Commentary on the current state of development and potential benefit of an artificial tobacco substitute.

676. _____: Smoking and cancer: Research in etiology and prevention at the National Cancer Institute. *Cancer* 30:1340-1343, 1972
General outline of the N.C.I. approaches to reducing cigarette smoking or altering its harmful effects.

677. Gorlich GM: Package inserts and noncompliance with doctors' orders (letter). *Pediatrics* 51:312, 1973
Letter suggesting that when physician samples are given to patients, the inserts intended for the physician tend to list adverse reactions in such detail that the patient will not be likely to comply.

678. Green LW, Levine DM, Deeds S: Clinical trials of health education for hypertensive outpatients—design and baseline data. *Prev Med* 4:417-425, 1975

Theoretical consideration of baseline data for experiments in health education to improve patient compliance.

679. Green LW: Evaluation and measurement: Some dilemmas for health education. *Am J Public Health* 67:155-161, 1977
Several problems of assessment posed by the nature of health education are described along with suggestions for their resolution.

680. _____: Site- and symptom-related factors in secondary prevention of cancer, pp 45-61, in Cullen JW, Fox BH, Isom RN (eds): *Cancer: The Behavioral Dimensions*. New York, Raven Press, 1976
This chapter discusses some of the factors involved in delay in seeking medical care for cancer.

681. _____: The potentital of health education includes cost effectiveness. *Hospitals* 50:57-61, 1976
Commentary on the potential benefits to be derived from formal health education programs.

682. Grissom RL: Patient self-care in hypertension: A physician's perspective, pp 105-113, in Barofsky I (ed): *Medication Compliance: A Behavioral Management Approach*. Thorofare, NJ, Slack, 1977
Discussion of self-care in the management of hypertension.

683. Gwinup G, Poucher R: A controlled study of thyroid analogs in the therapy of obesity. *Am J Med Sci* 254:416-420, 1967
Comparison of T4, T3, and placebo in inducing weight reduction. Not a compliance study per se, this study illustrates a potential avenue for obviating compliance problems.

684. Hackney RL: Treating tuberculosis in the poor black alcoholic male. *Am Rev Resp Dis* 112:150-151, 1975
Comment suggesting need for longer (four-eight weeks) initial hospitalization for TB therapy in poor black alcoholic males.

685. Haddon W: Perspective on a current public health controversy. *Am J Public Health* 65:1342-1344, 1975
Informative commentary on active and passive restraints for automobile safety and the legal wrangling involved in their implementation.

686. _____: Strategy in preventive medicine: Passive vs active approaches to reducing human wastage. *J Trauma* 14:353-354, 1974
Editorial outlining the differences between active and passive approaches to health-related activities and their relative potency in achieving cooperation.

687. Hall B: Mutual withdrawal: The non-participant in a therapeutic community. *Perspect Psychiatr Care* 14:75-77,93, 1976
Thoughtful commentary on active and passive participation in psychotherapy.

688. Halperin M, Rogot E, Gurian J, Ederer F: Sample sizes for medical trials with special reference to long-term therapy. *J Chron Dis* 21:13-24, 1968
Theoretical considerations concerning sample sizes for long-term studies allowing for withdrawals, dropouts, and nonadherence; includes tables.

689. Hannay D: Self-medication—developing a concept in future hospital pharmacy service. A report submitted to the pharmacy residency committee, Victoria Hospital, London, Ontario, Canada, 1973
Review of two inpatient programs of drug self-administration and a protocol for assessment of the effect of such programs on subsequent outpatient compliance.

690. Hauser R: Rapid smoking as a technique of behavior modification: Caution in selection of subjects. *J Consult Clin Psychol* 42:625-626, 1974
Comment on the potential risks of rapid smoking as an antismoking measure and a reply to the caution.

691. Hayes-Bautista D: Modifying the treatment: Patient compliance, patient control and medical care. *Soc Sci Med* 10:233-238, 1976
Theoretical formulation of routes to noncompliant behavior from the patient's reported perspective, focusing on the patient-therapist interaction.

692. Haynes R, Sackett D, Gibson E, Taylor D, Roberts R, Johnson A: Manipulation of the therapeutic regimen to improve patient compliance: Conceptions and misconceptions. *Clin Pharmacol Ther* 22:125-130, 1977
Analysis of factors related to the nature, frequency, duration, amount, cost, and side effects of the treatment and their bearing on compliance.

693. Haynes RB, Sackett DL: Appendix I: An Annotated Bibliography, pp 193-279, in Sackett DL, Haynes RB (eds): *Compliance with Therapeutic Regimens*. Baltimore, Johns Hopkins University Press, 1976
A bibliography of compliance research reports including annotations, assessment of scientific merit, and an extensive topic and content index.

694. Haynes RB: A critical review of the "determinants" of patient compliance with therapeutic regimens, pp 26-39, in Sackett DL, Haynes RB (eds): *Compliance with Therapeutic Regimens*. Baltimore, Johns Hopkins University Press, 1976
Methodologically derived description and review of the range of determinants of patient compliance.

695. _____: Strategies for improving compliance: A methodologic analysis and review, pp 69-82, in Sackett DL, Haynes RB (eds): *Compliance with Therapeutic Regimens*. Baltimore, Johns Hopkins University Press, 1976
Review of strategies for improving patient compliance and an assessment of their effectiveness.

696. Hecht A: Self-medication, inaccuracy, and what can be done. *Nurs Outlook* 18:30-31, 1970
Succinct review of the practical aspects of patient noncompliance from a nursing perspective.

697. Henderson J, Enelow A: The coronary risk factor problem: A behavioral perspective. *Prev Med* 5:128-148, 1976
Theoretical consideration and review of the behavioral aspects of achieving cooperation with preventive health measures.

698. Hewitt A: Significance of the "defaulter" in the assessment of efficiency of treatment in gonorrhea. *Br J Vener Dis* 45:40-41, 1969
Brief commentary urging inclusion of dropouts in the analysis of venereal disease studies.

699. Hieb E, Wang R: Compliance: The patient's role in drug therapy. *Wis Med J* 73:s152-s154, 1974
General advice on compliance, written in a journalistic style.

700. Hill M, Blane H: Evaluation of psychotherapy with alcoholics: A critical review. *Q J Stud Alcohol* 28:76-104, 1967
Methodologically oriented analysis of research on the use of psychotherapy to treat alcoholism.

701. Hingson RW: The physician's problems in identifying potentially noncompliant patients, pp 117-132, in Barofsky I (ed): *Medication Compliance: A Behavioral Management Approach*. Thorofare, NJ, Slack, 1977
Outline of the importance of finding reliable predictors of patient noncompliance.

702. Hochbaum G: Fear is not enough. *Am Lung Assoc Bulletin* :13-16, June 1975
Some practical and impractical suggestions for motivating smokers to quit.

703. Hogue C: Compliance in health care: Selected conceptual and methodologic issues. Paper presented at Regional Research Development Project Workshop, Chapel Hill, NC, September 1976
A brief review on the theory and practice of compliance management and research.

704. Hunt W, Bespalec D: An evaluation of current methods of modifying smoking behavior. *J Clin Psychol* 30:431-438, 1974
Methodological review of the relative success of various forms of antismoking therapy.

705. Hunt W, Matarazzo J: Three years later: Recent developments in the experimental modification of smoking behavior. *J Abnorm Psychol* 81:107-114, 1973
"State of the art" review of the (lack of) effectiveness of interventions for smoking, alcoholism, drug addiction with constructive comments for the future.

706. Hussar D: Patient noncompliance. *J Am Pharm Assoc* NS 15:183-190, 201, 1975
Thorough review of noncompliance with medications with a special focus on pharmacy aspects.

707. Inui T: Compliance with medical regimens: A problem in perspective. Unpublished article
Review of and commentary on compliance problems.

708. Jeffrey D: Some methodological issues in research on obesity. *Psychol Rep* 35:623-626, 1974
Call for greater scientific rigor in obesity studies with specific constructive criticisms of several methodologic inadequacies.

709. Jeffrey DB: Treatment outcome issues in obesity research, pp 20-29, in Williams B (ed): *Obesity: Behavioral Approaches to Dietary Management*. New York, Brunner-Mazel, 1976
This chapter discusses a number of treatment outcome issues, including compliance, that are relevant to the effectiveness of research in obesity.

710. Jellett LB: Patient compliance and drug therapy. *Aust J Pharm* 56:433-436, 1975
A review of factors influencing patient compliance and of methods for measuring compliance.

711. Jenkins CD: Cultural differences in concepts of disease and how this affects health behavior. Paper presented at compliance symposium, Mass College Pharmacy, Boston, February 1974
Discussion of various models of health behavior and their implications for predicting and dealing with noncompliance.

712. _____: Cultural differences in concepts of disease and how these affect health behavior, pp 9-18, in Barofsky I (ed): *Medication Compliance: A Behavioral Management Approach*. Thorofare, NJ, Slack, 1977
Discussion of health beliefs in different cultural and ethnic groups.

713. Johnson R: The ethical aspects of government intervention into individual behavior. Staff paper, Long Range Health Planning Branch, Ministry of Health, Ottawa, Canada, May 1976
Philosophical consideration of the ethical implications of government and medical attempts to alter unhealthy lifestyles.

714. Joubert P: Failure of therapeutic compliance—facts, fantasies and fallacies. *S Afr Med J* 52:254-255, 1977
A brief comment on the necessity of dealing with noncompliance in order to have successful therapies.

715. Joyce CR, Caple G, Mason M, Reynolds E, Mathews JA: Quantitative study of doctor-patient communication. *Q J Med* 38:183-194, 1969
Study of the information and instructions given by physicians to patients and the amount of information actually retained by the patient.

716. Kaplan NM: Achieving patient cooperation in the treatment of hypertension. *Hosp Formulary* 11:68-72, 1976
A discussion of the problems associated with hypertension therapy stressing the importance of maintaining patient compliance with effective medication regimens.

717. Kasachkoff AR: Group treatment and management of the hypertensive patient, pp 181-188, in Barofsky I (ed): *Medication Compliance: A Behavioral Management Approach*. Thorofare, NJ, Slack, 1977
Description of psychoeducational groups that can give patients mutual support and information.

718. Kasl SV, Cobb S: Health behavior, illness behavior and sick role behavior. *Arch Environ Health* 12:246-266, 1966
Review of scientific literature to 1964 concerning health behavior, illness behavior, and sick role behavior.

719. Keutzer C, Lichtenstein E, Mees H: Modification of smoking behavior: A review. *Psychol Bull* 70:520-533, 1968
Analytical review of behavior modification techniques compared to other methods of reducing cigarette smoking.
720. Kirscht JP: Communication between patients and physicians. *Ann Intern Med* 86:499-501, 1977
Editorial discussing the importance of doctor-patient interactions.
721. Komaroff A: The practitioner and the compliant patient. *Am J Public Health* 66:833-835, 1976
Editorial providing a brief but insightful review of compliance determinants and management.
722. Kratschmar A: An ergonomic patient instruction system for orthodontic appliances. *Quintessence International* 5:45-47, 1975
Description of printed instructions for children requiring orthodontic appliances, aimed at eight-nine-year-old level.
723. Kroll HW: Bibliography on behavioral approaches to modification of smoking: January 1964 through December 1973. *Psychol Rep* 35:435-440, 1974
Some 126 references on behavioral approaches to smoking modification are listed.
724. Laney F: Blood pressure and weight control programs. *Occup Health Nurs* 22:11-12, 1974
Informal pointers and advice on helping employees become thin and normotensive.
725. Lasagna L: Fault and default (editorial). *N Engl J Med* 289:267-268, 1973
Companion editorial to Blackwell's comprehensive review (*N Eng J Med* 289:249-253, 1973).
726. Lasky JJ: The problem of sample attrition in controlled treatment trials. *J Nerv Ment Dis* 135:332-337, 1962
General discussion of the effect of dropouts on study outcomes with specific examples and with some suggestions for avoiding or managing the problem.
727. Law SA: The patient's right to refuse treatment. *Hosp Med Staff* 5:1-7, 1976
A review of some of the legal aspects of a patient's refusal of treatment.
728. Leventhal H: Fear communications in the acceptance of preventive health practice. *Bull NY Acad Med* 41:1144-1168, 1965
Discussion of several studies concerning the ability of communications that induce fear to induce healthful behavioral change as well.
729. _____: Fear appeals and persuasions: The differentiation of a motivational construct. *Am J Public Health* 61:1208-1224, 1971
Review and discussion of the psychological effects of various types of health messages and their resultant effects on motivation and behavior.
730. Levy RL, Carter RD: Compliance with practitioner instigations. *Soc Work* 21:188-193, 1976

Review of methods for promoting compliance with a focus on social workers' behavioral instructions.

731. Lewis CE, Michnich M: Contracts as a means of improving patient compliance, pp 69-75, in Barofsky I (ed): *Medication Compliance: A Behavioral Management Approach*. Thorofare, NJ, Slack, 1977
Recommendation for use of contracts to increase patient compliance.

732. Ley P: Patient compliance—a psychologist's viewpoint. *Prescriber's J* 17:15-20, 1977
Practical pointers about the doctor-patient interaction and compliance.

733. _____: Towards better doctor-patient communications, pp 75-98, in Bennett AE (ed): *Communications between Doctors and Patients*. London, Oxford University Press, 1976
Comprehensive review of the relationships between medical communications and patients' memories, satisfactions, and compliance.

734. Liberman P, Swartz AJ: Prescription dispensing to the problem patient. *Am J Hosp Pharm* 29:163-166, 1972
Discussion of pharmacists' potential role in improving compliance with medications, with a case report as an example.

735. _____: A guide to help patients keep track of their drugs. *Am J Hosp Pharm* 29:507-509, 1972
Two types of medication calendars, designed to facilitate compliance, are described. Actual testing of the calendars was not reported.

736. Lichtenstein E, Danaher B: Modification of smoking behavior: A critical analysis of theory, research, and practice. *Prog Behav Mod* 3:79-132, 1976
Extensive review of behavior modification approaches (aversive and self-management techniques) to smoking cessation.

737. MacGregor FC: Uncooperative patients: Some cultural interpretations. *Am J Nurs* 67:88-91, 1967
Anecdotal account of some presumed cultural determinants of noncompliance.

738. MacHann W: A community hypertension-control program: Follow-up and patient compliance. *Bull NY Acad Med* 52:665-670, 1976
Description of the *modus operandi* of a public health approach for detecting and achieving optimal management of hypertension, with a major focus on proadherence maneuvers.

739. Mahoney A: Patient education: A nurse's perspective, pp 195-201, in Barofsky I (ed): *Medication Compliance: A Behavioral Management Approach*. Thorofare, NJ, Slack, 1977
The nurse's role in augmenting compliance to medication regimens.

740. Marston M: Nursing management of compliance with medication regimens, pp 139-164, in Barofsky I (ed): *Medication Compliance: A Behavioral Management Approach*. Thorofare, NJ, Slack, 1977
The role of the nurse in maintaining and enhancing medication compliance.

741. Marston MV: Compliance with medical regimens: A review of the literature. *Nurs Res* 19:312-323, 1970

Comprehensive review òf magnitude, measurement, and determinants of compliance.

742. Mason M: Some problems posed by out-patient trials with antirheumatic agents, pp 287-292, in Wagenhauser FJ (ed): *Chronic Forms of Polyarthritis*. Bern, Hans Huber, 1976
Review of some experimental work studying the determinants of outpatient cooperation with medication therapy for arthritis.

743. Mattar ME, Yaffe S: Compliance of pediatric patients with therapeutic regimens. *Postgrad Med* 56:181-188, 1974
Review article emphasizing practical aspects of managing noncompliance among pediatric patients.

744. Matthews D, Hingson R: Improving patient compliance: A guide for physicians. *Med Clin North Am* 61:879-889, 1977
A review of factors that influence compliance and interventions that have been used to improve compliance.

745. Matthews D: The noncompliant patient. *Primary Care* 2:289-294, 1975
General discussion of noncompliance, with practical suggestions for preventing and managing it.

746. May SJ, Kuller LH: Methodological approaches in the evaluation of alcoholism treatment: A critical review. *Prev Med* 4:464-481, 1975
Incisive critique of alcoholism programs and their evaluation.

747. Mazzullo J: Editorial: The nonpharmacologic basis of therapeutics. *Clin Pharmacol Ther* 13:157-158, 1972
Anecdotal account of reasons for using different, distinctive pill sizes, shapes, colors in prescribing in order to reduce medication errors.

748. Mazzullo JM, Lasagna L: Take thou . . . but is your patient really taking what you prescribed? *Drug Ther* 2:11-15, 1972
Proposed methods of improving compliance with medications are discussed.

749. Mazzullo JV, Lasagna L, Grinar PF: Variations in interpretation of prescription instructions: The need for improved prescribing habits. *JAMA* 227:929-931, 1974
Hospitalized patients were asked to interpret the instructions given on the prescription labels for ten commonly prescribed medications. Compliance was not studied, although the implication was that one source of noncompliance is misinterpretation of prescription instructions.

750. McAlister A, Farquhar J, Thoresen C, Maccoby N: Behavioral science applied to cardiovascular health: Progress and research needs in the modification of risk-taking habits in adult populations. *Health Educ Monogr* 4:45-74, 1976
A compendium of behaviorally oriented approaches to changing unhealthy lifestyles.

751. McKenney JM: The pharmacist's role in patient counselling. Paper presented to First International Congress on Patient Counselling. Amsterdam, Excerpta Medica Foundation, 1976

A review of some of the factors that affect adherence to drug prescriptions
in the treatment of hypertension.

752. McLeod DC: Contribution of clinical pharmacists to patient care. *Am J
Hosp Pharm* 33:904-911, 1976
A review of the literature concerned with the pharmacist's role in health
care.

753. Mecham vs McLeary, malpractice decisions you should know about.
Patient's contributing negligence. *Med Times* 104: 55-56, 1976
A malpractice suit that hinged upon "contributory negligence" by a
patient who failed to make and keep appointments.

754. Meenan RF: Improving the public's health—some further reflections.
N Engl J Med 294:45-47, 1976
Thoughtful consideration of some of the ethical issues in promoting com-
pliance with lifestyle changes.

755. Merrett RA, Clarke W: Auxiliary medication instructions: One way of
improving compliance. *Can Med Assoc J* 117:735, 1977
A letter containing a brief report on the use of instruction sheets for
prescription medications for outpatients.

756. Mikeal RL, Sharpe T: Patient compliance, pp 177-194, in Wertheimer A,
Smith M (eds): *Pharmacy Practice: Social and Behavioral Aspects*.
Baltimore, University Park Press, 1974
A comprehensive review of patient compliance with prescribed regimen
literature, including discussions of the problems related to methodology,
determinants and future research.

757. Morbidity and mortality in mild essential hypertension. United States
Public Health Service Hospitals Cooperative Study Group. *Circ Res*
30, Suppl 2:110-124, 1972
Preliminary results from a multicentred hypertension trial giving, additionally, a description of initial screening to eliminate noncompliers
from the study and an analysis of subsequent compliance.

758. Morris L, Gagliardi V: The patient package insert as drug education, pp
95-103, in Barofsky I (ed): *Medication Compliance: A Behavioral
Management Approach*. Thorofare, NJ, Slack, 1977
Advocates adequate medication information for the patient.

759. Moser M, Wood D: Management of hypertension—the problem of physician adherence. *JAMA* 235:2297-2298, 1976
A comment on the lack of physician motivation and enthusiasm in the
management of hypertension.

760. Moser M: Hypertension: A major controllable public health problem—
industry can help. *Occup Health Nurs* 25:19-26, 1977
Epidemiologic data and other factors related to hypertension are reported. Industry's role in helping hypertensive patients achieve better
results is discussed.

761. _____: Long-term management of hypertension. *NY State J Med* 77:76-
80, 1977
Reasons and suggested remedies for nonadherence to hypertension treatment programs, physician and patient oriented.

762. Moulding T: The realized and unrealized benefits from chemotherapy for tuberculosis. *Public Health Rep* 82:753-758, 1967
Review of identification, implications, and management of noncompliance in patients with tuberculosis.

763. Myers SA: Diabetes management by the patient and a nurse practitioner. *Nurs Clin North Am* 12:415-426, 1977
Discussion of problems related to compliance with programs of diabetes management.

764. Neeman RL, Neeman M: Complexities of smoking education. *J Sch Health* 45:17-23, 1975
A review of the effectiveness of public health education programs addressed to smoking prevention.

765. Neufeld VR: Patient education: A critique, pp 83-92, in Sackett DL, Haynes RB (eds): *Compliance with Therapeutic Regimens*. Baltimore, Johns Hopkins University Press, 1976
Review and analysis of the adequacy of educational principles and practice in reports of attempts to promote patient compliance through education.

766. Nies AS: Adverse reactions and interactions limiting the use of antihypertensive drugs. *Am J Med* 58:495-503, 1975
Review of the side effects of common antihypertensive drugs that may be responsible for patient compliance.

767. Patient's contributing negligence in malpractice decisions you should know about. *Med Times* 104:55-56, 1976
Malcompliance and malpractice: the law holds the patient responsible for failing to comply.

768. Pearson RM, Welsby PD: How not to do it: Prescribing. *Hosp Update* June:331-337, 1977
Advice to physicians on how to improve drug adherence by remaining knowledgeable about the drugs they prescribe and by checking patients' compliance.

769. Peck C: Current legislative issues concerning the right to refuse versus the right to choose hospitalization and treatment. *Psychiatry* 38:303-317, 1975
Consideration of current American legislation and legal controversy concerning the rights of patients to refuse and to seek psychiatric treatment.

770. Peto J: Price and consumption of cigarettes: A case for intervention? *Br J Prev Soc Med* 28:241-245, 1974
Statistical analysis and theoretical consideration of the effect of price, income, and antismoking publicity on cigarette consumption in England.

771. Pfeiffer FG: Analysis of the pharmacist's role in improving therapeutic compliance in ambulatory hypertensive outpatients. Master's thesis, University of Oklahoma, 1975
Introductory chapter reviewing the clinical pharmacist's role in promoting increased adherence to medication therapies.

772. Podell R: *Physician's Guide to Compliance in Hypertension.* Summit, NJ, Merck and Company, 1975
    Practical manual for the practitioner who wants to understand something about compliance and to become skilled in its management.

773. Podell RM, Gary LR: Hypertension and compliance: Implications for the primary physician. *N Engl J Med* 294:1120-1121, 1976
    Review and commentary on compliance problems and their management in hypertension with special focus on the need for research at the primary care level.

774. _____: Compliance: A problem in medical management. *Am Fam Physician* 13:74-80, 1976
    General review.

775. Polowich C, Elliott MR: The juvenile diabetic: In or out of control? *Can Nurse* 73:24-27, 1977
    Discussion of problems of noncompliance with diet restrictions in juvenile diabetics.

776. Pomerleau O, Bass F, Crown V: Role of behavior modification in preventive medicine. *N Engl J Med* 292:1277-1282, 1975
    Reviews behavior modification strategies used to improve compliance.

777. Porter AM: The problem of self-administration of drugs. Unpublished doctoral thesis, University of London, 1967
    The thesis describes at length the published findings concerning medication compliance among several groups of ambulatory private practice patients and also contains an extensive review of literature on compliance.

778. Porter RM: Patient assessment. *Bull Int Union Tuberc* 49:313:315, 1974
    Brief assessment of TB treatment in western Australia with emphasis on the use of objective measures, especially urine tests, to check drug compliance.

779. Pothier PD: Patient compliance in therapy. *Drug Intell Clin Pharm* 10:318-320, 1976
    A computer-generated bibliography of patient compliance from January 1973 to July 1975.

780. Potter R, Moots B: Reinsertion rates: A critique, in Hefnawi F, Segal SJ (eds): *Analysis of Intrauterine Contraception: Proceedings of Third International Conference on Intrauterine Contraception, Cairo, Egypt.* Amsterdam, North Holland, 1974
    A critical analysis of IUD continuation and reinsertion rates.

781. *Proceedings of the Nutritional-Behavioral Research Conference.* Bethesda Md, 1975
    Conference report containing a review of an ongoing project on compliance with dietary intervention therapy utilizing the health belief model of M.H. Becker. In addition, there is a workshop and discussion summary on the same topic.

782. Reichert P: Patients who won't take their medicine. *Consultant* :116-117, Jan 1976

Description of a practical method for patients to monitor their own compliance through a medication diary.

783. Reichman LB: Monitoring preventive therapy patients for liver disease as well as compliance. *Chest* 68:178-180, 1975
Description of a standardized surveillance protocol to detect, early on, patients who have toxicity from isoniazid prophylaxis for tuberculosis or who default from treatment.

784. Report of the task group on hypertension, pp 89-91, in Weiss SM (ed): *Proceedings of the National Heart and Lung Institute Working Conference on Health Behavior.* Bethesda, NIH, 1975
Recommendations for research on treatment regimens for hypertension and methods of determining and encouraging compliance.

785. Richards ND: Methods and effectiveness of health education: The past, present and future of social scientific involvement. *Soc Sci Med* 9:141-156, 1975
Thorough consideration of the definition, scope, strengths, and shortcomings of health education and attempts to evaluate it.

786. Roccella ET: Potential for reducing health care costs by public and patient education. *Public Health Rep* 91:223-224, 1976
Review of impact of patient education upon effectiveness of physician advocated maneuvers.

787. Rosenberg CM, Raynes AE: Dropouts from treatment. *Can Psychiatr Assoc J* 18:229-233, 1973
Review of characteristics of dropouts among general psychiatric patients, heroin addicts, and alcoholics.

788. Rosenberg SG: A case for patient education. *Hosp Formulary Management* 6:1-4, 1971
Review of the work of the author and others with respect to the efficacy of patient education methods designed to improve compliance and therapeutic outcomes.

789. _____: Patient education—an educator's view, pp 93-99, in Sackett DL, Haynes RB (eds): *Compliance with Therapeutic Regimens.* Baltimore, Johns Hopkins University Press, 1976
Chapter concerning patient education emphasizing the idea that educational efforts should be part of the total approach to care.

790. Rosenfield AG: The IUD in family planning programs: Programmatic issues, in Hefnawi F, Segal SJ (eds): *Analysis of Intrauterine Contraception*, Proceedings of the Third International Conference on Intrauterine Contraception, Cairo, Egypt, Amsterdam, North Holland, 1974
Review of some factors influencing IUD use and continuance in family planning programs.

791. Rosenstock IM: Patients' compliance with health regimens. *JAMA* 234:402-403, 1975
Summary article on the health belief model and its application in a Tay-Sachs screening project.

792. _____: Why people use health services. *Milbank Mem Fund Q* 44:94-124, 1966
     Review article of studies of relevance to the health belief model of pre-ventive health behavior.

793. Rosser WW: Does the family physician have a role in convincing people to stop smoking? Unpublished, University of Ottawa, 1977
     An outline of various techniques for helping patients reduce or stop smoking.

794. Sackett DL, Haynes RB (eds): *Compliance with Therapeutic Regimens.* Johns Hopkins University Press, Baltimore, 1976
     This book contains the plenary session presentations and annotated compliance bibliography from the first workshop/symposium on compliance held at McMaster University in May 1974.

795. Sackett DL: Introduction, pp 1-6, in Sackett DL, Haynes RB (eds): *Compliance with Therapeutic Regimens.* Baltimore, Johns Hopkins University Press, 1976
     Chapter introducing compliance terminology and airing recurring issues in compliance research and practice.

796. _____: Priorities and methods for future research, pp 169-189, in Sackett DL, Haynes RB (eds): *Compliance with Therapeutic Regimens.* Baltimore, Johns Hopkins University Press, 1976
     Chapter integrating the priorities for future research into compliance and a discussion of important methodological issues.

797. _____: The magnitude of compliance and noncompliance, pp 9-25, in Sackett DL, Haynes RB (eds): *Compliance with Therapeutic Regimens.* Baltimore, Johns Hopkins University Press, 1976
     Summary of representative studies documenting the magnitude of non-compliance.

798. Salkind MR: Assessment of drugs in general practice. *Br J Clin Pharm* 3:69-72, 1976
     Commentary on differences in compliance with tablet dosage and at-tendance between hospital and general practice.

799. Sarll DW: Patient co-operation in orthodontic treatment. *Br Dent J* 136:117-118, 1974
     A description of how satisfactory cooperation in orthodontic treatment may be obtained.

800. Sather M, Weber C, George J, Beilman A, Rasplica I, Sweeney T: Educa-ting patients on a spinal cord injury unit for self-medication. *Hosp Pharm* 11:14-21, 1976
     Comment on the importance of educating inpatients about their medica-tion therapy with the aim being improved compliance after dis-charge.

801. Schmidt DD: Patient compliance: The effect of the doctor as the thera-peutic agent. *J Fam Pract* 4:853-856, 1977
     A review of compliance research literature with 12 concrete suggestions for improving patient compliance.

802. Schoenberger JA, Stamler J, Shekelle RB, Shekelle S: Current status of

hypertension control in an industrial population. *JAMA* 222:559-562, 1972
Results of screening of 22,929 persons for hypertension at 76 work sites with descriptions of demographic features and therapeutic status (no direct measures of individual compliance per se).

803. Seeman M: Patients who abandon psychotherapy. *Arch Gen Psychiatry* 30:486-491, 1974
Classification of psychotherapy patients by relationship with parents is suggested as a method for detecting and preventing dropouts.

804. Sharpe TR, Mikeal RL: Patient compliance with prescription medication regimens. *J Am Pharm Assoc* 15:191-192, 197, 1975
A review of compliance with prescribed medication using Talcott Parson's "sick role" as a basis.

805. _____: Understanding your patient: Why your patient doesn't take his medicine. *Bull Bureau Pharm Services* 9:1-4, 1973
Trial comparing a group receiving standard dispensing with a group receiving additional written instructions.

806. SharpeTR: Identifying the noncompliant patient. *Apothecary* March/April: 8-10, 45-47, 1976
Review and commentary emphasizing the need for and methods of identifying noncompliance when it occurs and of predicting it before it occurs.

807. _____: The pharmacist's potential role as a factor in increasing compliance, pp 133-138, in Barofsky I (ed): *Medication Compliance: A Behavioral Management Approach*. Thorofare, NJ, Slack, 1977
Comment on the community pharmacist's potential contribution in achieving increased compliance with medication regimens among hypertensive patients.

808. Shewchuk LA: Problems of high-risk populations and high-risk non-responders: Smoking behavior, pp 93-99, in Cullen JW, Fox BH, Isom RN (eds:) *Cancer: The Behavioral Dimensions*. New York, Raven Press, 1976
A call for standardization of data collection and reporting of results in studies of smoking behavior.

809. _____: Special report: Smoking cessation programs of the American Health Foundation. *Prev Med* 5:454-474, 1976
Thirteen specific smoking cessation techniques are designed for various levels of smoking intervention. Future assessment plans are outlined.

810. Shorr GI, Nutting PA: A population-based assessment of the continuity of ambulatory care. *Med Care* 15:455-464, 1977
Description of a strategy to promote constructive evaluation of the health care system.

811. Simonds SK: Focusing on the issues. Paper presented at the Second Invitational Conference on Health Education in the Hospital, Chicago, 1969
Commentary on the current status of patient education and on priorities for validating and utilizing it in the future.

812. Sinaiko AR, Mirkin BL: Therapeutic agents for pediatric hypertension. *Pediatr Ann* 6:401-409, 1977
     Noncompliance is noted as a major obstacle to effective drug therapy for hypertension in children.
813. Smith DL: Patient compliance with medication regimens. *Drug Intell Clin Pharm* 10:386-393, 1976
     Review of and commentary on literature dealing with drug compliance.
814. Smith SE: Patients do not always take their drugs. *Nurs Times* 72:72-73, 1976
     General editorial on noncompliance.
815. Smoking: Successes and failures. Editorial. *Lancet* 2:759-760, 1971
     Conference report giving recommendations for action against smoking from the British Royal College of Physicians, the World Health Organization, and the Second World Conference on Smoking.
816. Sobel R, Ingalls A: Resistance to treatment: Explorations of the patient's sick role. *Am J Psychother* 18:562-573, 1964
     A questionnaire was administered to 588 physicians and patients to examine the interpretation of sick roles and to define further the parameters affecting the sick role of psychiatric, surgical, and medical patients.
817. Spiegel AD: Programmed instructional materials for patient education. *J Med Educ* 42:958-962, 1967
     Field test of a programmed learning package for diabetic patients. Compliance and outcomes other than knowledge were not assessed.
818. Stern S, Moore S, Gross S: A reply to Garfield. *J Consult Clin Psychol* 45:486-488, 1977
     A note on the confounding of personality and social class characteristics in research on premature termination.
819. Stewart RB, Cluff LE: A review of medication errors and compliance in ambulant patients. *Clin Pharmacol Ther* 13:463-468, 1972
     Review of articles concerned with the determinants of medication errors and compliance among outpatients.
820. Stimson G: Obeying doctors' orders: A view from the other side. *Soc Sci Med* 8:97-104, 1974
     Compliance viewed from the patient's perspective as seen by a sociologist.
821. *Strategies for Patient Education*, Chairman's Report on the Second Invitational Conference on Patient Education in Hospitals. Chicago, 1969
     Handbook with a political focus that outlines strategies for implementing patient education programs.
822. Stunkard A: Studies on TOPS: A self-help group for obesity, pp 387-391, in Bray G (ed): *Obesity in Perspective*. Bethesda, DHEW Publication NIH 75-708, 1976
     A summary of three studies dealing with the TOPS program for treatment of obesity.
823. Stunkard AJ, Mahoney MJ: Behavioral treatment of the eating disorders,

pp 45-73, in Leitenberg H (ed): *Handbook of Behavior Modificiation.*
Englewood Cliffs, NJ, Prentice-Hall, 1976
Comprehensive review of behavioral approaches to overeating and under-
eating.
824. Stunkard AJ: Presidential address—1974: From explanation to action in
psychosomatic medicine: The case of obesity. *Psychosom Med* 37:
195-236, 1975
An interesting historical perspective on the development of successful behaviorally oriented programs for treating obesity, with an extensive review of the pertinent literature.
825. Svarstad BL: Physician-patient communication and patient conformity
with medical advice, pp 220-238, in Mechanic D (ed): *The Growth
of Bureaucratic Medicine.* New York, Wiley, 1976
An overview of some of the factors influencing patient compliance and
of strategies physicians can use to improve compliance.
826. Swezey R, Swezey A: Educational theory as a basis for patient education.
J Chron Dis 29:417-422, 1976
Brief survey of educational principles from a behavioral perspective.
827. Tempero KF: Biological variability and drug response variability as factors
influencing patient compliance: Implications for drug testing and
evaluation, pp 45-52, in Barofsky I (ed): *Medication Compliance: A
Behavioral Management Approach*, Thorofare, NJ, Slack, 1977
An assessment of some of the pharmaceutical factors affecting medication
compliance.
828. Thornburg H, Thornburg E: How to motivate patients to care. *Dental
Survey* :36-39, Feb 1975
Description of educational and psychological principles which might be
used to improve dental hygiene.
829. Thorner N: Nurses violate their patients' rights. *J Psychiatr Nurs* 14:7-12,
1976
Report on nurses' impressions and violations of patients' legal rights to
refuse medication.
830. Tilson E: Organization for long-term management of hypertension: The
trade union as a compliance mechanism in the treatment of hypertension. *Bull NY Acad Med* 52:714-717, 1976
Description of the role played by the United Storeworkers Union in promoting and organizing the participation of members in a successful
work site based hypertension program.
831. Trinca GW, Dooley BJ: The effects of mandatory seat belt wearing on the
mortality and pattern of injury of car occupants involved in motor
vehicle crashes in Victoria. *Med J Aust* 1:675-678, 1975
Compliance is reported but noncentral in this study of the effectiveness
of mandatory seat belt use in reducing injury in car accidents.
832. Tso Y: Drug dosing for pediatric patients. *Nurse Pract* 2:35-37, 1977
Description of a method of estimating pediatric dosage with a brief note
about the psychosocial factors affecting compliance.

833. Vaisrub S: You can lead a horse to water——. Editorial. *JAMA* 234:80-81, 1975

Commentary on the failure of educational programs to improve compliance in hypertension and coronary prevention projects.

834. Vanputten T: Why do patients with manic-depressive illness stop their lithium. *Comp Psychiatr* 16:179-183, 1975

Six case studies of manic depressives who have stopped their lithium.

835. Vernon SM, Pratt LL: Motivation in hearing aid acceptance. *Laryngoscope* 87:1413-1417, 1977

The use of an interview plus three personality tests is suggested as a predictor of acceptance of a hearing aid.

836. Waller PF, Barry PZ: *Seat belts: A Comparison of Observed and Reported Use.* Chapel Hill, NC, University of North Carolina Highway Safety Research Center, 1969

Abstract of a study of seat belt use on short and long trips.

837. Ward G: How the pharmacist can help in long-term maintenance of antihypertensive therapy. *J Am Pharm Assoc* 17:301-302, 1977

Outline of ways the pharmacist can improve patients' compliance with drug therapy for hypertension.

838. Wari K, Wigley SC: Defaulter and abscondee: A Melanesian miscellany. *Bull Int Union Tuberc* 49:51-60, 1974

Descriptive account of nonadherence to tuberculosis treatment programs in New Guinea.

839. Warner K: The effects of the anti-smoking campaign on cigarette consumption. *Am J Public Health* 67:645-650, 1977

An analysis of cigarette consumption data from 1947 to 1970 noting the effects of various events of the antismoking campaign.

840. Weber C, Sather M: Discharge medication counseling—how to enhance patient compliance with prescribed medication regimens. *Hosp Top* 54:39-42, 1976

Brief review of some factors affecting compliance with medication regimens and a description of a program designed to improve compliance through pharmacist-patient consultation.

841. Weinstein M, Stason W: *Hypertension: A Policy Perspective.* Cambridge, Mass, Harvard University Press, 1976

Cost-effectiveness and cost-benefit analyses of hypertension management, with inclusion of compliance considerations.

842. Weintraub M: Promoting patient compliance. *NY State J Med* 75:2263-2266, 1975

Commentary on the role of health professionals, government, and the pharmaceutical industry in improving compliance.

843. _____: The role of industrial nurses in improving patients' adherence to therapeutic plans. *Occup Health Nurs* 23:16-17, 1975

Editorial comment outlining the potential contribution of occupational health nurses to improving the compliance of employee-patients.

844. West KM: Diet therapy of diabetes: An analysis of failure. *Ann Intern Med* 79:425-434, 1973
An emphasis on the extent of noncompliance with the diabetic diet and on possible causes of failure to adhere to the regimen.
845. Whelan EM: Compliance with contraceptive regimens. *Stud Fam Plann* 5:349-355, 1974
Comprehensive report on determinants of compliance with contraceptive regimens.
846. Whiston WB: Some economic issues in medication compliance, pp 21-27, in Barofsky I (ed): *Medication Compliance: A Behavioral Management Approach*, Thorofare, NJ, Slack, 1977
Review of the associations between costs and compliance.
847. Wilber JA, Millward D, Baldwin A, Capron B, Silverman D, Levy LM, Wolbert T, McCombs NJ: Atlanta community high blood pressure program methods of community hypertension screening. *Circ Res* 30 (suppl 11): 101-109, 1972
Discussion of various methods of community hypertension screening based on the experience at Atlanta, Georgia, giving degree of cooperation received and treatment status of those found hypertensive.
848. Wilson JT: Compliance with instructions in the evaluation of therapeutic efficacy. *Clin Pediatr* 12:333-340, 1973
Review article concerning the implications of compliance for establishing effective treatment.
849. _____: Noncompliance contributing to apparent drug failure in status epilepticus. *Pediatrics* 53:938-940, 1974
Case study of failure of staff to deliver proper medication dosage to an epileptic seven-year-old girl.
850. Yurchak P: One physician's approach to the teaching of patients, pp 203-208, in Barofsky I (ed): *Medication Compliance: A Behavioral Management Approach*. Thorofare, NJ, Slack, 1977
A brief comment on educating the patient.
851. Zifferblatt SM, Curry PJ: Patient self-management of hypertension medication, pp 77-93, in Barofsky I (ed): *Medication Compliance: A Behavioral Management Approach*. Thorofare, NJ, Slack, 1977
Discussion on self-control and the maintenance of motivation in compliance with medicaton regimens.
852. Zifferblatt SM: Increasing patient compliance through the applied analysis of behavior. *Prev Med* 4:173-182, 1975
Theoretical considerations of behavior modification techniques applied to compliance problems.
853. Zola IK: Taking your medication—problem for doctor or patient, pp 3-8, in Barofsky I (ed): *Medication Compliance: A Behavioral Management Approach*. Thorofare, NJ, Slack, 1977
General discussion of patient-doctor problems in medication compliance.

CATEGORICAL TABLES OF FACTORS
STUDIED IN RELATION TO COMPLIANCE

TABLE 1. Disease features

Feature	Association with compliance		
	Positive	Negative	None
Diagnosis	Association found: 7*, 15, 27, 29*, 92, 113*, 126, 204*, 260*, 270, 351*, 359, 368, 369, 424*, 444*, 497, 510, 528, 529		15, 63, 95, 126, 135, 178, 187, 188, 192*, 222*, 223, 258, 272, 302, 306, 312, 377, 454
Severity	240*, 342, 368 497	57, 65, 66, 141, 269, 280	56, 91, 95, 128, 135, 192*, 204*, 222*, 258, 272, 327, 362, 377, 393, 403, 408, 414, 437*, 447, 459
Symptoms		19, 260*, 277, 315	95, 233*, 321
Degree of disability	138, 235, 240*	19, 471	53*, 258
Duration	385*	369	7*, 17*, 56, 121, 192*, 258, 269, 272, 342, 359, 368, 376, 393, 441
Previous bouts	33	359	95, 127, 235, 327, 368, 486, 487
Recency of last attack			235
Previous hospitalization	29*, 200, 377	315	223, 235, 330, 408, 536
Length of hospitalization		414	327, 377, 428
Prognosis	315		135
Clinical improvement	29*	192*, 323*	340, 341
Concurrent conditions	Association found: 56, 328		258, 414
Previous detection	204*, 537		

*Compliance with appointments only.

TABLE 2. Features of referrals and appointments

Feature	Association with compliance		
	Positive	Negative	None
Referrals:			
Time between screening and referral		169*, 194*, 243*	
Referral source	Association found: 240*, 259*, 497		17*, 368, 417*
Method of referral	Association found: 259*, 520		
Specificity of referral	243*		
Appointments:			
Waiting time		7*, 186, 417*	
Method of scheduling	Association found: 434*		

TABLE 2. (*continued*)

Feature	Association with compliance		
	Positive	*Negative*	*None*
Time of day of visit		243*	184*, 243*, 341, 375*, 453*
Time between visits		260*	184*, 375*, 453*
Day of week of visit	Association found: 453*		184*, 260*
Distance to clinic	224*	369	53*, 167, 240*, 243*, 260*, 327, 350*, 368, 512
Having to leave work	Association found: 463*		260*
Weather	17*		220
Mobile facilities	450		
Particular clinic	Association found: 167, 345		
Assignment of specific therapist	7*		
Patient load of therapist			260*
Type of visit	Association found: 224*		502*

*Compliance with appointments only.

TABLE 3. Features of the therapeutic regimen

Feature	Association with compliance		
	Positive	*Negative*	*None*
Type of treatment:			
For the same condition	Association found: 23, 97, 112, 150, 162, 170, 205, 263, 265, 266, 272, 285, 298, 326, 381, 388, 405, 407, 415, 424*, 427, 435, 477, 523		53*, 95, 124, 158, 188, 192*, 223, 246, 310, 315, 336, 345, 355, 414, 435, 448, 516
For different conditions	Association found: 66, 103, 236, 258, 397		395
Duration of therapy	134	42, 55, 95, 192*, 202, 245, 246, 265, 348, 433, 436, 489, 524*	127, 133, 137, 155, 188, 322, 328, 405, 441
Number of drugs/treatments	113*, 362	65, 91, 102, 127, 174, 236, 258, 376, 395	236, 322, 329
Frequency of dosing		65	312, 336, 395, 403
Dosage	192*, 377		405, 441
Side effects		56, 302, 377, 425, 513, 535	188, 192*, 321, 523
Cost	105, 507	7*, 65, 126, 236	312, 330
Health insurance	7*		
Safety-lock dispensers		300	
Pharmacy dispensing			377
Prior therapy	315	163	115, 121, 192*, 362
Co-therapy	53*		

*Compliance with appointments only.

TABLE 4. Features of the patient-therapist interaction

Feature	Association with compliance		
	Positive	Negative	None
Patient-therapist interaction	134, 176		129, 155
Difficulty with communication		168	132, 186, 256, 257
Amount of time with therapist	322	176	
Patient agreement with therapist	132		176
"Tension-release" in meetings	132		
Malintegrative patient behavior		131	
Patient seeking suggestions for action	132		
Patient satisfaction—general	7*, 32, 33, 135, 291, 295, 311, 322		
Patient's appraisal of therapist	260*		287
Patient's attitudes toward therapist/care	Association found: 11*		108, 128, 129, 200, 247, 248, 439
Patient's attitudes toward hospital			423
Patient's belief in diagnosis	32		
Patient's belief in therapist's ability	32*, 377		
Patient's expectations met	81*, 155, 174, 283, 295, 448		
Patient's perception of therapist's expectation	490		
Patient perceives therapist as friendly	174, 295, 497		127
Patient perceives therapist as businesslike		186	
Patient feels that therapist is interested	377		
Number of pieces of advice received	490		291
Asking for medication for psychological problem		207*, 232*	
Resisting therapy (children)		100, 340	12
Resisting therapy (adults)		19, 138	

TABLE 4. (continued)

Patient's intention to take therapy	128		95, 122, 137, 364, 370, 371
Level of supervision	117*, 223, 266, 479, 512*, 536		95
Therapist's prediction of compliance	55, 133, 368, 428, 439		
Interviewer's prediction of compliance	133, 503		
Therapist's prediction of prognosis	459		
Therapist's attitude toward efficacy of therapy			266, 362
Particular physician	Association found: 89, 143*	520	95, 209, 275, 314
Private versus public physician			7*, 95, 426, 513
GP versus psychiatrist for psychiatric patients			394
Regular versus substitute physician	32, 33, 35, 95, 220*		12, 95, 209, 312
Failure of therapist to give feedback	Association found:459	132	
Therapist's attitude toward patient			315, 330
Therapist's perception of patient's attitude			138
Empathy of therapist	439		494*
Therapist showing positive regard			494*
Genuineness of therapist			494*
Friendliness of therapist	176		490
Self-disclosure by therapist			494*
Concreteness of suggestions	494*		467*, 506*
Development of a structured plan			494*
Identification of specific problems		494*	
Amount of demonstration by therapist	498		
Therapist appeals to reason	490		
Therapist's discussion of diagnosis	497		
Patient cooperation with treatment team	328		176
Age of physician	260*		
Use of authority by physician	490		

*Compliance with appointments only.

TABLE 5. Patient characteristics: General

Feature	Association with compliance		
	Positive	*Negative*	*None*
Health belief model—patient's perception of:			
The disease as serious	32, 34, 37, 56, 95, 174, 215*, 287*, 376, 495*	36*, 278*	91, 104, 287*, 323*, 340, 341, 413
Personal specific susceptibility	32, 33, 34, 36*, 37, 144, 215*, 278*, 287*, 487, 516	495*	247, 413
General susceptibility to disease	32, 33, 37, 504*		34
Efficacy of therapy	32, 33, 138, 186, 215*, 287, 377, 487		34, 200, 232, 287*, 291, 302, 413, 495*
Therapy as painful		287*, 413	186
Therapy as unpleasant, difficult			395
Attitudes toward illness			
Favorable or coping	328, 525		91, 329
Supernatural cause		135, 287*	12, 127, 128, 423
General worry	32*, 33, 34, 37		108, 128, 261, 168, 278*
Knowledge of disease, therapy	5, 58, 63, 100, 104, 144, 302, 311, 335, 428, 439, 471, 479, 491*, 495*, 504*, 511, 516		11*, 34, 42, 54, 55, 56, 91, 138, 149, 200, 331, 340, 341, 349, 395, 403, 428, 449, 487, 505, 513, 535
Previous awareness of problem	100, 104, 222*		14, 168, 223, 324, 523, 530
Intelligence	326, 445, 446		281
Signs of organic brain damage			
Method of remembering medication	142, 179, 345		326, 376
Number of places where medication kept			376
Exposure to media	487, 504*		

TABLE 5. *(continued)*

Duration of local residence	143*, 144		408
Number of years registered with clinic			275
Telephone in home	461*, 517*		220*
Compliance with other aspects of regimen	55, 129, 142, 153, 245, 302, 339, 411, 428, 443, 503		34, 89, 115
Previous compliance	240*, 269, 287*, 357	307	247, 375*
Attendance at appointments	61, 198, 366, 428		34, 126, 129, 443
Immunization rate	7*	220*	
Patient's attitude toward therapy			91
Own car			350*
Hypnotic susceptibility	400		
Postdischarge contact with clinic	519		

*Compliance with appointments only.

TABLE 6. Patient characteristics: Sociodemographic features

Feature	Association with compliance		
	Positive	Negative	None
Age	1*, 15, 17*, 37, 54, 63, 113*, 126, 184*, 194*, 200, 206*, 224*, 240*, 260*, 302, 306, 346, 373, 433, 446, 447, 455, 487, 489, 495* 504*, 510, 516	11*, 36*, 104, 115, 141, 146*, 152, 204*, 224*, 278*, 294*, 357, 412, 457	12, 32, 33, 46, 53*, 55, 56, 58, 61, 65, 66, 74*, 78, 81*, 91, 95, 102, 108, 121, 127, 128, 131, 135, 138, 142, 152, 167, 174, 188, 192*, 197, 209, 215*, 220*, 222*, 223, 229, 247, 252, 258, 269,272, 275*, 305, 327, 329, 330, 331, 340, 341, 342, 350*, 359, 368, 369, 374*, 375*, 376, 377, 383*, 395, 405, 408, 411, 414, 431, 432, 445, 448, 453*, 471, 483, 503, 513, 523, 526, 536
Sex	Association found: 1*, 14, 31, 55, 56, 78, 146*, 200, 243*, 260*, 280, 284, 288, 294*, 306, 329, 368, 369, 408, 476, 479, 486, 495*, 504* 505, 510, 516, 535		3*, 12, 27, 37, 46, 53*, 58, 63, 65, 66, 74*, 81*, 91, 95, 108, 113*, 121, 126, 128, 131, 135, 137, 138, 141, 142, 177*, 184, 188, 192*, 194*, 209, 215*, 223, 240*, 252, 258, 272, 290, 302, 310, 323*, 327, 330, 342, 364, 374*, 376, 395, 405, 412, 417*, 431, 432, 433, 447, 448, 453*, 455, 471, 483, 494*, 503, 523, 526, 536
Education	3*, 5, 29*, 36*, 65, 66, 100, 108, 121, 152, 224*, 278*, 287*, 340, 350*, 416, 439, 445, 455, 457, 480*, 495*, 504*, 517*	19, 55, 349	11*, 12, 32, 33, 37, 46, 56, 58, 61, 63, 91, 92, 95, 113*, 127, 128, 129, 131, 138, 144, 174, 194*, 200, 207*, 215, 229, 235, 247, 252, 258, 269, 287*, 302, 329, 330, 331, 341, 342, 362, 364, 368, 369, 376, 383*, 395, 471, 503, 505, 526

TABLE 6. (*continued*)

Socioeconomic status	5, 7*, 17*, 208, 222*, 224*, 233*, 243*, 260*, 269, 278*, 416, 464, 476, 500, 529	143*	14, 55, 63, 142, 144, 152, 174, 200, 206*, 207*, 223, 243, 247, 258, 302, 314, 357, 377, 395, 405, 412, 448, 450
Occupational status	3*, 5, 30, 61, 91, 272, 287*, 329, 380, 408, 445, 476, 510, 526	450	11*, 46, 92, 121, 128, 131, 135, 138, 167, 192*, 194*, 207*, 229, 235, 240*, 280, 287*, 330, 342, 359, 376, 503
Income	65, 66, 108, 322, 364, 487	321*, 368	3*, 37, 46, 91, 92, 135, 138, 144, 167, 168, 194*, 207*, 229, 238, 287*, 350, 364, 369, 471, 495*
Marital status	Association found: 3*, 11*, 29*, 37, 61, 66, 121, 141, 240*, 269, 280, 340, 408, 455, 457, 487, 504*, 505		32, 33, 46, 58, 65, 115, 128, 131, 135, 138, 167, 192*, 206*, 258, 267, 294*, 302, 330, 341, 368, 369, 376, 405, 445, 503, 526
Race (white versus others)	7*, 17*, 108, 144, 275*, 374*, 431, 495*, 517	288, 457	37, 46, 58, 63, 113*, 121, 128, 141, 220*, 222*, 229, 244, 247, 252, 260*, 294*, 305, 327, 364, 408, 412, 433, 453*, 471, 526
Ethnic background	Association found: 11*, 476		3*, 135, 167, 174, 194*, 229, 240*, 376, 536
Religion	Association found: 143*, 146*, 224*		14, 128, 131, 135, 192*, 445
Urban versus rural	495*	480*	64*, 229

*Compliance with appointments only.

TABLE 7. Patient characteristics: Psychosocial factors

Feature	Association with compliance		
	Positive	Negative	None
Influence of family	5, 14, 50, 64*, 112, 138, 234, 280, 377, 384, 394, 399, 428, 516, 523		91, 129, 155, 258, 368, 526
Influence of friends	50, 208*, 394, 428	11*	127, 129, 155, 526
Family stability	7*, 135, 144, 263, 327, 423, 480*, 517*		14, 200, 414
Family size		7*, 36*, 104, 200, 224*, 260*, 278*, 409, 457	37, 152, 323*
Family fails to show upward mobility		104, 144	
Pretreatment home satisfaction			261
Concurrent illness in family		19, 327	95
Intrafamily identity	399		
Interpersonal relationships	373, 526		247
"Good" social environment	408		
Social isolation	487	19, 377, 455	376, 395, 405
Social participation/integration	390, 504*, 526		233*, 261, 448
Parenthood status			192*
Parity	405		
Welfare status			121, 306
Prior criminal conviction		518	121, 526
Alcoholism		270, 408, 522*	
Ever abuse alcohol		11*, 153, 263	121, 526
Concurrent drug abuse	121	14, 270	526
Pretreatment level of function	530		
Pretreatment job satisfaction			261
Resolution of conflicts			428
Family orientation toward tradition		11*	
Tobacco use/smoking		11*	
Sports participation			11*

*Compliance with appointments only.

462

TABLE 8. Patient characteristics: Psychological factors

Feature	Association with compliance		
	Positive	Negative	None
Self-confidence about ability to comply	49, 384	153, 261, 409	
Dependency	320	281	128
Primary gain		261	
Secondary gain		383*	55, 135
Locus of control (active versus passive)	232, 247		
Futuristic orientation	135, 487		200
Obstructive		128	153, 206*
Anxiety/nervousness	84*, 305, 445	135, 287*, 487	81*, 92, 211*, 274, 296, 305, 448, 486
Personality (MMPI, etc.)		254	
Stable personality	27, 270, 516		
Unreliable personality type		19, 192*	
Aesthetic concern (dental)			
For child	287*		
For self			287*
View of disease as stigma	54	261	
Self-concept		71	233*
Low self-esteem		464	261, 423
Blames others for problem		207*	
Reason for referral			
Personal crisis		207*	
Intolerable emotional crisis		207*	
Nonspecific discomfort		207*	
Acting out behavior		122	281
Denial of sick role, illness			281, 403

TABLE 8. (continued)

Feature	Association with compliance		
	Positive	Negative	None
Acceptance of diagnosis	377		
High work orientation		527	127
Low frustration tolerance		122, 281	
Feeling of loneliness		261	
Feeling of alienation			200, 206*
Motivation	19, 138, 467*, 506*		
Pretreatment somatization			152, 192*
Immaturity		21	
Avoiding responsibility		21	
Impulsivity		21	
Neuroticism		78, 217	
Extroversion	362		78, 217
Responsive, cooperative, grateful	128		
Authoritarian, overbearing, demanding		128	
Articulate, intelligent, formal	128		
Impulsive, defiant, distressed		269	
Constricted, guarded, isolated		269	
Demanding, cold, harsh mother		269	
Acceptance of sick role	153		
Strength of sexual identity	Association found: 14		11*
Depression	133	133	

*Compliance with appointments only.

464

TABLE 9. Features of the patient-therapist interaction
and family of the patient in pediatrics

Feature	Association with compliance		
	Positive	*Negative*	*None*
Description of mother's personality	Association found: 95		
Amount of social conversation	176, 295		
Time spent with physician	497		
Mother feels concern not understood		144	
Patient accompanied to clinic	200		
"Always do what doctor advises"	32, 33, 247		
Follow-up visits given only when necessary	32		
Therapist's status/seniority	497		
Position of child in family	224*, 497		95, 269
Working mother		7*, 12	
Social activity of father			480*
Mother's attitude toward child's daily behavior	480*		
Seek care for symtoms with no delay	32		247
Use special foods to keep child healthy	32		
Family has clinical thermometer	32*		
Child's illness affects mother's social role		32	
Mother's perception of own health	32*		
High expectations for child's future	32		
Anxious about being a good mother	32		
Adults other than mother at home	32*		
Mother feels "can get through the day"	32, 37		
Number of people giving child therapy			340
Child "stubborn"	152		
Mother desires understanding of problem	152		
Mother's belief about cause of problem			152
Grades in school	50		
Child's anxiety	451		
Parental permissiveness			451
Parents' understanding of therapy	497		
Parents' expectations met	497		
Parental satisfaction	497		
Both parents attending child	497		
Child given vitamins regularly			33

*Compliance with appointments only.

TABLE 10. Reasons patients give for noncompliance

Reasons	Citations
Dissatisfaction with therapy	1*, 82, 100, 125, 220*, 240*, 274, 277, 288, 302, 420, 423, 424*, 487
Feeling better, well	12, 82, 124, 220*, 224*, 236, 274, 302, 323, 329, 385*, 420, 424*, 425, 499, 513
Forgetting	7*, 17*, 124, 220*, 224*, 288, 291, 302, 316, 329, 424*, 513
Side effects	23, 56, 82, 124, 192*, 236, 240*, 274, 288, 291, 302, 323, 425, 489, 499, 513, 532
Waiting time at clinic	17*, 168*, 224*
Financial need	7*, 82, 125, 291, 385*, 513
Sickness, disability	220*, 240*, 424*
Poor instruction	82, 302, 351*
Confusion over medication	125, 288, 291, 302, 513
Clinic scheduling error	7*, 146*
Confusion over appointment	17*, 220*
Lost appointment slip	224*
Difficulty getting appointment	499
Poor patient-therapist relationship	168*, 291
Feeling worse, no better	124, 192*, 288, 316, 425, 499
Indifference	7*, 123, 288, 424*
Lack of willpower	291
Never intended to return	7*
Out of town	1*, 17*, 123, 125, 240*
No babysitter	7*, 64*, 424*
No transportation	1*, 7*, 123, 125, 224*, 313, 351*, 424*
Weather	123, 276*, 351*
Asleep at pill-taking time	420
Employment	1*, 64*, 192*, 291, 450, 499
Thought extra dose needed	302
Lack of family support	125, 192*
Child threw tablets away	124
Contradictory advice from friends	288, 291
Another doctor stopped treatment	124, 385*
Concurrent illness in family	7*, 17*, 220*
"Too much" medication	192*, 513
Antagonism toward medication	92, 192*
Access to another doctor	1, 220*, 224*
Occupied with housework	64*, 224*
Bothered by questions/tests	224*, 450
Delay in seeking care for breast cancer	195

*Compliance with appointments only.

TABLE 11. Objective methods of measuring compliance

Treatment/substance being measured	Method of measurement	Citations
Oral medications	Pill counts	12, 42, 63, 75, 90, 95, 96, 97, 101, 102, 107, 136, 142, 160, 162, 174, 179, 185, 228, 229, 249, 253, 262, 277, 300, 302, 304, 310, 312, 315, 322, 329, 336, 339, 340, 341, 348, 349, 370, 371, 382, 392, 395, 419, 426, 441, 442, 443, 449, 460, 483, 490, 509, 563, 616, 738, 757
	Pharmacy records	6, 40, 144, 178, 217, 265, 330, 348, 403, 443, 496, 510, 734
	Medication monitors	364, 365, 366, 419, 567, 568, 569
	Direct observation	16, 22
Penicillins	Bioassay (urine)	32, 33, 42, 95, 106, 124, 198, 199, 200, 202, 209, 304, 354
Rifampicin	Bioassay (urine)	566
Nitrofurantoin	Bioassay (urine)	124
Nalidixic acid	Bioassay (urine)	124
Cephalexin	Bioassay (urine)	124
Gentamicin	Bioassay (urine)	124
Chloramphenicol	Bioassay (urine)	124
Sulfamethoxazole	Bioassay (urine)	124
Isoniazid	Biochemical (urine)	45, 46, 114, 229, 330, 345, 410, 512, 536, 538, 574, 581, 664
Para-aminosalicylate	Biochemical (urine)	6, 45, 46, 137, 186, 203, 272, 330, 398, 410, 535, 536, 541, 542, 580, 664
Atropine	Biochemical (urine)	443
Iron	Biochemical (stool)	57
Phenothiazines	Biochemical (urine)	22, 223, 266, 344, 377, 378, 423, 528, 550, 551, 573
	Gas chromatography	543
	Paper chromatography	523
	Colorimetry	523
Imipramine	Biochemical (urine)	22, 344, 550
Amitryptiline		22
Diphenylhydantoin	Biochemical (serum)	59, 189, 297, 427, 544, 553, 561, 564, 582
	Gas chromatography	22, 59, 548
	Biochemical (urine)	297
Mesantoin	Biochemical (serum)	427
Phenobarbitol	Biochemical (serum)	22, 427, 532, 548, 564
Benzodiazepines	Colorimetry (urine)	22
Ethosuximide	Biochemical (serum)	462
Primidone	Chromatography (urine)	22
Heroin	Bioassay (urine)	552
Ethanol	Enzymatic (blood)	196
Disulfiram	Breath test	571
Nicotine	Gas chromatography	447
Carboxyhemoglobin	Biochemical (blood)	267, 447, 575
Carbon monoxide	Breath test	298
Digoxin	Biochemical (serum)	93, 189, 213, 513, 578
Thiazides	Biochemical (urine)	319

TABLE 11. (*continued*)

Treatment/substance being measured	Method of measurement	Citations
Propranolol	Biochemical (serum)	68
Alphamethyldopa	Biochemical (urine)	319, 556, 630
Chlorthalidone	Chromatography	147
Theophylline	Gas chromatography	145
Paracetemol	Biochemical (urine)	22, 339
Mefenamic acid	Fluorescence (urine)	339
Flufenamic acid	Fluorescence (urine)	339
Phenylbutazone	Biochemical (urine)	339
Tolbutamide	Spectometry (urine)	549
	Chromatography	549
Chloral compounds	Biochemical (urine)	22
Diet	Biochemical:	479
	Lipids (serum)	73, 171, 205, 361, 558
	Ketones (urine)	539
	Endpoints (weight)	37, 38, 40, 55, 112, 116, 133, 182, 191, 196, 203, 205, 216, 225, 281, 292, 307, 325, 399, 422, 465, 468, 477, 481, 485, 508, 524
	Tissue biopsy	356, 361
	Bowel biopsy	20
	Diabetic control	481
	Serum antibodies	20
	Potassium (serum)	55, 133, 281, 328
	Phosphorus (serum)	133
	Sodium (urine)	438
	Direct observation	89, 112, 511, 562
Dental care	Dye wafers	149, 547
	Direct assessment	26, 446, 500
Post-MI activity	Direct observation	527
Physical activity	Pedometer	196
Stroke rehab	Direct observation	135
Diabetic self-care	Direct observation	333, 511
Seat belt use	Direct observation	430, 431, 432, 433
Psychotherapy	Tape recordings	242
Markers/tracers	Riboflavin	46, 366, 405, 543, 545, 550, 554, 555, 565, 579
	Bromide	442
	Phenol red	277, 576
	Radioisotape	443
	Quinine	187, 188
Acetylsalicylate	Biochemical (urine)	22, 162, 339
	Biochemical (serum)	162, 285
	Platelet test	162
Dapsone	Biochemical (urine)	316

TABLE 12. Strategies for improving compliance

Strategy	Citations
Information/instruction:	
Patient/health education	5, 26, 27, 30, 31, 51, 55, 61, 79, 86, 91, 96, 100, 101, 104, 118, 123, 136, 148, 149, 150, 156, 165, 166, 170, 181, 193, 203, 210, 212, 214, 215, 216, 219, 229, 242, 248, 259, 262, 264, 267, 278, 288, 289, 303, 304, 310, 317, 326, 329, 331, 341, 348, 350, 357, 372, 397, 401, 407, 413, 415, 419, 430, 435, 438, 449, 471, 477, 479, 481, 493, 515, 516, 585, 586, 609, 616, 617, 624, 628, 632, 650, 651, 653, 660, 678, 679, 680, 681, 721, 722, 738, 739, 751, 755, 758, 760, 761, 764, 765, 768, 783, 789, 793, 800, 825, 826, 833, 837, 839, 840, 850
Written instructions	91, 101, 106, 136, 170, 203, 204, 304, 310, 312, 314, 329, 341, 342, 397, 440, 460, 509, 540, 722, 745, 751, 755, 758, 805, 840
Special counseling	24, 27, 30, 47, 55, 79, 97, 106, 115, 133, 139, 182, 205, 210, 219, 241, 242, 245, 267, 288, 307, 326, 329, 342, 351, 357, 372, 388, 400, 404, 406, 407, 419, 448, 468, 471, 477, 479, 484, 524, 610, 616, 717, 745, 787
Increased communication	176, 311, 654, 720, 721, 761, 774, 801, 825
Fear arousal	37, 150, 435
Mass media health campaigns	5, 51, 181, 278, 294, 429, 430, 479, 487, 586, 588, 651, 674, 770, 839
Education for physicians	123, 264, 421, 609, 652, 734
Compliance reminders/cues:	
Telephone appointment reminders	8, 24, 114, 134, 167, 168, 169, 184, 204, 259, 290, 308, 359, 453, 461
Mailed appointment reminders	109, 167, 184, 204, 259, 323, 352, 359, 375, 391, 424, 453, 461, 472
Medication calendars	136, 179, 326, 341, 456, 509, 735, 782, 800, 840
Medication monitors	364, 567, 568, 569, 581, 751
Pill containers with alarms	16, 525
Tailoring to daily routine	228, 456, 734, 748, 852
Starter-interlock seat belts	433
Reducing barriers to compliance:	
Alternative methods of treatment	23, 106, 159, 255, 273, 381, 387, 433, 436, 447, 463, 465, 469, 484, 489, 528, 651, 683, 692
Reducing the cost of treatment	57, 105, 262, 473, 680, 692, 738, 770

TABLE 12. (*continued*)

Strategy	Citations
Decreasing waiting time	168, 351, 434, 534, 660
Alternative referral methods	94, 169, 172, 488, 489, 520, 585
Community disease register	499
Drug treatment (obesity)	465, 683
Drug treatment (smoking)	80, 447, 516
Drug treatment (alcoholism)	60, 115, 571, 787
Decentralized clinics	117, 167, 203, 255, 259, 387, 680
Comprehensive versus specialty care	166, 168, 202
Prepaid care	380
Problem solving	61, 118, 166
Hospital leaves	118
Change of clinic hours	117
Treatment at worksite	4, 51, 449, 473, 724, 830, 843
Passive versus active treatments	23, 252, 685, 686
Enlist family support	60, 91, 112, 234, 328, 384
Gratifying dependency needs	94
Social support	86, 91, 115, 182, 245, 602
Telephone support	47, 112, 263
Reduced regimen complexity	23, 381, 396, 589, 663, 692, 768
Reduced clinic complexity	10, 24, 660
Pills with unique appearance	456, 608, 663, 747, 748
Uniform measures for liquids	253

Behavior modification strategies:

General and mixed	5, 28, 38, 44, 47, 48, 49, 51, 98, 116, 216, 225, 228, 280, 292, 299, 307, 353, 468, 479, 485, 524, 597, 653, 697, 736, 750, 822, 823, 852
Compliance monitoring	24, 83, 114, 145, 182, 189, 213, 324, 452, 462, 512, 653, 669
Legal coercion	60, 118, 181, 237, 255, 387, 437, 662, 831
Self-monitoring/biofeedback	38, 88, 150, 196, 228, 283, 292, 298, 458, 485, 508
Monetary reinforcement	67, 116, 216, 228, 292, 299, 586
Peer group pressure	119, 182, 401, 508, 524, 602
Role playing	334
Self-reinforcement	38, 388
Verbal/written commitments	67, 85, 98, 225, 309, 418, 477, 731
Threat of stopping therapy	24
Induced expectancy	283
Aversive conditioning	28, 119, 298, 448, 452

Increased supervision:

General	60, 79, 83, 94, 114, 117, 123, 134, 145, 166, 173, 189, 201, 213, 214, 228, 245, 262, 273, 299, 317, 324, 325, 387, 391, 465, 512, 515, 531, 628, 738
Home visits and follow-up	8, 79, 91, 117, 118, 165, 166, 201, 203, 240, 241, 255, 259, 285, 328, 359, 387, 438, 473, 512, 517, 521
Continuity of care	35, 94, 113, 115, 117, 168, 201, 203, 263, 387, 484, 810

TABLE 12. (*continued*)

Strategy	Citations
Special clinics	10, 189, 201, 202, 262
Hospitalization	203, 325
Smaller treatment groups	47
Doctor versus hospital prescriptions	142
Pharmacy interventions:	
Consultation	40, 101, 107, 136, 178, 210, 312, 314, 322, 326, 329, 331, 341, 348, 377, 419, 460, 496, 509, 616, 706, 734, 751, 755, 807, 840
Special prescription labels	312, 314, 460, 616, 748, 751
Special pill packaging	147, 314, 326, 419
In-hospital self-treatment	377, 689, 800
Nursing interventions	77, 123, 165, 166, 229, 285, 474, 475, 493, 696, 739, 740, 763, 843
Ward psychologist	135

TABLE 13. Clinical perspectives of compliance studies

Condition	Citations
Medicine:	
General medicine	10, 63, 65, 69, 96, 98, 101, 103, 107, 128, 131, 132, 138, 142, 173, 184, 224, 236, 260, 270, 275, 276, 288, 291, 311, 322, 329, 347, 349, 350, 351, 358, 370, 371, 395, 397, 405, 421, 424, 440, 453, 491, 492, 493, 509, 540, 598, 617, 625, 642, 660, 715, 745, 756, 840
Hypertension	1, 4, 41, 68, 82, 86, 87, 88, 123, 147, 156, 168, 169, 172, 179, 183, 228, 230, 262, 264, 301, 319, 336, 348, 403, 419, 422, 449, 473, 477, 493, 499, 520, 521, 556, 584, 596, 610, 614, 630, 636, 646, 647, 650, 657, 682, 707, 716, 717, 724, 751, 757, 759, 760, 761, 771, 772, 773, 784, 803, 807, 812, 830, 833, 837, 841, 848, 851
Cardiac	11, 41, 54, 93, 97, 109, 125, 127, 129, 156, 213, 256, 258, 293, 356, 361, 381, 479, 513, 522, 578, 697, 750, 833
Myocardial infarction	54, 74, 171, 272, 407, 527, 533
Congestive heart failure	335, 438
Rehabilitation (general)	51, 84, 135, 320, 420, 509
Rehabilitation (stroke)	162, 261, 407, 478
Lipids	52, 73, 97, 156, 205, 479, 531, 558, 781

TABLE 13. (*continued*)

Condition	Citations
Diabetes mellitus	61, 148, 153, 154, 214, 256, 257, 258, 333, 481, 493, 511, 525, 549, 630, 763, 775, 844
Infections (adults)	312, 314, 405, 460, 805
Tuberculosis	6, 45, 46, 83, 114, 117, 118, 137, 141, 203, 229, 255, 265, 330, 345, 364, 365, 366, 374, 385, 387, 398, 402, 408, 410, 483, 512, 535, 536, 538, 541, 542, 545, 566, 574, 580, 645, 664, 665, 684, 762, 778, 783, 838
Venereal disease	284, 359, 629, 698
Leprosy	197, 240, 316
Renal failure/hemodialysis	55, 58, 122, 133, 281, 328, 399, 501, 530
Cancer	9, 104, 167, 195, 212, 259, 429, 680
Arthritis	91, 140, 186, 277, 285, 339, 362, 382, 384, 393, 498, 742
Peptic ulcer	89, 90, 441, 442, 443
Cirrhosis of the liver	196
Coeliac disease	20
Glaucoma	53, 56, 193, 194, 505
Geriatrics	66, 179, 326, 349, 558, 587, 628, 663
Epilepsy	537, 546, 548

Pediatrics:

Condition	Citations
General pediatrics	7, 8, 17, 35, 75, 112, 165, 166, 174, 176, 177, 201, 220, 222, 227, 295, 308, 313, 352, 375, 461, 480, 497, 517, 621, 654, 832
Infections (general)	12, 42, 95, 124, 136, 166, 268, 312, 341
Acute otitis media	32, 33, 34, 340
Streptococcal pharyngitis	106, 209, 253, 304, 360
Rheumatic fever (prophylaxis)	144, 157, 158, 159, 160, 198, 199, 200, 202, 235, 289, 323, 327, 412, 507, 669
Immunizations	25, 100, 208, 247, 396, 413, 500, 641
Epilepsy	59, 189, 297, 324, 462, 544, 553, 561, 564, 849
Enuresis	474, 475
Asthma	110, 145, 444
Cystic fibrosis	354
Febrile convulsions	532
Preschool development	177
Well-child care	77, 201, 313

Psychiatry:

Condition	Citations
General psychiatry	3, 15, 22, 29, 81, 92, 113, 126, 133, 146, 151, 155, 163, 206, 207, 223, 231, 232, 242, 243, 250, 251, 266, 270, 290, 306, 344, 355, 363, 367, 368, 369, 372, 373, 378, 390, 406, 417, 423, 424, 439, 445, 454, 484,

TABLE 13. (*continued*)

Condition	Citations
	488, 518, 523, 557, 585, 591, 593, 611, 627, 652, 668, 687, 769, 787, 803, 818
Schizophrenia	105, 126, 245, 246, 273, 338, 377, 394, 528, 529
Anxiety neurosis	252, 286, 310, 315, 425, 426, 427, 502
Depression	134, 187, 188, 192, 274, 310, 372, 392, 405, 589, 726
Adolescents and children	152, 241, 459
Crisis intervention	206, 467, 494
Anorexia nervosa	823
Obstetrics and gynecology:	
Contraception	21, 23, 64, 436, 457, 463, 466, 469, 489, 780, 790, 845
Prenatal care	57, 317, 318, 405
Postnatal care	248
Ophthalmology:	
Glaucoma	56, 193, 194, 471, 505
Amblyopia	332
Dentistry	26, 149, 195, 287, 380, 416, 446, 451, 464, 472, 476, 495, 500, 515, 547, 594, 621, 624, 632, 722, 799, 828
Lifestyle problems:	
General	754
Smoking	27, 28, 44, 47, 48, 49, 50, 76, 78, 79, 80, 119, 139, 150, 156, 212, 218, 219, 226, 267, 269, 280, 283, 298, 299, 303, 334, 342, 343, 388, 400, 401, 404, 415, 435, 447, 448, 452, 469, 516, 575, 586, 588, 607, 644, 651, 653, 666, 675, 676, 690, 702, 704, 705, 719, 723, 736, 745, 764, 770, 793, 808, 809, 815, 839
Obesity	27, 37, 38, 40, 76, 116, 156, 182, 191, 216, 225, 292, 307, 325, 422, 465, 468, 485, 486, 508, 524, 539, 540, 607, 618, 638, 683, 708, 709, 724, 781, 822, 823, 824
Alcoholism	2, 18, 19, 27, 51, 60, 61, 67, 76, 94, 114, 115, 211, 212, 233, 244, 254, 263, 270, 279, 296, 383, 391, 409, 414, 428, 437, 458, 503, 571, 591, 602, 626, 634, 645, 648, 649, 684, 700, 705, 746, 787
Drug addiction	14, 27, 71, 72, 76, 111, 121, 305, 526, 534, 591, 705, 787
Car seat belts	5, 30, 181, 237, 357, 430, 431, 432, 433, 637, 662, 685, 686, 831, 836
Health and fitness	234, 353, 386, 522

TABLE 13. (*continued*)

Condition	Citations
Screening:	
Periodic health examination	215, 450
Multiphasic	204, 294, 680
Genetic	31, 36, 278, 504, 791
Vision, glaucoma	193, 194, 222, 505
Speech and hearing	24, 222
Clinical trial methods	18, 470, 590, 667, 688
Economics of compliance	238, 680, 761, 841, 846
Legal aspects of compliance	727, 767, 769, 829
Ethics of intervention	713, 754, 820
Clinical pharmacology	63, 97, 178, 210, 326, 349, 496, 616, 619, 659, 667, 710, 730, 751, 752, 800, 827, 837
Child-resistant packaging	346
Social work	730
Patient's view of compliance	820

Appendix II:
Additional
Chapter References

ADDITIONAL REFERENCES—
CHAPTER 1 (Citations 1-853 listed in Appendix I)

854. Illich I: *Medical Nemesis*. London, Calder and Boyars, 1975
855. Sackett DL: Patients and therapies: Getting the two together. *N Engl J Med* 298:278-279, 1978

ADDITIONAL REFERENCE—
CHAPTER 2 (Citations 1-853 listed in Appendix I)

856. Sackett DL, Haynes RB, Gibson ES, Taylor DW, Roberts RS, Johnson AL, Hackett BC, Turford C, Mossey J: Randomized trials of compliance-improving strategies in hypertension, pp 1-19, in Lasagna L (ed): *Patient Compliance*. Mount Kisco, NY, Futura, 1976

ADDITIONAL REFERENCES—
CHAPTER 3 (Citations 1-853 listed in Appendix I)

857. Brodie BB, Weiner M, Burns JJ, Simson G, Yale EK: The physiological disposition of ethyl biscoumacetate (tromexan) in man and a method for its estimation in biological material. *J Pharm Exp Ther* 106: 453-463, 1952
858. Chasseaud LF, Taylor T: Bioavailability of drugs from formulations after oral administration. *Annu Rev Pharmacol* 14:35-46, 1974
859. Gordis L, Desi L, Schmerler HR: Treatment of acute sore throats: A comparison of pediatricians and general physicians. *Pediatrics* 57:422-424, 1976
860. Lindenbaum J, Mellow MH, Blackstone MO, Butler BP: Variation in biologic availability of digoxin from four preparations. *N Engl J Med* 285:1344-1346, 1971
861. Markowitz M: Eradication of rheumatic fever: An unfilled hope. *Circulation* 41:1077-1084, 1970

862. Markowitz M, Gordis L: A mail-in technique for detecting penicillin in urine: Application to the study of maintenance of prophylaxis in rheumatic fever patients. *Pediatrics* 41:151-153, 1968

863. Vessell ES: Factors causing interindividual variations of drug concentrations in blood. *Clin Pharmacol Ther* 16:135-148, 1974

ADDITIONAL REFERENCES— CHAPTER 5 (Citations 1-853 listed in Appendix I)

864. Griffith W: Educating your patients about medications. Presentation at the Duke Forum for Primary Care: Compliance in Therapy, Doctors and Patients, Durham NC, 2 April, 1977

865. Hulka BS, Kupper LL, Cassel JC, Thompson SJ: A method for measuring physicians' awareness of patients' concerns. *HSMHA Health Reports* 86:741, 1971

866. Hulka BS, Kupper LL, Cassel JC, Babineau RA: Practice characteristics and quality of primary medical care: The doctor-patient relationship. *Med Care* 13:808-820, 1975

867. Hulka BS, Kupper LL, Daly M, Cassel JC, Schoen F: Correlates of satisfaction and dissatisfaction with medical care: A community perspective. *Med Care* 13:648-658, 1975

868. Hulka BS, Zyzanski SJ, Cassel JC, Thompson SJ: Scale for the measurement of attitudes toward physicians and primary medical care. *Med Care* 8:429-435, 1970

869. _____ : Satisfaction with medical care in a low income population. *J Chron Dis* 24:661-673, 1971

870. Korsch BM, Gozzi EK, Francis V: Gaps in doctor-patient communication 1. Doctor-patient interaction and patient satisfaction. *Pediatrics* 42:855-871, 1968

871. Kupper LL, Hulka BS, Cassel JC: Statistical considerations based on an instrument for measuring advisor perceptions. *Br J Math and Stat Psychol* 26:177, 1973

872. Zyzanski SJ, Hulka BS, Cassel JC: Scale for the measurement of 'satisfaction' with medical care: Modifications in content, format and scoring. *Med Care* 12:611-620, 1974

ADDITIONAL REFERENCES— CHAPTER 6, PART I (Citations 1-853 listed in Appendix I)

873. Aho WR: Relationship of wives' preventive health orientation to their beliefs about heart disease in husbands. *Public Health Rep* 92:65-71, 1977

874. Becker MH, Rosenstock IM: Social-psychological research on determinants of preventive health behavior, pp 25-35, in *The Behavioral Sciences and Preventive Medicine: Opportunities and Dilemmas*, Washington, DHEW

publication (NIH) 76-878, 1977
875. Becker MH, Maiman LA: Sociobehavioral determinants of compliance with health and medical care recommendations. *Med Care* 13:10-24, 1975
876. Campbell DA: A study of the preventive health behavior of a group of men with increased risk for the development of coronary heart disease. Doctoral dissertation, Ohio State University, Columbus, 1971
877. D'Onofrio CA: Motivational and promotional factors associated with acceptance of a contraceptive method in the postpartum period. Doctoral dissertation, University of California, Berkeley, 1973
878. Hochbaum GM: Public participation in medical screening programs: A socio-psychological study. Washington, PHS publication 572, 1958
879. Kirscht JP: Research related to the modification of health beliefs. *Health Educ Monogr* 2:455-469, 1974.
880. Maiman LA, Becker MH: The health belief model: Origins and correlates in psychological theory. *Health Educ Monogr* 2:336-353, 1974
881. Rosenstock IM: Historical origins of the health belief model. *Health Educ Monogr* 2:328-335, 1974
882. Simonds SK: Emerging challenges in health education. *Int J Health Educ* 19 (suppl): 1-19, 1976

ADDITIONAL REFERENCES–CHAPTER 6, PART II

883. Aday L, Eichhorn RC: The utilization of health services: Indices and correlates—a research bibliography. Washington, DHEW publication (HSM) 73-3003, 1972
884. Berkowitz L, Cottingham D: The interest value and relevance of fear-arousing communications. *J Abnorm Soc Psychol* 60:37-43, 1960
885. Bruch H: Psychological aspects of reducing. *Psychosom Med* 14:337-346, 1952
886. Freeman HE, Lambert C Jr: Preventive dental behavior of urban mothers. *J Health Hum Behav* 6:141-147, 1965
887. Friedman J: Weight problems and psychological factors. *J Couns Psychol* 23:524-527, 1959
888. Gill DJ: The role of personality and environmental factors in obesity. *J Am Diet Assoc* 22:398-400, 1946
889. Hammar SL, Campbell MM, Campbell VA, Moores NL, Sareen C, Gareis FJ, Lucas B: An interdisciplinary study of adolescent obesity. *J Pediatr* 80:373-383, 1972
890. Janis I: Vigilance and decision making in personal crises, pp 139-175, in Coelho G, Hamburg D, Adams RJ (eds): *Coping and Adaptation.* New York, Basic Books, 1974
891. Kegeles SS: A field experiment attempt to change beliefs and behavior of women in an urban ghetto. *J Health and Soc Behav* 10:115-124, 1969
892. Kerlinger FN: *Foundations of Behavioral Research.* New York, Holt, Rinehart and Winston, 1973

893. Kriesberg L, Treiman BR: Preventive utilization of dentists' services among teenagers. *J Am Coll Dent* 29:28-45, 1962

894. Leventhal H: Findings and theory in the study of fear communications, pp 119-186, in Berkowitz L (ed): *Advances in Experimental Social Psychology*, vol 5, New York, Academic Press, 1970

895. _____ : Changing attitudes and habits to reduce risk factors in chronic disease. *Am J Cardiol* 31:571-581, 1973

896. Litman TJ: The family as a basic unit in health and medical care: A social-behavioral overview. *Soc Sci Med* 8:495-519, 1974

897. Maddox GL, Anderson CF, Bogdonoff MD: Overweight as a problem of medical management in a public outpatient clinic. *Am J Med Sci* 252:394-403, 1966

898. Mayer J: Obesity during childhood, pp 73-80, in Winick M (ed): *Childhood Obesity*. New York, Wiley, 1975

899. McGuire W: The nature of attitudes and attitude change, pp 136-314, in Lindzey G, Aronson E (eds): *The Handbook of Social Psychology*. Reading, Mass, Addison-Wesley, 1968

900. Mechanic D: The influence of mothers on their children's health attitudes and behavior. *Pediatrics* 33:444-453, 1964

901. Mendelsohn H: Some reasons why information campaigns succeed. *Public Opinion Q* 37:50-61, 1973

902. Rimm IJ, Rimm AA: Association between juvenile onset obesity and severe adult obesity in 73,532 women. *Am J Public Health* 66:479-481, 1976

903. Rogers RW: A protection motivation theory of fear appeals and attitude change. *J Psychol* 91:93-114, 1975

904. Seaton DA, Rose K: Defaulters from a weight reduction clinic. *J Chron Dis* 18:1007-1111, 1965

905. Stunkard A, Levine H, Fox S: The management of obesity: Patient self-help and medical treatment. *Arch Intern Med* 125:1067-1072, 1970

906. Zborowski M: Cultural components in responses to pain. *J Soc Issues* 8:16-30, 1952

ADDITIONAL REFERENCES—
CHAPTER 7 (Citations 1-853 listed in Appendix I)

907. Korsch B, Gozzi EK, Francis V: Gaps in the doctor-patient relationship. *Pediatrics* 42:855-869, 1969

ADDITIONAL REFERENCES—
CHAPTER 8 (Citations 1-853 listed in Appendix I)

908. Haynes RB, Sackett DL, Taylor DW, Gibson ES, Johnson AL: Inceased absenteeism from work after detection and labeling of hypertensive patients. *N Eng J Med* 299:741-744, 1978

ADDITIONAL REFERENCES—
CHAPTER 9 (citations 1-853 listed in Appendix I)

909. Ayd FJ Jr (ed): Once-a-day neuroleptic and tricyclic antidepressant therapy. *Int Drug Ther Newsletter* 7:33-40, 1972.
910. _____: Once-a-day drug therapy. *Int Drug Ther Newsletter* 8: 1-4, 1973
911. Blackwell B: Antidepressant drugs, pp 10-16, in Dukes NMG (ed): *Meyler's Side Effects of Drugs*, Vol 9. Amsterdam, Exerpta Medica, 1976
912. Blackwell B: Rational drug use in the management of anxiety. *Ration Drug Ther* 9:1, 1975
913. Caldwell JR: Drug regimens for long-term therapy of hypertension. *Geriatrics* 31:115-119, 1976
914. David NA, Welborn S, Pierce HI: Comparison of multiple and combination tablet drug therapy in hypertension. *Curr Ther Res* 18:741-754, 1975
915. DiMascio A: Innovative drug administration regimens and the economics of mental health care, pp 118-130, in Ayd JR (ed): *Rationale Psychopharmacotherapy and the Right to Treatment*. Baltimore, Ayd Medical Communications Ltd., 1974
916. Materson BJ, Oster JR, Michael UF, Perez-Stable EC: Antihypertensive effectiveness of oxprenolol administered twice daily. *Clin Pharmacol Ther* 19:325-332, 1976
917. Mendels J, Schless A: A controlled comparison of doxepin h.s. and doxepin q.i.d. *J Clin Pharmacol* 15:534-539, 1975
918. Stetler CJ: Unpublished material submitted by Pharmaceutical Manufacturers Association to Department of Health, Education and Welfare, 1971
919. Winstead D, Blackwell B, Eilers MK, Anderson A: Psychotropic drug use in five city hospitals. *Dis Nerv System* 37:504-509, 1976
920. Wright CJ, Hook RH, Blackwell B: Metabolic and clinical observations on metiapine in humans, pp 445-455, in Forrest IS, Carr CJ, Usdine E (eds): *The Phenothiazines and Structurally Related Drugs*. New York, Raven Press, 1974
921. Wright JM, McLeod PJ, McCullougy W: Antihypertensive efficacy of a single bedtime dose of methyldopa. *Clin Pharmacol Ther* 20:733-737, 1976

ADDITIONAL REFERENCES—
CHAPTER 10 (Citations 1-853 listed in Appendix I)

922. Abramson EE: A review of behavioral approaches to weight control. *Behav Res Ther* 11:547-555, 1973
923. Aiken L, Aiken JL: A systematic approach to the evaluation of interpersonal relationships. *Am J Nurs* 73:863-867, 1973
924. Alpert JJ: Slave patients and free physicians. *N Engl J Med* 284:667-668, 1971

925. Andersen R: A behavioral model of families' use of health services. University of Chicago Center for Health Administration Studies Research Series 25, 1968
926. Anthony WA: Human relations training and rehabilitation counseling: Further implications. *Rehabil Coun Bull* 17:171-175, 1974
927. Antonovsky A, Hartman H: Delay in the detection of cancer: A review of the literature. *Health Educ Monogr* 2:98-128, 1974
928. Atwater JB: Adapting the veneral disease clinic to today's problem. *Am J Public Health* 64:433-437, 1974
929. Baric L: Recognition of the "at-risk" role: A means to influence health behavior. *Int J Health Educ* 12:24-34, 1969
930. Bauman HE: What does the consumer know about nutrition? *JAMA* 225:61-62, 1973
931. Becker MH, Maiman LA: Sociobehavioral determinants of compliance with health and medical care recommendations. *Med Care* 13:10-24, 1975
932. Berkanovic E, Reeder L: Ethnic, economic and social psychological factors in the source of medical care. *Soc Prob* 21:246-259, 1973
933. Bernstein L, Headlee R, Jackson B: Changes in acceptance of others resulting from a course in the physician-patient relationship. *Br J Med Educ* 4:65-66, 1970
934. Bossé R, Rose CL: Age and interpersonal factors in smoking cessation. *J Health Soc Behav* 14:381-387, 1973
935. Boyle CM: Differences between patient's and doctor's interpretation of some common medical terms. *Br Med J* 2:286-289, 1970
936. Burt R: Differential impact of social integration on participation in the diffusion of innovations. *Soc Sci Res* 2:1-20, 1973
937. Canfield RE: The physician as a teacher of patients. *J Med Educ* 48:79-87, 1973
938. Carrera MA, Rosenburg G: Inservice education in human sexuality for social work practitioners. *Clin Soc Work J* 1:261-267, 1973
939. Cauffman JG, Lloyd JS, Lyon ML: Health information and referral services within Los Angeles County. *Am J Public Health* 63:872-877, 1973
940. Crawford TJ: Theories of attitude change and "beyond family planning" debate: The case for the persuasion approach in population policy. *J Soc Issues* 30:211-234, 1974
941. Danaher BG: Theoretical foundations and clinical applications of the Premack Principle: Review and critique. *Behav Ther* 5:307-324, 1974
942. Deeds S: A *Guidebook for Family Planning Education*. Rockville MD, DHEW publication (HSA) 74-16002, 1973
943. Dodge JS: What patients should be told: Patients' and nurses' beliefs. *Am J Nurs* 72:1852-1854, 1972
944. D'Onofrio CN: Aides—pain or panacea? *Public Health Rep* 85:788-801, 1970
945. Eaton D: NIE attacks the reading and language skills problem, in *Research*

Developments. Reprinted by the National Institute of Education from *Am Educ*, May 1974

946. Fass MF, Green LW, Deeds S: The effect of family education on patient adherence to antihypertensive regimens. Paper presented at the National High Blood Pressure Control Conference, Washington, April 1977

947. Feldman JJ: *The Dissemination of Health Information: A Case Study in Adult Learning*. Chicago, Aldine, 1966

948. Finlayson A: Social networks as coping resources: Lay help and consultation patterns used by women in husband's post-infarction career. *Soc Sci Med* 10:97-103, 1976

949. Fleckenstein L, Joubert P, Lawrence R, Pastner B, Mazzullo JM, Lasagna L: Oral contracpetive patient information: A questionnaire study of attitudes, knowledge and preferred information sources. *JAMA* 235: 1331-1336, 1976

950. Fox LA: Written reinforcement of auxiliary directions for prescription medications. *Am J Hosp Pharm* 26:334-341, 1969

951. Garner JL, Mulcahy MJ: MIC project: Another kind of dietetics outreach program. *Hospitals* 47:96-97, 1973

952. Green LW, Lewis C: The placebo effect in self-care. Presented at the Association for the Advancement of Health Education, Seattle, April 1977

953. Green LW, Faden RR: The potential effects of patient package inserts on patients and drug consumers. *Drug Info J* 11 (supplement): 645-705, 1977

954. Green LW: Should health education abandon attitude change strategies? Some perspectives from recent research. *Health Educ Monogr* 1(30): 25-48, 1970

955. ____: Toward cost-benefit evaluations of health education: some concepts, methods and examples. *Health Educ Monogr* 2 (suppl 1): 34-64, 1974

956. ____: Theory and research vs practice (editorial). *Health Educ Monogr* 3:352-358, 1975

957. ____: Diffusion and adoption of innovations related to cardiovascular risk behavior in the public, pp 84-108, Enelow A, Henderson JB (eds): *Applying Behavioral Science to Cardiovascular Risk*. New York, American Heart Association, 1975

958. ____: Change-process models in health education. *Public Health Rev* 5:5-33, 1976

959. ____: Methods available to evaluate the health education components of preventive health programs, pp 162-171, in John E Fogarty International Center for Advanced Study in Health Science, *Preventive Medicine USA*. New York, Prodist, 1976

960. Green LW and Brooks-Bertram P: Peer review and quality control in health education. *Health Values* 3:1978, in press.

961. Green LW, Figà-Talamanca I: Suggested designs for evaluation of patient education programs. *Health Educ Monogr* 2:54-71, 1974

962. Green LW, Fisher AA, Amin R, Shafiullah A: Paths to the adoption of family planning: A time-lagged correlation analysis of the Dacca experiment in Bangladesh. *Int J Health Educ* 18:85-96, 1975

963. Green LW, Green PF: Intervening in social systems to make smoking education more effective, pp 393-401, in Steinfeld J, Griffiths W, Ball K, Taylor RM (eds): *Proceedings of the Third World Conference on Smoking and Health*. Washington, DHEW Publication (NIH) 77-1413, 1977

964. Green LW, Kalmer H: *Selecting an Evaluation Design for a Patient Education Program: Options for the Practitioner without Research Funds*, Proceedings, Maryland Workshop on Patient Education. Baltimore, Md Dept of Health and Mental Hygiene, 1976

965. Green LW, Roberts BJ: The research literature on why women delay in seeking medical care for breast symptoms. *Health Educ Monogr* 2:129-177, 1974

966. Green LW, Werlin SH, Schauffler H, Avery CH: Research and demonstration issues in self-care: Measuring the decline of mediocentrism. *Health Educ Monogr* 5:161-189, 1977

967. Hall SM, Hall RG: Outcome and methodological considerations in behavioral treatment of obesity. *Behav Ther* 5:352-364, 1974

968. Harris L and Associates: *The Public and High Blood Pressure: A Survey Conducted for the National Heart and Lung Institute*. Bethesda, Md, DHEW publication (NIH) 74-356, 1973

969. Hazell JW, Hodges FB, Cunningham GC: Intermediate benefit analysis— Spencer's dilemma and school health services. *Am J Public Health* 62:560-565, 1972

970. Heagarty MC, Robertson LS: Slave doctors and free doctors—a participant observer study of the physician-patient relation in a low-income comprehensive care program. *N Engl J Med* 284:636-641, 1971

971. Hingson R: Obtaining optimal attendance at mass immunization programs. *Health Serv Rep* 89:53-64, 1974

972. Hoff W: The importance of training for effective performance. *Public Health Rep* 85:760-766, 1970

973. Jacobs D, Charles E, Jacobs T, Weinstein H, Mann D: Preparation for treatment of the disadvantaged patient: Effects on disposition and outcome. *Am J Orthopsychiatry* 42:666-674, 1972

974. Jordan HA, Levitz LS: Behavior modification in a self-help group. *J Am Diet Assoc* 62:27-29, 1973

975. Joubert P, Lasagna L: Patient package inserts I: Nature, notions and needs. *Clin Pharmacol Ther* 18:507-513, 1975

976. _____: Patient package inserts II: Toward a rational patient package insert. *Clin Pharmacol Ther* 18:663-669, 1975

977. Kalba K: Communicable medicine: Cable television and health services. *Socio-Econ Plann Sci* 7:611-632, 1973

978. Kalmer H: Member-professional agreement related to use of a prepaid adult ambulatory care setting. Paper presented at American Public Health Association, Chicago, November 1975

979. Kar SB: Community interventions in health and family planning programs:

A conceptual framework. *Int J Health Educ* 20 (suppl): 1-15, 1977

980. _____: Consistency between fertility attitudes and behavior: A conceptual model. Paper presented at the American Psychological Assoc, Washington, 1976

981. Kasl SV: The health belief model and behavior related to chronic illness. *Health Educ Monogr* 2:433-454, 1974

982. Kazdin AE: *Behavior Modification in Applied Settings*. Homewood, Ill, Dorsey Press, 1975

983. Kerri JN: Anthropological studies of voluntary associations and voluntary action: A review. *J Vol Action Res* 3:10-25, 1974

984. Kupst MJ, Dresser K, Schulman JL, Paul MH: Evaluation of methods to improve communications in the physician-patient relationship. *Am J Orthopsychiatr* 45: 420-429, 1975

985. Levin LS, Katz AH, Holst E: *Self-care: Lay Initiatives in Health*. New York, Prodist, 1976

986. Levin LS. Forces and issues in the revival of interest in self-care: Impetus for redirection in health. *Health Educ Monogr* 5:115-120, 1977

987. Levine DM, Bonito AJ: Impact of clinical training on attidues of medical students: Self-perpetuating barrier to change in the system? *Br J Med Educ* 8:13-16, 1974

988. Levoy RP: Do questions from your patients bug you? *Dental Economics* 67:95-100, 1977

989. Ley P: Communication in the clinical setting. *Br J Orthod* 1:173-177, 1974

990. _____: The measurement of comprehensibility. *J Inst Health Educ* 11:17-20, 1973

991. Ley P, Bradshaw PW, Eaves D, Walker CM: A method for increasing patients' recall of information presented by doctors. *Psychol Med* 3:217-220, 1973

992. Ley P, Spelman MS: *Communicating with the Patient*. London, Staples Press, 1967

993. Ley P: Primacy, rated importance, and the recall of medical statements. *J Health Soc Behav* 13:311-317, 1972

994. _____: The use of techniques and findings from social and experimental psychology to improve doctor-patient communications, pp 14-35, in *Health Education and Primary Care: Conference Report*. Leeds, Department of Community Medicine and Leeds Polytechnic, 1975

995. Lin N: *The Study of Human Communication*. Indianapolis, Bobbs-Merrill, 1973

996. Lin N, Burt RS: Role of differential information channels in the process of innovation diffusion. Albany, International Center for Social Research, State University of New York, Monograph 001, 1973

997. Lin N, Hingson R: Diffusion of family planning innovations: Theoretical and practical issues. *Stud Fam Plann* 5:189-194, 1974

998. Linde TF, Patterson CH: Influence of orthopedic disability on conformity behavior. *J Abnorm Soc Psychol* 68:115-118, 1964

999. Mackie M: Lay perception of heart disease in an Alberta community. *Can J Public Health* 64:444-454, 1973

1000. Mahoney MJ: *Cognition and Behavior Modification.* Boston, Ballinger, 1974

1001. Mahoney MJ, Thoresen CE: *Self-control: Power to the Person.* Monterey, Calif, Brooks-Cole Publishing, 1974

1002. Marketing Economics Division: *Impact of the Expanded Food and Nutrition Education Program on Low-Income Families: An In-depth Analysis.* Washington, US Department of Agriculture, Economic Research Service, Report 220, 1972

1003. McAlister A: Helping people quit smoking: Current progress, pp 147-165, in Enelow A, Henderson JB (eds): *Applying Behavioral Sciences to Cardiovascular Risk,* New York, American Heart Association, 1975

1004. Meichenbaum D: Toward a cognitive theory of self control, pp 223-255, in Schwartz G, Shapiro D (eds): *Consciousness and Self-regulation: Advances in Research.* New York, Plenum, 1976

1005. Meichenbaum D, Cameron R: The clinical potential of modifying what clients say to themselves, pp 263-290, in Mahoney MJ, Thoresen CE (eds): *Self-control: Power to the Person.* Monterey, Calif, Brooks-Cole, 1974

1006. Meichenbaum D, Turk D: The cognitive-behavioral management of anxiety, anger and pain, pp 1-34 in Davidson PO (ed): *The Behavioral Management of Anxiety, Depression and Pain.* New York, Brunner-Mazel, 1976

1007. Mico PR, Ross HS: *Health Education and Behavioral Science.* Oakland, Third Party Associates, 1975

1008. Minkler M: The use of incentives in family planning programmes: A study of competing theories regarding their influence on attitude change. *Int J Health Educ* 19 (suppl):1-12, 1976

1009. Mitchell JH: Compliance with medical regimens: An annotated bibliography. *Health Educ Monogr* 2:75-87, 1974

1010. National Clearinghouse for Smoking and Health: *Adult Use of Tobacco, 1970.* Atlanta, Center for Disease Control, DHEW publication (HSM) 73-8727, 1973

1011. Neumann AK, Neumann CG, Ifekwunigwe AE: Evaluation of small-scale nutrition programs. *Am J Clin Nutr* 26:445-452, 1973

1012. Nichaman M, Collins G: Nutrition programs in state health agencies. *Nutr Rev* 32:65-69, 1974

1013. Pyrczak F, Roth DH: The readability of directions on non-prescription drugs. *J Am Pharm Assoc* 16:242-243, 267, 1976

1014. Rogers EM: *Communication Strategies in Family Planning.* New York, Free Press, 1973

1015. Rogers EM, Shoemaker FF: *Communication of Innovations.* New York, Free Press, 1971

1016. Ross J: Influence of experts and peers upon Negro mothers of low socioeconomic status. *J Soc Psychol* 89:79-84, 1973

1017. Roter D: Patient participation in the patient-provider interaction: The effects of patient question-asking on the quality of interaction, satisfaction and compliance. Doctoral dissertation, Johns Hopkins University School of Hygiene and Public Health, Baltimore, 1977

1018. Schwartz JL, Dubitzsky M: Expressed willingness of smokers to try ten smoking withdrawal methods. *Public Health Rep* 82:855-861, 1967

1019. Simons HW, Bertowitz NN, Moyer RJ: Similarity, credibility, and attitude change: A review and a theory. *Psychol Bull* 73:1-16, 1970

1020. Smith FA, Trivax G, Zuehlke DA et al: Health information during a week of television. *N Engl J Med* 286:516-620, 1972

1021. Stahl S, Lawrie T, Neill P, Kelley C: Motivational interventions in community hypertension screening. *Am J Public Health* 67:345-352, 1977

1022. Stamler J: *High Blood Pressure in the U.S.—An Overview of the Problem and the Challenge.* Proceedings of the National Conference on High Blood Pressure Education. Rockville, National Heart and Lung Institute, DHEW Publication (NIH) 73-486, 1973

1023. Steele J, McBroom WH: Conceptual and empirical dimensions of health behavior. *J Health Soc Behav* 13:382-392, 1972

1024. Stunkard AJ: The success of TOPS, a self-help group. *Postgrad Med* 51:143-147, 1972

1025. Ubell E: Health behavior change: A political model. *Prev Med* 1:209-221, 1972

1026. Udry R Clark LT, Chase CL, Levy M: Can media advertising increase contraceptive use? *Fam Plann Perspect* 4:37-44, 1972

1027. Wang VL, Ephross PH, Green LW: The point of diminishing returns in nutrition education through home visits by aides: An evaluation of EFNEP. *Health Educ Monogr* 3:70-88, 1975

1028. Weiss RL, Swearingen RV: *Chairside Psychology in Patient Education: A Self-instruction Course.* San Francisco, Dental Health Center, 1973

1029. Williams AF, Wechsler H: Interrelationship of preventive actions in health and other areas. *Health Serv Rep* 87:969-976, 1972

1030. Williamson JW, Aronovitch SE, Simonson L, Ramirez C, Kelly D: Health accounting: An outcome-based system of quality assurance: Illustrative application to hypertension. *Bull NY Acad Med* 51:727-738, 1975

1031. Wolle JM: Multidisciplinary teams develop programming for patient education. *Health Serv Rep* 89:8-12, 1974

1032. World Health Organization: Training and preparation of teachers for schools of medicine and allied health sciences. Geneva technical report series 521, 1973

1033. Young MAC: Review of research and studies related to health education communication: Methods and materials. *Health Educ Monogr* 1:63-70, 1967

1034. Zifferblatt SM, Wilbur CS: Dietary counseling: Some realistic expectations and guidelines. *J Am Diet Assoc* 70:591-595, 1977

1035. Zimmerman RR, Munro N: Changing Head Start mothers' food attitudes and practices. *J Nutr Educ* 4:66-68, 1972

1036. Zola IK: Pathways to the doctor—from person to patient. *Soc Sci Med* 7:677-689, 1973

ADDITIONAL REFERENCES—
CHAPTER 11 (Citations 1-853 listed in Appendix I)

1037. Alderman MH: Organization for long-term management of hypertension. *Bull NY Acad Med* 52:697-717, 1976

1038. ____: Three years of work-site based hypertensive treatment. Paper presented at the National Conference on High Blood Pressure Control, Washington, 1977

1039. Bandura A: *Social Learning Theory*. Englewood Cliffs, Prentice-Hall, 1977

1040. Barlow D: Self-report measures. Paper presented at the High Blood Pressure Education Research Program meeting, New Orleans, 1976

1041. Bellak AS, Rozensky R, Schwartz JA: A comparison of two forms of self-monitoring in a behavioral weight reduction program. *Behav Ther* 5:523-530, 1974

1042. Bigelow G, Strickler D, Leisbon I, Griffiths R: Maintaining disulfiram ingestion among outpatient alcoholics: A security-deposit contingency contracting procedure. *Behav Res Ther* 14:378-381, 1976

1043. Brigg EH, Mudd EH: An exploration of methods to reduce broken first appointments. *Fam Coord* 17:41-46, 1968

1044. Brosens IA, Robertson WB, Van Assche FA: Assessment of incremental dosage regimen of combined oestrogen-progestogen oral contraceptive. *Br Med J* 4:643-645, 1974

1045. Brownell KD, Heckerman CL, Westlake RJ, Hayes SC, Monti R: Couples training and spouse cooperativeness in the behavioral treatment of obesity. Presented at the Eleventh Annual Convention of the Association for the Advancement of Behavior Therapy, Atlanta, 1977

1046. Dinoff M, Rickard NC, Colwick J: Weight reduction through successive contracts. *Am J Orthopsychiatr* 42:110-113, 1972

1047. Dunbar JM: Adherence to medication regimen: An intervention study with poor adherers. Unpublished dissertation, Stanford University, 1977

1048. Fass MF, Green LW, Deeds SG: The effect of family education on patient adherence to antihypertensive regimens. Presented at the National Conference on High Blood Pressure Control, Washington, 1977

1049. Hallburg JC: Teaching patients self-care. *Nurs Clin North Am* 5:223-231, 1970

1050. Hladek WB, White SJ: Evaluation of written reinforcements used in counseling cardiovascular patients. *Am J Hosp Pharm* 33:1277-1280, 1976

1051. Jeffery RW, Wing RR, Stunkard AJ: Behavioral treatment of obesity: The state of the art—1976. *Behav Ther* 9:189-199, 1978

1052. Johnson SM, White G: Self-observation as an agent of behavioral change. *Behav Ther* 2:488-497, 1971

1053. Kanfer FH: Self-monitoring: Methodological limitations and clinical applications. *J Consult Clin Psychol* 35:148-152, 1970

1054. Kanfer FH: Cox LE, Gruner JM, Karoly P: Contracts, demand characteristics and self-control. *J Pers Soc Psychol* 30:605-619, 1974

1055. Kanfer FH, Phillips JS: *Learning Foundations of Behavior Therapy.*
New York, Wiley, 1970

1056. Mahoney MJ: Self-reward and self-monitoring techniques for weight
control. *Behav Ther* 5:48-57, 1974

1057. Mahoney MJ, Moura NGM, Wade TC: The relative efficacy of self-
rewards, self-punishment, and self-monitoring techniques for weight
loss. *J Consult Clin Psychol* 40:404-407, 1973

1058. Mahoney MJ, Thoresen CE: *Self-control: Power to the Person.* Monterey,
Calif, Brooks-Cole, 1974

1059. Maletzky BM: Behavior recording as treatment: A brief note. *Behav
Ther* 5:107-111, 1974

1060. Mann RA: The behavior-therapeutic use of contingency contracting to
control an adult-behavior problem: Weight control. *J Appl Behav Anal*
5:99-109, 1972

1061. Marshall GD, Agra WS, Rotchstein N: The use of medication dispensers
in improving adherence. Unpublished manuscript, Stanford University
Laboratory for the Study of Behavioral Medicine, 1976

1062. Marston AR: Imitation, self-reinforcement, and reinforcement of another
person. *J Pers Soc Psychol* 2:255-261, 1965

1063. Nelson RO, Lipinski DP, Black JL: The relative reactivity of external
observations and self-monitoring. *Behav Ther* 7:314-321, 1976

1064. Rimanczyk RG: Self-monitoring in the treatment of obesity: Parameters
of reactivity. *Behav Ther* 5:531-540, 1974

1065. Seybold ME, Drachman DB: Gradually increasing doses of prednisone
in myasthenia gravis. *N Engl J Med* 290:81-84, 1974

1066. Shmarak KL: Reduce your broken appointment rate: How one children
and youth project reduced its broken appointment rate. *Am J Public
Health* 61:2400-2404, 1971

1067. Thoresen CE, Mahoney MJ: *Behavioral Self-Control.* New York, Holt,
Rinehart and Winston, 1974

1068. Turner AJ, Vernon JC: Prompts to increase attendance in a community
mental-health center. *J Appl Behav Anal* 9:141-145, 1976

ADDITIONAL REFERENCES—
CHAPTER 12 (Citations 1-853 listed in Appendix I)

1069. Adler J, Kuehn AA: How advertising works in market experiments,
pp 63-70, in Hale WS (ed): *Proceedings of the Fifteenth Annual Conference of the Advertising Research Foundation.* New York, Advertising Research Foundation, 1969

1070. Brown N, Gatty R: Designing experiments with TV advertising labora-
tories, pp 120-129, *Proceedings of the Business and Economic Statistics
Section.* Washington, American Statistical Association, 1969

1071. Bruskin RH: *Seat Belt Usage Remains at Low Level Despite $51 Million Ad Effort*. New Brunswick, NJ, R.H. Bruskin Associates, 1969

1072. Council FM: *Seat Belts: A Follow-up Study of Their Use under Normal Driving Conditions*. Chapel Hill, University of North Carolina Highway Safety Research Center, 1969

1073. Fleischer GA: *An Experiment in the Use of Broadcast Media in Highway Safety: Systematic Analysis of the Effect of Mass Media Communications in Highway Safety*. Los Angeles, Department of Industrial and Systems Engineering, University of Southern California, 1972

1074. Galton L: New and better ways to take medication, pp. 14-15, in *Parade Magazine, Washington Post*, supplement, May 29, 1977

1075. Haddon W Jr, Goddard JL: *An Analysis of Highway Safety Strategies: Passenger Car Design and Highway Safety*. New York, Association for the Aid of Crippled Children and Consumers Union of the US, 1962

1076. Haddon W Jr: A logical framework for categorizing highway safety phenomena and activity. *J Trauma* 12:193-207, 1972

1077. Haskins JB: Effects of safety communication campaigns: A review of the research evidence. *J Safety Res* 1:58-66, 1969

1078. _____: Evaluative research on the effects of mass communication safety campaigns: A methodological critique. *J Safety Res* 2:86-96, 1970

1079. Howard B: The Advertising Council: Selling lies . . . *Ramparts* 10:5, 1975

1080. Kelley AB: Passive vs active=life vs death. Presented at the Automotive Engineering Congress, Detroit, Mich. 1975

1081. Klein D, Waller JA: *Causation, Culpability and Deterrence in Highway Crashes*. Washington, US Government Printing Office, 1970

1082. Levine DN, Campbell BJ: *Effectiveness of Lap Seat Belts and the Energy Absorbing Steering System in the Reduction of Injuries*. Chapel Hill, University of North Carolina Highway Safety Research Center, 1971

ADDITIONAL REFERENCES–
CHAPTER 13 (Citations 1-853 listed in Appendix I)

1083. Andrews DA: Aversive Treatment Procedures in the Modification of Smoking. Unpublished doctoral dissertation, Queen's University, 1970

1084. Azrin NH, Powell J: Behavioral engineering: The reduction of smoking behavior by a conditioning apparatus and procedure. *J Appl Behav Anal* 1:193-200, 1968

1085. Bandura A: *Principles of Behavior Modification*. New York, Holt, Rinehart and Winston, 1969

1086. Berecz J: Modification of smoking behavior through self-administered punishment of imagined behavior: A new approach to aversion therapy. *J Consult Clin Psychol* 38:244-250, 1972

1087. _____: Reduction of cigarette smoking through self-administered aversion conditioning: A new treatment model with implications for public health. *Soc Sci Med* 6:57-66, 1972

1088. _____: Treatment of smoking with cognitive conditioning therapy: A self-administered aversion technique. *Behav Ther* 7:341-348, 1976

1089. _____: Punishment, placebos, psychophysiology and polemics in aversion therapy: A reply to Danaher and Lichtenstein. *Behav Ther* 4:117-122, 1974

1090: _____: Smoking, stuttering, sex and pizza: Is there commonality? Presented at the annual meeting of the Association for the Advancement of Behavior Therapy, Chicago, 1974

1091. Bernstein D: Modification of smoking behavior: An evaluative review. *Psychol Bull* 71:418-440, 1969

1092. _____: The modification of smoking behavior: Some suggestions for programmed "symptom substitution." Presented to the annual meeting of the Association for the Advancement of Behavior Therapy, Chicago, 1974

1093. Bernstein D, McAlister A: The modification of smoking behavior: Progress and problems. *Addict Behav* 1:89-102, 1976

1094. Best JA, Bloch M, Owen LE: The effects of written instructions on compliance and outcome in a self-managed smoking cessation program. Manuscript, University of British Columbia, 1977

1095. Best JA, Hakstian R: A situation-specific model for smoking behavior. *Addict Behav*, in press

1096. Best JA, Steffy RA: Smoking modification tailored to subject characteristics. *Behav Ther* 2:177-191, 1971

1097. _____: Smoking modification procedures for internal and external locus of control clients. *Can J Behav Sci* 7:155-165, 1975

1098. Bloch M, Best JA: Cognitive versus behavioral strategies in the maintenance of smoking cessation. Manuscript, University of British Columbia, 1977

1099. Bornstein PH, Carmody TP, Relinger H, Zohn CJ, Devine DA, Bugge ID: Reduction of smoking behavior: A multivariable treatment package and the programming of response maintenance. *Psychol Rec* 27:733-741, 1977

1100. Bowers KS: Situationism in psychology: An analysis and critique. *Psychol Rev* 80:307-336, 1973

1101. Bozzetti LP: Group psychotherapy with addicted smokers. *Psychother Psychosom* 20:172-175, 1972

1102. Brantmark B, Ohlin P, Westling H: Nicotine-containing chewing gum as an anti-smoking aid. *Psychopharmacol* 31:191-200, 1973

1103. Brengelmann JC, Sedlmayr E: Experiments in the reduction of smoking behavior and health. Presented to the Third World Conference on Smoking, New York, 1975

1104. Cautela JR: Treatment of smoking by covert sensitization. *Psychol Rep* 26:415-420, 1970

1105. Chapman RF, Smith JW, Layden TA: Elimination of cigarette smoking by punishment and self-management training. *Behav Res Ther* 9:255-264, 1971

1106. Claiborn WL, Lewis P, Humble S. Stimulus satiation and smoking: A revisit. *J Clin Psychol* 28:416-419, 1972

1107. Conway JB: Self-management and aversive conditioning in the control of smoking. Presented at the annual meeting of the Canadian Psychological Association, Windsor, Ontario, 1974

1108. Crasilneck HB, Hall JA: The use of hypnosis in controlling cigarette smoking. *South Med J* 61:999-1002, 1968

1109. Danaher BG: Coverant control of cigarette smoking, pp. 117-137, in Krumboltz JD, Thoresen CE (eds): *Counseling Methods*. New York, Holt, Rinehart and Winston, 1976

1110. Danaher BG, Lichtenstein E: An experimental analysis of coverant control: Cueing and consequation. Presented at the annual meeting of the Western Psychological Association, San Francisco, 1974

1111. Danaher BG, Lichtenstein E, Sullivan JM: Comparative effects of rapid and normal smoking on heart rate and carboxyhemoglobin. *J Consult Clin Psychol* 44:556-563, 1976

1112. Davidson PO: Therapeutic compliance. *Can Psychol Rev* 17:247-259, 1976

1113. Davison GC, Rosen RC: Lobeline and reduction of cigarette smoking. *Psychol Rep* 31:443-456, 1972

1114. Dawley HH Jr: Minimizing the risks in rapid smoking treatment. *J Behav Ther Exper Psychiatry* 6:174, 1975

1115. Dawley HH Jr., Ellithorpe DB, Tretola R: Aversive Smoking: Carboxyhemoglobin levels before and after rapid smoking. *J Behav Ther Exper Psychiatry* 7:13-15, 1976

1116. Dawley HH Jr, Sardenga PB: Aversive cigarette smoking as a smoking cessation procedure. *J Clin Psychol* 33:234-239, 1978

1117. Delahunt J, Curran JP: Effectiveness of negative practice and self-control techniques in the reduction of smoking behavior. *J Consult Clin Psychol* 44:1002-1007, 1976

1118. Delarue NC: A study in smoking withdrawal. *Can J Public Health* 64 (Smoking and Health Supplement): S5-S19, 1973

1119. Devine DA, Fernald PS: Outcome effects of receiving a preferred randomly assigned or non preferred therapy. *J Consult Clin Psychol* 41:104-107, 1973

1120. Dunn WL Jr: *Smoking Behavior: Motive and Incentives*. Washington, Winston and Sons, 1973

1121. Edwards G: Double blind trial of lobeline in an anti-smoking clinic. *Med Offic* 111:158-160, 1964

1122. Eisinger RA: Psychosocial predictors of smoking recidivism. *J Health Soc Behav* 12:355-362, 1971

1123. Elliott R, Tighe T: Breaking the cigarette habit: Effects of a technique involving loss of money. *Psychol Rec* 18:503-513, 1968

1124. Eysenck HG: Personality and the maintenance of the smoking habit, pp. 113-146, in Dunn WL Jr (ed): *Smoking Behavior: Motives and Incentives*, Washington, Winston and Sons, 1973

1125. Ferraro DP: Self-control of smoking: The amotivational syndrome.

J Abnorm Psychol 81:152-157, 1973

1126. Flaxman J: Smoking cessation: Gradual vs abrupt quitting, timing, and self-control. Presented at the annual meeting of the Association for the Advancement of Behavior Therapy, Chicago, 1974

1127. Ford S, Ederer F: Breaking the cigarette habit. *JAMA* 194:139-142, 1965

1128. Frederiksen LW, Peterson GL: Short and long-term effects of three methods of smoking cessation. Presented to the annual meeting of the South Eastern Psychological Association, New Orleans, 1973

1129. ____: Modification of smoking by stimulus saturation. Presented to the annual meeting of the South Eastern Psychological Association, Hollywood, Fla, 1974

1130. ____: Controlled smoking: An alternative to abstinence. Presented at the annual meeting of the South Eastern Psychological Association, New Orleans, 1976

1131. ____: Controlled smoking: The case for a new treatment goal. Presented to the annual meeting of the Association for the Advancement of Behavior Therapy, New York, 1976

1132. Frederiksen LW, Peterson GL, Murphy WD: Controlled smoking: Development and maintenance. *Addict Behav* 1:193-196, 1976

1133. Gerson P, Lanyon RI: Modification of smoking behavior with an aversion-desensitization procedure. *J Consult Clin Psychol* 38:399-402, 1972

1134. Glad WR, Adesso VJ: The relative effects of socially induced tension and behavioral contagion for smoking behavior. *J Abnorm Psychol* 85:119-121, 1976

1135. Glad WR, Tyre TE, Adesso VJ: A multidimensional model of cigarette smoking. *Am J Clin Hypn* 19:82-90, 1976

1136. Goldfriend MR, Trier CS: Effectiveness of relaxation as an active coping skill. *J Abnorm Psychol* 83:348-355, 1974

1137. Gordon SP, Katz RC: A comparison of three maintenance procedures following treatment by rapid smoking. Presented to the annual meeting of the Western Psychological Association, Seattle, 1977

1138. Guilford JS: Group treatment versus individual initiative in the cessation of smoking. *J Appl Psychol* 56:162-167, 1972

1139. Gutmann M, Marston A: Problems of S's motivation in a behavioral program for reduction of cigarette smoking. *Psychol Rep* 20:1107-1114, 1967

1140. Hall RG, Sachs DPL, Hall SM: Medical risk of rapid smoking. Presented to the annual meeting of the Western Psychological Association, Seattle, 1977

1141. Harris DE, Lichtenstein E: Contribution of nonspecific social variables to a successful behavioral treatment of smoking. Presented at the annual meeting of the Western Psychological Association, San Francisco, 1971

1142. Harris MG, Rothberg C: A self-control approach to reducing smoking. *Psychol Rep* 31:165-166, 1972

1143. Hildebrandt DE, Feldman SE: The impact of commitment and change tactics training on smoking. Presented to the annual meeting of the Association for the Advancement of Behavior Therapy, San Francisco, 1975

1144. Hunt WA, Barnett LW, Branch LG: Relapse rates in addiction programs. *J Clin Psychol* 27:455-456, 1971

1145. Hunt WA, Matarazzo JD: Habit mechanisms in smoking, pp. 65-90, in Hunt WA, Matarazzo JD (eds): *Learning Mechanisms in Smoking*. Chicago, Aldine, 1970

1146. Hunt WA, Matarazzo JD, Weiss SM: Habit and the maintenance of behavior: Implications for compliance behavior in medical regimens. Unpublished manuscript, 1976

1147. Ikard FF, Green DE, Horn D: A scale to differentiate between types of smoking as related to the management of effect. *Int J Addict* 4:649-659, 1969

1148. Jacobs MA, Spilken AZ, Norman MM, Wohlberg GW, Knapp PH: Interaction of personality and treatment conditions associated with success in a smoking control program. *Psychosom Med* 33:545-556, 1971

1149. Janis IL, Hoffman D: Facilitating effects of daily contact between partners who make a decision to cut down on smoking. *J Pers Soc Psychol* 17:25-35, 1970

1150. Janis IL, Mann L: Effectiveness of emotional role-playing in modifying smoking habits and attitudes. *J Exper Res Per* 1:84-90, 1965

1151. Jenks R, Schwartz JL, Dubitsky M: Effect of the counselor's approach to changing smoking behavior. *J Counsel Psychol* 16:215-222, 1969

1152. Johnston JM: Punishment of human behavior. *Am Psychol* 27:1033-1054, 1972

1153. Kanfer FH, Karoly P: Self-control: A behavioristic excursion into the lion's den. *Behav Ther* 3:398-416, 1972

1154. Kantorowitz DA, Walters J: Positive versus negative self-monitoring in the self-control of smoking. Presented to the annual meeting of the Western Psychological Association, Seattle, 1977

1155. Kazdin AE: Self-monitoring and behavior change, pp. 218-246, in Mahoney MJ, Thoreson CE (eds): *Self-control: Power to the Person*. Monterey, Calif, Brooks-Cole, 1974

1156. Keutzer CS, Lichtenstein E, Mees HL: Modification of smoking behavior: A review. *Psychol Bull* 70:520-533, 1968

1157. Kline MV: The use of extended group hypnotherapy sessions in controlling cigarette habituation. *Int J Clin Exp Hypn* 18:270-282, 1970

1158. Koenig KP, Masters J: Experimental treatment of habitual smoking. *Behav Res Ther* 3:235-243, 1965

1159. Kopel SA: The effects of self-control, booster sessions, and cognitive factors on the maintenance of smoking reduction. *Dis Abst Internat* 35:4182B-4183B, 1975

1160. Lalonde M: *A New Perspective on the Health of Canadians: A Working Document*. Ottawa, National Health and Welfare, 1974

1161. Lando HA: Self-pacing in eliminating chronic smoking: Serendipity revisited? *Behav Ther* 7:634-640, 1976

1162. Lando HA, Davison GC: Cognitive dissonance as a modifier of chronic smoking behavior: A serendipitous finding. *J Consult Clin Psychol* 43:750, 1975

1163. Lawson DM, May RB: Three procedures for the extinction of smoking behavior. *Psychol Rec* 20:151-157, 1970

1164. Levenberg SB, Wagner MK: Smoking cessation: Long-term irrelevance of mode of treatment. *J Behav Ther Exper Psychiatry* 7:93-95, 1976

1165. Leventhal H: Experimental studies of anti-smoking communications, pp. 95-121, in Borgatta EF, Evans RR (eds): *Smoking, Health and Behavior*. Chicago, Aldine, 1968

1166. Levine BA: Effectiveness of contingent and non-contingent electric shock in reducing cigarette smoking. *Psychol Rep* 34:223-226, 1974

1167. Levinson BL, Shapiro D, Schwartz GE, Tursky B: Smoking elimination by gradual reduction. *Behav Ther* 2:477-487, 1971

1168. Lewittes DJ, Israel AC: Responsibility contracting for the maintenance of reduced smoking: A technique innovation. *Behav Ther* 6:696-698, 1975

1169. Lichtenstein E, Antonuccio DO, Rainwater G: Unkicking the habit: The resumption of cigarette smoking. Presented to the annual meeting of the Western Psychological Association, Seattle, 1977

1170. Lichtenstein E, Glasgow RE: Rapid smoking: Side effects and safeguards. *J Consult Clin Psychol* 45:815-821, 1977

1171. Lichtenstein E, Harris DE, Birchler GR, Wahl JM, Schmahl DP: A comparison of rapid smoking, warm, smoky air, and attention-placebo in the modification of smoking behavior. *J Consult Clin Psychol* 40:92-98, 1973

1172. Lichtenstein E, Keutzer CS: Modification of smoking behavior: A later look, in Rubin RD, Fensterheim H, Lazarus AA, Franks CM (eds): *Advances in Behavior Therapy*. New York, Academic Press, 1971

1173. Lichtenstein E, Keutzer CS, Himes KH: Emotional role-playing and changes in smoking attitudes and behavior. *Psychol Rep* 25:379-387, 1969

1174. Logan FA: The smoking habit, in Hunt WA (ed): *Learning Mechanisms in Smoking*. Chicago, Aldine, 1970

1175. ____: Self-control as habit, drive and incentive. *J Abnorm Psychol* 81:127-136, 1973

1176. McAlister A: Helping people quit smoking: Current progress, in Enelow A, Henderson J (eds): *Applying Behavioral Science to Cardiovascular Disease*. New York, American Heart Association, 1975

1177. McCallum RN: The modification of smoking behavior: A comparison of treatment techniques. Presented to the annual meeting of the Southwestern Psychological Association, San Antonio, 1971

1178. McFall RM, Hammen CL: Motivation, structure and self-monitoring: Role of nonspecific factors in smoking reduction. *J Consult Clin Psychol* 37:80-86, 1971

1179. McGrath MJ, Hall SM: Self-management treatment of smoking behavior. *Addict Behav* 1:287-292, 1976

1180. McKennell AC: Smoking motivation factors. *Br J Soc Clin Psychol* 9:8-22, 1970

1181. McKennell AC: *A Comparison of Two Smoking Typologies*. London, Tobacco Research Council, 1973

1182. Mahoney MJ: *Cognition and Behavior Modification*. Cambridge, Mass, Ballinger, 1974

1183. Marrone RL, Merksamer MA, Salzberg PM: A short-duration group treatment of smoking behavior by stimulus saturation. *Behav Res Ther* 8:347-352, 1970

1184. Marston AR, McFall RM: A comparison of behavior modification approaches to smoking reduction. *J Consult Clin Psycho* 36:153-162, 1971

1185. Mausner B: Some comments on the failure of behavior therapy as a technique for modifying cigarette smoking. *J Consult Clin Psycho* 36:167-170, 1971

1186. Mausner B, Platt ES: *Smoking: A Behavioral Analysis*. Toronto, Pergamon, 1971

1187. Meichenbaum D: Self-instructional methods, pp. 357-391, in Kanfer F, Goldstein A (eds): *Helping People Change*. New York, Pergamon, 1975

1188. ____: Towards a cognitive theory of self-control, pp. 223-255, in Schwartz G, Shapiro D (eds): *Consciousness and Self-regulation: Advances in Research*. New York, Plenum, 1976

1189. Merry J, Preston G: The effect of buffered lobeline sulphate on cigarette smoking. *Practitioner* 190:629-631, 1963

1190. Mischel W: *Personality and Assessment*. New York, Wiley, 1968

1191. Morrow JE, Sachs LB, Gmeinder S, Burgess H: Elimination of cigarette smoking behavior by stimulus satiation, self-control techniques, and group therapy. Paper presented at the meeting of the Western Psychological Association, Anaheim, Calif, 1973

1192. National Interagency Council on Smoking and Health. *Guidelines for Research on the Effectiveness of Smoking Cessation Programs: A Committee Report*. Chicago, American Dental Association, 1974

1193. Nehemkis AM, Lichtenstein E: Conjoint social reinforcement in the treatment of smoking. Presented at the meeting of the Western Psychological Association, San Francisco, April 1971

1194. Nolan JD: Self-control procedures in the modification of smoking behavior. *J Consult Clin Psychol* 32:92-93, 1968

1195. Norton GR, Barske B: The role of aversion in the rapid-smoking treatment procedure. *Addict Behav* 2:21-25, 1977

1196. Nuland W, Field PB: Smoking and hypnosis: A systematic clinical approach. *Int J Clin Exper Hypn* 18:290-306, 1970

1197. Ober DC: Modification of smoking behavior. *J Consult Clin Psychol* 32:543-549, 1968

1198. Ochsner A, Damrau F: Control of cigarette habit by psychological aversive conditioning: Clinical evaluation in 53 smokers. *J Am Geriatr Soc* 18:365-369, 1970

1199. Pechacek TF: Specialized treatments for highly anxious smokers. Presented to the annual meeting of the Association for the Advancement of Behavior Therapy, New York, 1976

1200. Pederson LL, Scrimgeour WG, Lefcoe NM: Comparison of hypnosis plus counseling, counseling alone, and hypnosis alone in a community service smoking withdrawal program. *J Consult Clin Psychol* 43:920, 1975

1201. Platt ES, Krassen E, Mausner B: Individual variation in behavior change following role playing. *Psychol Rep* 24:155-170, 1969

1202. Pomerleau OF, Ciccone P: Preliminary results of a treatment program for smoking cessation using multiple behavior modification techniques. Presented at the annual meeting of the Association for the Advancement of Behavior Therapy, Chicago, 1974

1203. Powell J, Azrin N: The effects of shock as a punisher for cigarette smoking. *J Appl Behav Anal* 1:63-71, 1968

1204. Pyke S, Agnew NMcK, Kopperud J: Modification of an overlearned maladaptive response through a relearning program: A pilot study on smoking. *Behav Res Ther* 4:197-203, 1966

1205. Pyszka RH, Ruggels WL, Janowicz LM: *Health Behavior Change: Smoking Cessation.* Stanford, Stanford Research Institute, Institute Research and Development Report, December 1973

1206. Rapp GW, Dusza BT, Blanchet L: Absorption and utility of lobeline as a smoking deterrent. *Am J Med Sci* 237:287-292, 1959

1207. Relinger H, Bornstein PH, Bugge ID, Carmody TP, Zohn CJ: Utilization of adverse rapid smoking in groups: Efficacy of treatment and maintenance procedures. *J Consult Clin Psychol* 45:245-249, 1977

1208. Resnick JH: Effects of stimulus satiation on the overlearned maladaptive response of cigarette smoking. *J Consult Clin Psychol* 32:500-505, 1968

1209. ____: The control of smoking behavior by stimulus satiation. *Behav Res Ther* 6:113-114, 1968

1210. Roberts AH: Self-control procedures in modification of smoking behavior: Replication. *Psychol Rep* 24:675-676, 1969

1211. Rogers RW, Thistlethwaite DL: Effects of fear arousal and reassurance on attitude change. *J Pers Soc Psychol* 15:227-233, 1970

1212. Rosen GM, Lichtenstein E: A workers' incentive program for the reduction of cigarette smoking. *J Consult Clin Psychol* 45:957, 1977

1213. Rozensky RH: The effect of temporal location of self-monitoring behavior on reducing cigarette consumption. *J Behav Ther Exper Psychiatry* 5:301-303, 1974

1214. Russell MAH: Effect of electric aversion on cigarette smoking. *Br Med J* 1:82-86, 1970

1215. Russell MAH, Peto J, Patel UA: The classification of smoking by factorial structure of motives. *J Rl Statist Soc* (series A) 137:313-346, 1974

1216. Sachs LB, Bean H, Morrow JE: Comparison of smoking treatments. *Behav Ther* 1:465-472, 1970

1217. St Pierre R, Lawrence PS: Reducing smoking using positive self-management. *J Sch Health* 45:7-9, 1975

1218. Schlegel RP, Kunetsky M: Immediate and delayed effects of the five-day plan to stop smoking including factors affecting recidivism. *Prev Med* 6:454-461, 1977

1219. Schmahl DP, Lichtenstein E, Harris DE: Successful treatment of habitual smokers with warm, smoky air and rapid smoking. *J Consult Clin Psychol* 38:105-111, 1972

1220. Schwartz JL: A critical review and evaluation of smoking control methods. *Public Health Rep* 84:483-506, 1969

1221. Schwartz JL, Dubitsky M. The results of helping people fight cigarettes. *Calif Health* 24:78-83, 1967

1222. Severson HH, Hynd GW: A comparison of the effectiveness of rapid smoking, modeling and covert sensitization in smoking cessation. Presented to the annual meeting of the Western Psychological Association, Seattle, 1977

1223. Shapiro D, Tursky B, Schwartz GE, Shnidman SR: Smoking on cue: A behavioral approach to smoking reduction. *J Health Soc Behav* 12:108-113, 1971

1224. Shewchuk LA, Dubren R, Burton D, Forman M, Clark RR, Jaffin AR: Preliminary observations on an intervention program for heavy smokers. *Int J Addict* 12:323-337, 1977

1225. Sipich JF, Russell RK, Tobias LL: A comparison of covert sensitization and "nonspecific" treatment in the modification of smoking behavior. *J Behav Ther Exper Psychiatr* 5:201-203, 1974

1226. Spiegel H: A single-treatment method to stop smoking using auxillary self-hypnosis. *Int J Clin Exper Hypn* 18:235-250, 1970

1227. Steffy RA, Meichenbaum D, Best JA: Aversive and cognitive factors in the modification of smoking behavior. *Behav Res Ther* 8:115-125, 1970

1228. Streltzer NE, Koch GV: Influence of emotional role-playing on smoking habits and attitudes. *Psychol Rep* 22:817-820, 1968

1229. Suedfeld P: Sensory deprivation used in the reduction of cigarette smoking: Attitude change experiments in an applied context. *J Appl Soc Psychol* 3:30-38, 1973

1230. Suedfeld P, Best JA: Satiation and sensory deprivation combined in smoking therapy: Some case studies and unexpected side-effects. *Int J Addict* 12:337-359, 1977

1231. Suedfeld P, Ikard FF: Attitude manipulation in restricted environments: IV. Psychologically addicted smokers treated in sensory deprivation. *Br J Addict* 68:170-176, 1973

1232. Suedfeld P, Ikard FF: Use of sensory deprivation in facilitating the reduction of cigarette smoking. *J Consult Clin Psychol* 42:888-895, 1974

1233. Suedfeld P, Landon PB, Pargament R, Epstein YM: An experimental attack on smoking: Attitude manipulation in restricted environments, III. *Int J Addict* 7:721-733, 1972

1234. Sushinsky LW: Expectation of future treatment, stimulus satiation, and smoking. *J Consult Clin Psychol* 39:343, 1972

1235. Sutherland A, Amit Z, Golden M, Roseberger Z: Comparison of three behavioral techniques in the modification of smoking behavior. *J Consult Clin Psychol* 43:443-447, 1975

1236. Tighe T, Elliott RA: A technique for controlling behavior in natural life settings. *J Appl Behav Anal* 1:263-266, 1968

1237. Tomkins SS: Psychological model for smoking behavior. *Am J Public Health* 56:17-20, 1966

1238. Tomkins SS: A modified model of smoking behavior, in Borgatta EF, Evans RR (eds): *Smoking, Health and Behavior*. Chicago, Aldine, 1968

1239. Thompson DS, Wilson TR: Discontinuance of cigarette smoking: "Natural" and with "therapy". *JAMA* 196:1048-1052, 1966

1240. United States Public Health Service: *Adult Use of Tobacco: 1975*. Washington, US Department of Health, Education and Welfare, 1976

1241. Upper D, Meredith L: A stimulus control approach to the modification of smoking. *Proceedings of the Seventeenth American Psychological Association Convention* 5:739-740, 1970

1242. Von Dedenroth TEA: The use of hypnosis in 1000 cases of "tobacco-maniacs." *Am J Clin Hypn* 8:194-197, 1968

1243. Wagner MK, Bragg RA: Comparing behavior modification approaches to habit decrement—smoking. *J Consult Clin Psychol* 34:258-263, 1970

1244. Watkins HH: Hypnosis and smoking: A five-session approach. *Int J Clin Exper Hypn* 24:381-390, 1976

1245. Weinrobe PA, Lichtenstein E: The use of urges as termination criterion in a rapid smoking program for habitual smokers. Presented at the annual meeting of the Western Psychological Association, Sacramento, 1975

1246. Weir JM, Dubitsky M, Schwartz JL: Counselor style and group effectiveness in a smoking withdrawal study. *J Psychother* 23:106-118, 1969

1247. Whitman TL: Modification of chronic smoking behavior: A comparison of three approaches. *Behav Res Ther* 7:257-263, 1969

1248. _____: Aversive control of smoking behavior in a group context. *Behav Res Ther* 10:97-104, 1972

1249. Winett RA: Parameters of deposit contracts in the modification of smoking. *Psychol Rec* 23:49-60, 1973

1250. Wisocki PA, Rooney EJ: A comparison of thought-stopping and covert sensitization techniques in the treatment of smoking. Presented to the annual meetings of the Association for the Advancement of Behavior Therapy, Washington, 1971

ADDITIONAL REFERENCES—
CHAPTER 14 (Citations 1-853 listed in Appendix I)

1251. Addiction Research Foundation Information Center, Toronto, Canada: Statistics on alcohol and other drug use in Canada and Ontario, data available in 1976. Information Review, revised, October 1976

1252. Azrin NH: Improvements in the community reinforcement approach to alcoholism. *Behav Res Ther* 14:339-348, 1976

1253. Baekeland F, Lundwall L, Kissin B: Methods for the treatment of chronic alcoholism: A critical appraisal, pp 247-327, in Gibbins RJ, Israel Y, Kalant H, Popham RE, Schmidt W, Smart R (eds): *Recent Advances in Alcohol and Drug Problems*. New York, Wiley, 1975

1254. Baekeland F, Lundwall K: Engaging the alcoholic in treatment and keeping him there, pp 161-195, in Kissin AB, Begleiter H, (eds): *The Biology of Alcoholism, Vol 5, Treatment and Rehabilitation of the Chronic Alcoholic*. New York, Plenum, 1976

1255. Bigelow G, Cohen M, Leibson I, Faillace LA: Abstinence or moderation? Choice by alcoholics. *Behav Res Ther* 10:209-214, 1972

1256. Bigelow G, Griffiths R, Liebson I: Experimental human drug self-administration: Methodology and application to the study of sedative abuse. *Pharmacol Rev* 27:523-531, 1976

1257. Brunn K, Edwards G, Lumio M, Makala K, Pan L, Popham R: Alcohol control policies in public health perspective, Helsinki. *The Finnish Foundation for Alcohol Studies* 25:1-106, 1975

1258. Cobby J, Mayersohn M, Selliah S: The rapid reduction of disulfiram in blood and plasma. *Pharmacol Exp Ther* 202:724-731, 1977

1259. Cohen M, Liebson IA, Faillace LA, Speers W: Alcoholism: Controlled drinking and incentive for abstinence. *Psychol Rep* 28:575-580, 1971

1260. Cutler SJ, Ederer F: Maximum utilization of the life table method in analyzing survival. *J Chron Dis* 8:699-712, 1958

1261. De Leon G, Rosenthal M, Bordney K: Therapeutic community for drug addicts; long-term measurement of emotional changes. *Psychol Rep* 29:595-600, 1971

1262. De Leon G, Skodol A, Rosenthal MS: Phoenix House: Changes in psychopathological signs of resident drug addicts. *Arch Gen Psychiatr* 28:131-135, 1973

1263. De Lint J, Schmidt W: Control laws and price manipulation as preventive strategies. *Addiction Research Foundation* Substudy 705, 1975

1264. Gerrein JR, Rosenberg CM, Manohar V: Disulfiram maintenance in outpatient treatment of alcoholism. *Arch Gen Psychiatr* 28:298-802, 1973

1265. Glaser FB: Splittings: Attrition from a drug-free therapeutic community. *Am J Drug Alcohol Abuse* 1:329-348, 1974

1266. ____: The treatment of drug abuse in the rural south: Application of the Core-Shell treatment system model. *South Med J* 67:580-586, 1974

1267. ____: Testimony given February 5, 1976 before the Subcommittee on Alcoholism and Narcotics of the Committee on Labor and Public Health, US Senate, 1976

1268. Goldstein A: Heroin addiction and the role of methadone in its treatment. *Arch Gen Psychiatr* 26:291-297, 1972

1269. Griffiths R, Bigelow G, Liebson I: Suppression of ethanol self-administration by contingent time-out from social interactions. *Behav Res Ther* 12:327-334, 1974

1270. Israelstam SM: Some statistics concerning consumption of alcoholic beverages and deaths by liver cirrhosis, for Ontario and Canada 1945-1974, with international comparisons. *Addiction Research Foundation* Substudy 846, 1977

1271. Isselbacher KJ: Metabolic and hepatic effects of alcohol. *N Engl J Med* 297:612-616, 1977

1272. Larkin EJ: Voluntary termination of out-patient treatment by alcoholics. Unpublished doctoral dissertation, York University, Toronto, 1972

1273. ____: *The Treatment of Alcoholism: Theory, Practice and Evaluation.* Toronto, Addiction Research Foundation Program Report 1, 1974

1274. Liebson I, Bigelow G, Flamer R: Alcoholism among methadone patients: A specific treatment method. *Am J Psychiatr* 130:483-485, 1973

1275. Malcolm MT, Madden JS: The use of disulfiram implantation in alcoholism. *Br J Psychiatr* 123:41-55, 1973

1276. Miller PM: the use of behavioral contracting in the treatment of alcoholism: A case report. *Behav Ther* 3:593-596, 1972

1277. Miller PM, Hersen M: Quantitative changes in alcohol consumption as a function of electrical aversive conditioning. *J Clin Psychol* 28:590-593, 1972

1278. Miller PM, Hersen M, Eisler R, Elkin TE: A retrospective analysis of alcohol consumption on laboratory tasks as related to therapeutic outcome. *Behav Res Ther* 12:73-76, 1974

1279. Mottin JL: Drug-induced attenuation of alcohol consumption. A review and evaluation of claimed, potential or current therapies. *Q J Stud Alcohol* 34:444-472, 1973

1280. Nathan PE, Briddell DW: Behavioral assessment and treatment of alcoholism, pp 301-349, in Kissin B, Begleiter H (eds): *The Biology of Alcoholism, Vol 5, Treatment and Rehabilitation of the Chronic Alcoholic.* New York, Plenum, 1976

1281. Pattison EM: Rehabilitation of the chronic alcoholic, pp 587-658, in Kissin B, Begleiter H (eds): *The Biology of Alcoholism, Vol 3, Clinical Pathology.* New York, Plenum, 1974

1282. Popham RE, Schmidt W: The effectiveness of legal measures in the prevention of alcohol problems. *Addiction Research Foundation*, Substudy 664, 1975

1283. Rankin JG, Orrego-Matte H, Deschenes J, Medline A, Findlay J: Diagnostic problems in alcoholic liver disease, in Seixas F (ed): *Currents in Alcoholism.* In press, 1978

1284. Sellers EM, Kalant H: Pharmacotherapy of acute and chronic alcoholism and the alcohol withdrawal syndrome, *Psychopharmacologia*, 3rd edition. In press, 1978

1285. Shaw S, Stimmel B, Lieber CS: Plasma alpha amino-n-butyric acid to leucine ratio: An empirical biochemical marker of alcoholism. *Science* 194:1057-1058, 1976

1286. Shaw S, Lue SL, Lieber CS: Diagnosis of alcoholism by a two step biochemical test, in Seixas F (ed): *Currents in Alcoholism.* In press, 1978

1287. Silberfeld M, Glaser FB: Unpublished observations.
1288. Sobell MB, Sobell LC: The need for realism, relevance and operational assumptions in the study of substance dependence, pp 133-167, in Cappell H,Le Blance AE (eds): *Biological and Behavioral Approaches to Drug Dependence*. Toronto, Addiction Research Foundation, 1975
1289. Vander Voort R, Phillips M, Becker C: A method for quantifying alcohol consumption, in Seixas F (ed): *Currents in Alcoholism*. In press, 1978
1290. Wren JC, Line NS, Cooper TB, Varga E, Canal O: Evaluation of lithium therapy in chronic alcoholism. *Clin Med* 81:33-36, 1974

ADDITIONAL REFERENCES—
CHAPTER 15 (Citations 1-853 listed in Appendix I)

1291. Argyris C: *Integrating the Individual and the Organization*. New York, Wiley, 1964
1292. Bessman AN: Comparison of medical care in nurse clinician and physician clinics in medical school affiliated hospitals. *J Chron Dis* 27:115-125, 1974
1294. Brill NI: *Teamwork: Working Together in the Human Services*. Philadelphia, Lippincott, 1976
1293. Bloch, D: Evaluation of nursing care in terms of process and outcome. *Nurs Res* 24:256-263, 1975
1295. Cassel JC: Psychological processes and "stress:" Theoretical formulation. *Int J Health Services* 4:471-482, 1974
1296. Caplan G: *Support Systems and Community Mental Health*. New York, Behavioral Publications, 1974
1297. Charney E, Kitzman H: The child-health nurse (pediatric nurse practitioner) in private practice. A controlled trial. *N Engl J Med* 285:1353-1358, 1971
1298. Combs AW, Avila DL, Purkey WW: *Helping Relationships: Basic Concepts for the Helping Professions*. Boston, Allyn and Bacon, 1971
1299. Davies J: Impact of the system on the patient-practitioner relationship, pp 137-144, in Cullen JW, Fox BH, Isom RN (eds): *Cancer: The Behavioral Dimension*. New York, Raven Press, 1976
1300. Davis F: *Passage through Crisis*. Indianapolis, Bobbs-Merrill, 1963
1301. Egan G: *The Skilled Helper: A Model for Systematic Helping and Interpersonal Relating*. Monterey, Calif, Brooks Cole, 1975
1302. Finlayson A, McEwan J: *Coronary Heart Disease and Patterns of Living*. New York, Prodist, 1977
1303. Flynn BC: The effectiveness of nurse clinicians' service delivery. *Am J Public Health* 64:604-611, 1974
1304. Ford LC, Silver HK: The expanded role of the nurse in child care. *Nurs Outlook* 15:43-45, 1967
1305. German PS, Chwalow AJ: Conflicts in ethical problems of patient education. Strategies for hypertension control explore contractual approach. *Int J Health Educ* 19:105-111, 1976

1306. Gerson EM, Strauss AL: Time for living: Problems in chronic illness care. *Social Policy* 6:12-18, 1975

1307. Goffman E: *Asylums.* Chicago, Aldine, 1961

1308. Green LW: Toward cost-benefit evaluations of health education: Some concepts, methods and examples. *Health Educ Monogr* 2:34-65, 1974

1309. Hall, JE: Nursing as process, pp 173-191, in Hall JE, Weaver BR (eds): *Distributive Nursing Practice: A Systems Approach to Community Health.* Philadelphia, Lippincott, 1977

1310. Hogue CC: Support systems: A model for research and practice. Presented at Gerontological Society Meetings, New York, October 1976

1311. ____: Support systems for health promotion, pp 65-80, in Hall JE, Weaver BR (eds): *Distributive Nursing Practice: A Systems Approach to Community Health.* Philadelphia, Lippincott, 1977

1312. ____: Professional teamwork: Implementation of a good idea. Presented at the Duke University Center for the Study of Aging and Human Development Conference, Asheville, NC, May 1977

1313. Horowitz JJ: *Team Practice and the Specialist.* Springfield, Ill, Thomas, 1970

1314. Hyman MD: Social isolation and performance in rehabilitation. *J Chron Dis* 25:85-97, 1972

1315. Jeanes JR, Grant JR: Children's retention of dental hygiene instruction. *Nurs Res* 25:452-454, 1976

1316. Johnson DE: One conceptual model of nursing. Presented at Vanderbilt University, Nashville, Tenn, April 1968

1317. Katz S, Halstead L, Wierenga M: A medical perspective of team care, pp 213-252, in Sherwood S (ed): *Long-Term Care.* New York, Spectrum, 1975

1318. Keith RA: The need for a new model in rehabilitation. *J Chron Dis* 21: 281-286, 1968

1319. King I: *Toward a Theory for Nursing.* New York, Wiley, 1971

1320. Leininger M: An open health care system model. *Nurs Outlook* 21:171-175, 1973

1321. Levine E: What do we know about nurse practitioners? *Am J Nurs* 77:1799-1803, 1977

1322. Lewis CE, Cheyovich TK: Who is a nurse practitioner? Processes of care and patients' and physicians' perceptions. *Med Care* 14:365-371,

1323. Lewis CE, Resnick BA: Nurse clinics and progressive ambulatory patient care. *N Engl J Med* 277:1236-1241, 1967

1324. Lewis CE, Resnick BA, Schmidt G, Waxman D: Activities, events and outcomes in ambulatory patient care. *N Engl J Med* 280:645-649, 1969

1325. Lewis CE, Lorimer A, Lindeman C, Palmer B, Lewis MA: An evaluation of the impact of nurse practitioners. *J Sch Health* 44:331-335, 1974

1326. Litman EJ: The family as a basic unit in health and medical care: A social-behavioral overview. *Soc Sci Med* 8:495-519, 1974

1327. Morgan B: The health action model: Correlates of compliance in preventive health behavior. Presented at the second Eastern Conference on Nursing Research, April 1976

1328. Orem DE: *Nursing: Concepts of Practice.* New York, McGraw Hill, 1971, p 13

1329. Powers MJ, Ford LC: The best kept secret: Consumer power and nursing's potential, pp 48-63, in Lasagna L (ed): *Patient Compliance.* Mount Kisco, NY, Futura, 1970

1330. Rogers ME: *An Introduction to Theoretical Bases of Nursing.* Philadelphia, FA Davis, 1970

1331. Roth J: *Timetables.* Indianapolis, Bobbs-Merrill, 1963

1332. Sheridan A, Smith RA: Student-family contracts. *Nurs Outlook* 23:114-117, 1975

1333. Sills GM: Research in the field of psychiatric nursing, 1952-1977. *Nurs Res* 26:201-207, 1977

1334. Silver HK, Ford L, Stearly S: A program to increase health care for children: The pediatric nurse practitioner program. *Pediatrics* 39:756-760, 1967

1335. Skipper JK: The role of the hospital nurse: Is it instrumental or expressive? pp 40-48, in Skipper JK, Leonard RC (eds): *Social Interaction and Patient Care.* Philadelphia, Lippincott, 1965

1336. Smith BC: Compliance of epileptics with anticonvulsant medication. Unpublished report, Durham, NC, April 1977

1337. Springer B: Health belief model to explain compliant/noncompliant smoking. Unpublished report, Durham, NC, April 1977

1338. Stillman MJ: Women's health beliefs about breast cancer and breast self-examination. *Nurs Res* 26:121-127, 1977

1339. Strauss AL: *Chronic Illness and the Quality of Life.* Saint Louis, Mosby, 1975

1340. Triplett JL: Characteristics and perceptions of low-income women and use of preventive health services. *Nurs Res* 19:140-146, 1970

1341. Twaddle AC: The concept of health status. *Soc Sci Med* 8:29-38, 1974

1342. US Health Resources Administration. *Longitudinal Study of Nurse Practitioners, Phase 1.* Washington, DHEW 76-43, US Government Printing Office, 1976

1343. Williams TF, Martin D, Hogan M, Watkins JD, Ellis EV: The clinical picture of diabetic control studied in four settings. *Am J Public Health* 57:441-451, 1967

1344. Although we have no empirical evidence, we speculate that people who describe themselves in ways that suggest they are lifelong isolates might benefit from carefully structured professional supervision with simple techniques such as those suggested by A. Hecht (696).

1345. The author acknowledges the thoughtful advice of Mary-Vesta Marston, PhD, in the planning of this chapter.

ADDITIONAL REFERENCES—
CHAPTER 16 (Citations 1-853 listed in Appendix I)

1346. Ascione FJ, Ravin RL: Physicians' attitudes regarding patients' knowledge of prescribed medications. *J Am Pharm Assoc* NS15: 386-390, 1975

1347. Avery C, Green LW, Kreider S: Reducing emergency visits of asthmatics: An experiment in patient education. Pittsburgh, Pa, Testimony, President's Committee on Health Education, 1972

1348. Becker MH: The health belief model and sick role behavior. *Health Educ Monogr* 2:409-419, 1974

1349. Becker MH, Maiman LA: Sociobehavioral determinants of compliance with health and medical care recommendations. *Med Care* 13:10-24, 1975

1350. Clark GM, Troop RC: One-tablet combination drug therapy in the treatment of hypertension. *J Chron Dis* 25:57-64, 1972

1351. Davis MS, von der Lippe RP: Discharge from hospital against medical advice: A study of reciprocity in the doctor-patient relationship. *Soc Sci Med* 1:336-342, 1968

1352. Eisey RD, Goldstein EO: Compliance of chronic asthmatics with oral administration of theophylline as measured by serum and salivary levels. *Pediatrics* 57:513-517, 1976

1353. Fleckenstein L, Joubert P, Lawrence R, Pastsner B, Mazzullo J, Lasagna L: Oral contraceptive patient information. *JAMA* 235:1331-1336, 1976

1354. Fleckenstein L: Attitudes toward the patient package insert—a survey of physicians and pharmacists. *Drug Info J* 11:23-29, 1977

1355. Fox LA: Written reinforcements of auxiliary directions for prescription medications. *Am J Hosp Pharm* 26:334-341, 1969

1356. Griffith HW: *Instructions for Patients*. Philadelphia, WB Saunders, 1975

1357. Gurwich EL, Swanson LN: Clinical pharmacy practice in an outpatient clinic. *J Am Pharm Assoc* NS15:392-399, 1975

1358. Hladik WB, White SJ: Evaluation of written reinforcements used in counselling cardiovascular patients. *Am J Hosp Pharm* 33:1277-1280, 1976

1359. Joubert P, Lasagna L: Patient package inserts I. Nature, notions and needs. *Clin Pharmacol Ther* 18:507-513, 1975

1360. ____: Patient package inserts II. Toward a rational patient package insert. *Clin Pharmacol Ther* 18:663-669, 1975

1361. Ley P, Spelman MS: Communication in an outpatient setting. *Br J Soc Clin Psychol* 4:114-116, 1965

1362. Liberman P: A guide to help patients keep track of their drugs. *Am J Hosp Pharm* 29:507-509, 1972

1363. Liberman P, Swartz AJ: Prescription dispensing to the problem patient. *Am J Hosp Pharm* 29:163-166, 1972

1364. Morris RW, Burkhart VP, Lamy PP: Technical and theoretical aspects of patient counselling using audiovisual aids. *Drug Intell Clin Pharm* 9:485-488, 1975

1365. Powell JR, Cali TJ, Linkewich JA: Inadequately written prescriptions. *JAMA* 226:999-1000, 1973

1366. Sapovsky A: Relationship between doctor-patient compatability, mutual perception and outcome or treatment. *J Abnorm Psychol* 70:70-76, 1965

1367. Smith DL: *Medication Guide for Patient Counselling*. Philadelphia, Pa,

Lea and Febiger, 1977
1368. Smith DL, Hill DS, Page EA, Pylatuk K: A patient information system in an outpatient clinic. *Can J Hosp Pharm* 27:165-169, 1974
1369. Soflin D, Young WW, Clayton BD: Development and evaluation of an individualized patient education program about digoxin. *Am J Hosp Pharm* 34:367-371, 1977
1370. Solomon DK, Baumgartner RP, Glascock LM, Glascock S, Briscoe M, Billups N: Use of medication profiles to detect potential therapeutic problems in ambulatory patients. *Am J Hosp Pharm* 31:348-354, 1974
1371. Stewart, RB: A study of outpatients' use of medication. *Hosp Pharm* 7:108-117, 1972
1372. Waitzkin H, Stoeckle JD: The communication of information about illness. *Adv Psychosom Med* 8:180-215, 1972
1373. Welk PC, Burkhart VP, Lamp PP: A comparison study of methods to educate patients. *Hosp Pharm* 10:240-248, 1975
1374. Wickware DS: What practitioners think about PPIs. *Pat Care* 11:50-57, 1977
1375. Statement on Pharmacist-conducted Patient Counselling. Approved by the ASHP Board of Directors at its meeting of November 1975 and by the ASHP House of Delegates on 7 April 1976
1376. Department of Health, Education and Welfare, Food and Drug Administration: Labelling of prescription drugs for patients. *Fed Reg* 40:52-75, 1975

ADDITIONAL REFERENCES–
CHAPTER 17 (Citations 1-853 listed in Appendix I)

1377. Charlebois AJ: Evaluation of an Industrial Rehabilitation Program. MSc thesis, Program in Design, Measurement and Evaluation, McMaster University, 1976
1378. Gibson ES: Problems with compliance, physician and patient. Paper presented at Cleveland Clinic, February 1976
1379. Gibson ES, Haynes RB, Martin RH: Vascular diseases in employed males. *J Occup Med* 17:425-429, 1975
1380. Greer CD, Cole SG: Organizational structure in hospital and community based clinics. *Am J Public Health* 65:714-719, 1975
1381. Harris L and Associates: *The Public and High Blood Pressure: A Survey.* Bethesda, DHEW publication 74-356, 1973
1382. Haynes RB, Sackett DL, Taylor DW, Gibson ES, Johnson AL: Increased absenteeism from work after detection and labeling of hypertensive patients. *N Eng J Med* 299:741-744, 1978
1383. Kirscht JP, Becker MH, Eveland JP: Psychological and social factors as predictors of medical behavior. *Med Care* 14:422-431, 1976
1384. Monk M: Personal communication.
1385. Mossey J: Psychosocial consequences of blood pressure intervention. *Am J Epid* 104:319, 1976

1386. Piore N, Lewis D, Seeliger J: *The Statistical Profile of Hospital Out-
       Patient Services in the United States: Present Scope and Potential
       Role*. New York, New York Association for the Aid of Crippled
       Children, 1971
1387. Sackett DL, Haynes RB, Gibson ES, Taylor DW, Roberts RS, Johnson
       AL: Clinical determinants of the decision to treat primary hyper-
       tension. *Clin Research* 24:648, 1977
1388. Stason WB, Weinstein MC: Allocation of resources to manage hyperten-
       sion. *N Engl J Med* 296:732-739, 1977
1389. Taylor DW, Sackett DL, Haynes RB, Gibson ES, Roberts RS, Johnson
       AL: Increased absenteeism among working men following the labelling
       and treatment of their hypertension. Presented to the American
       Federation of Clinical Research, Washington, May 1977
1390. Ontario Council of Health Task Force on Hypertension. Final Report.
       Sackett DL (Chairman). Toronto, Canada, 1978
1391. *Screening for Disease*. A series from *Lancet*. London. Lancet, 1974

ADDITIONAL REFERENCES–
CHAPTER 18 (Citations 1-853 listed in Appendix I)

1392. Sackett DL, Haynes RB, Gibson ES, Johnson A. The problem of com-
       pliance with antihypertensive therapy. *Practical Cardiology* 2:35-39,
       1976
1393. Sackett DL. How can we improve patient compliance? In Lasagna L
       (ed): *Controversies in Therapeutics*. Philadelphia, WB Saunders, in press

ADDITIONAL REFERENCES–
CHAPTER 19 (Citations 1-853 listed in Appendix I)

1394. Armitage P: *Statistical Methods in Medical Research*. New York, Wiley,
       1971
1395. Cox DR: *Planning of Experiments*. New York, Wiley, 1958
1396. Davies OL (ed): *The Design and Analysis of Industrial Experiments*.
       2nd edition. New York, Hafner, 1963
1397. Feinstein AR: Prognostic stratification series. *Clin Pharmacol Ther*
       13:285-297, 442-457, 609-624, 755-768, 1972

ADDITIONAL REFERENCES–
CHAPTER 20 (Citations 1-853 listed in Appendix I)

1398. Chalmers TC: Quoted in *Internal Medicine News* p 4, 11 Oct. 1973
1399. Feinstein AR: Clinical biostatistics: X. Sources of 'transition bias' in
       cohort statistics. *Clin Pharmacol Ther* 12:704-721, 1971

1400. ____: Clinical biostatistics: XI. Sources of 'chronology bias' in cohort statistics. *Clin Pharmacol Ther* 12:864-879, 1971

1401. Freis ED: Organization of a long-term multiclinic therapeutic trial in hypertension, pp 345-354, in Gross F (ed), with the assistance of Naegeli SR, Kirkwood AH: *Antihypertensive Therapy. Principles and Practice, An International Symposium.* New York, Springer-Verlag, 1966

1402. Kaebler CT: Quoted in *Medical News. JAMA* 227:1243-1244, 1974

1403. Lorenz KZ: The fashionable fallacy of dispensing with description. *Naturwissenschaften* 60:1-9, 1973

1404. University Group Diabetes Program: A study of the effects of hypoglycemic agents on vascular complications in patients with adult-onset diabetes. Part I: Design, methods, and baseline characteristics. Part II: Mortality results. *Diabetes* 19 (suppl 2): 747-830, 1970

1405. Veterans Administration Cooperative Study Group on Antihypertensive Agents: Effects of treatment on morbidity in hypertension. II. Results in patients with diastolic blood pressure averaging 90 through 114 mm Hg. *JAMA* 213:1143-1152, 1970

ADDITIONAL REFERENCES–
CHAPTER 21 (Citations 1-853 listed in Appendix I)

1406. Armitage P: The construction of comparable groups, pp 14-18, in Armitage, P: *Controlled Clinical Trials.* Oxford, Blackwell, 1960

1407. Feinstein AR: Clinical biostatistics: X. Sources of 'transition bias' in cohort statistics. *Clin Pharmacol Ther* 12:704-721, 1971

1408. ____: Clinical biostatistics: XI. Sources of 'chronology bias' in cohort statistics. *Clin Pharmacol Ther* 12:864-879, 1971

1409. ____: *Clinical Judgment.* Huntington, NY, Krieger, 1974

1410. ____: *Clinical Biostatistics.* Saint Louis, Mosby, 1977

1411. Hill AB: *Principles of Medical Statistics,* 9th ed. London, Lancet, 1971, pp 254-257

1412. ____: *Principles of Medical Statistics,* 9th ed. London, Lancet, 1971

1413. Mainland D: *Elementary Medical Statistics.* Philadelphia, WB Saunders, 1964

1414. Medawar PB: *Induction and Intuition in Scientific Thought.* Philadelphia, American Philosophical Society, 1969, p 59

1415. Murphey EA: *The Logic of Medicine.* Baltimore, Johns Hopkins University Press, 1976

1416. Sackett DL: Cigarettes, alcohol, hospitals and atherogenesis. *Am Heart J* 78:423-424, 1969

1417. ____: Data requirements of users of hospital discharge abstracts for epidemiologic research. *Med Care* 8:205-208, 1970

1418. ____: Design, measurement and analysis in clinical trials, pp 219-225, in Hirsh J (ed): *Platelets, Drugs and Thrombosis.* Basel, S Krager, 1975

1419. ____: Periodic examination of patients at risk, pp 437-456, in Schotten-feld D (ed). *Cancer Epidemiology and Prevention*. Springfield, Illinois, Thomas, 1975
1420. ____: Possible risk factors in the development of venous thrombosis. *Milbank Mem Fund Quart* 50, Part 2:105-120, 1972
1421. Sackett DL, Haynes RB, Gibson ES, Taylor DW, Roberts RS, Johnson AL, Hackett BC, Turford C, Mossey J: Randomized trials of compliance-improving strategies in hypertension, pp 1-19, in Lasagna L (ed): *Patient Compliance*. Mount Kisco, NY, Futura, 1976
1422. Sackett DL, Chambers LW, Macpherson AS, Goldsmith CH, McAuley RG: The development and application of indexes of health. I. General methods and a summary of results. *Am J Public Health* 67:423-428, 1977

Index

THE JOHNS HOPKINS UNIVERSITY PRESS

This book was set in IBM Selectric Press Roman by Culpeper Publishing. It was printed on 50-lb. #66 Eggshell Offset Cream and bound by Univeral Lithographers.

Library of Congress Cataloging in Publication Data

Main entry under title:
Compliance in health care.

Previous ed. published under title: Compliance
with therapeutic regimens.
Includes index.
Bibliography: pp. 337-507
1. Patient compliance–Congresses. I. Haynes,
R. Brian. II. Taylor, D. Wayne. III. Sackett,
David L. IV. Compliance with therapeutic
regimens. [DNLM: 1. Patient compliance–
Congresses. 2. Patients–Education–Congresses.
W3 W0512T 1977c]
R726.5.C65 1979   613   78-20527
ISBN 0-8018-2162-2